Community Integration
following Traumatic Brain Injury

Community Integration
following Traumatic Brain Injury

edited by

Jeffrey S. Kreutzer, Ph.D.
Associate Professor
Departments of Rehabilitation Medicine
and Neurological Surgery
Medical College of Virginia
Virginia Commonwealth University
Richmond

and

Paul Wehman, Ph.D.
Professor
Department of Rehabilitation Medicine
and Special Education
Medical College of Virginia
Director
Rehabilitation Research and Training Center on
Supported Employment for Persons with Severe Disabilities
Virginia Commonwealth University
Richmond

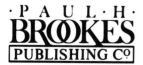
·P A U L·H·
BROOKES
PUBLISHING C?

Baltimore · London · Toronto · Sydney

Paul H. Brookes Publishing Co.
P.O. Box 10624
Baltimore, Maryland 21285-0624

Typeset by The Composing Room, Grand Rapids, Michigan.
Manufactured in the United States of America by
The Maple Press Company, York, Pennsylvania.

Library of Congress Cataloging-in-Publication Data
Community integration following traumatic brain injury / edited by
    Jeffrey S. Kreutzer and Paul H. Wehman.
        p.   cm.
    Includes bibliographical references.
    ISBN 1–55766–045–X
    1. Brain damage—Patients—Rehabilitation.   2. Brain damage—Patients—Long
term care.   I. Kreutzer, Jeffrey S., 1953—   .   II. Wehman, Paul.
    [DNLM: 1. Brain Injuries—rehabilitation.   WL 354 C7337]
RC387.5.C65   1990
617.4′8103—dc20
DNLM/DLC
for Library of Congress   89–7087
                                                                                                    CIP

Contents

v

Contributors

Janet K. Anderson-Parenté, Ph.D.
Associate Professor
Department of Psychology
Towson State University
Towson, MD 21204

Christine A. Baser, Ph.D.
Assistant Clinical Professor
Division of Neurosurgery
University of California at San Diego
San Diego, CA 92103

Corwin Boake, Ph.D.
Clinical Director
Challenge Program
The Institute for Rehabilitation and Research
1333 Moursund Avenue
Houston, TX 77030

Catherine F. Bontke, M.D.
Assistant Professor
Departments of Rehabilitation and Physical
  Medicine
Baylor College of Medicine
and
Director
Head Injury Program
The Institute for Rehabilitation and Research
1333 Moursund Avenue
Houston, TX 77030

Patricia Stiles Camplair, M.S.
Predoctoral Fellow in Neuropsychology
Department of Rehabilitation Medicine
Medical College of Virginia
Virginia Commonwealth University
Box 677, MCV Station
Richmond, VA 23284

Jeffrey Chase, Ph.D.
Department of Psychology
Radford University
Radford, VA 24142

David C. Clemmons, Ph.D.
Director, Vocational Services Unit
Regional Epilepsy Center
Harborview Medical Center
and
Assistant Professor
Department of Neurological Surgery
University of Washington School of Medicine
Seattle, WA 98104

Eloise Cobb, Ph.D.
Coordinator, Child Development Services
Children's Specialty Services
State Department of Health
Richmond, VA

Janice L. Cockrell, M.D.
Associate Professor
Departments of Rehabilitation and Pediatrics
Medical College of Virginia
Virginia Commonwealth University
Richmond, VA 23298
and
Director
Physical Medicine and Rehabilitation
Children's Hospital
2924 Brook Road
Richmond, VA 23227

Kathleen R. Doherty, B.A.
Psychology Staff
Department of Rehabilitation Medicine
Medical College of Virginia
Virginia Commonwealth University
Box 677, MCV Station
Richmond, VA 23298

Randall W. Evans, Ph.D.
Program Director, Learning Services
Carolina Community Reentry Program
707 Morehead Avenue
Durham, NC 27707

Robert T. Fraser, Ph.D., C.R.C.
Associate Professor
Departments of Neurological Surgery
  and Rehabilitation Medicine
Harborview Medical Center, ZA-05
325 9th Avenue
Seattle, WA 98104
and
President, Division of Rehabilitation Psychology
American Psychological Association
and
Community Re-entry Services of Washington
Mountlake Terrace, WA 98043

Jennifer A. Harris, M.A.
Psychology Staff
Department of Rehabilitation Medicine
Medical College of Virginia
Virginia Commonwealth University
Richmond, VA 23298

Jeffrey S. Kreutzer, Ph.D.
Associate Professor
Departments of Rehabilitation Medicine and
    Neurological Surgery
Medical College of Virginia
Virginia Commonwealth University
Box 677, MCV Station
Richmond, VA 23298-0677

Ellen Lehr, Ph.D.
Clinical Director of Pediatrics
New Medico Community Re-Entry Services of
    Washington
6911 226th Place, S.W.
Mountlake Terrace, WA 98043

Bruce E. Leininger, M.S.
Predoctoral Fellow in Clinical Neuropsychology
Department of Rehabilitation Medicine
Medical College of Virginia
Virginia Commonwealth University
Box 677, MCV Station
Richmond, VA 23298

Catherine A. Mateer, Ph.D., A.B.C.N.
Director of Neuropsychological Services
Good Samaritan Hospital
1322 Third Street, S.E.
Suite 250
Puyallup, WA 98372

Brian T. McMahon, Ph.D., C.R.C.
Midwest Regional Director of Operations
New Medico Head Rehabilitation Service
    of Chicago
1307 Butterfield
Suite 412
Downers Grove, IL 60515

Robin McNeny, O.T.R.
Occupational Therapist
13201 Groveton Terrace
Midlothian, VA 23113

Gregory J. O'Shanick, M.D.
Associate Professor of Psychiatry
    and Rehabilitation Medicine
Medical College of Virginia
Virginia Commonwealth University
Box 710, MCV Station
Richmond, VA 23298-0710

Rick Parenté, Ph.D.
Chairman, Experimental Psychology
and
Associate Professor
Department of Psychology
Towson State University
Towson, MD 21204

Brian K. Preston, M.S., C.R.C.
Vocational Coordinator
Carolina Community Reentry Program
707 Morehead Avenue
Durham, NC 27707

Ronald M. Ruff, Ph.D.
Director, UCSD Head Injury Center
    and Learning Services Institute
Associate Clinical Professor
Departments of Psychiatry
    and Division of Neurosurgery
University of California at San Diego
420 Walnut Avenue
San Diego, CA 92103

Ronald C. Savage, Ed.D.
Associate Professor of Education
Castleton State College
Castleton, VT 05735

Robert J. Sbordone, Ph.D., A.B.C.N.
Private Practice
Orange County Neuropsychology Group
8840 Warner Avenue, Suite 301
Fountain Valley, CA 92703
and
Departments of Neurosurgery, Physical Medicine,
    and Rehabilitation
College of Medicine
University of California, Irvine
Irvine, CA 92716

McKay Moore Sohlberg, M.Sc., C.C.C., Ph.D.
Good Samaritan Hospital Center for Cognitive
    Rehabilitation
319 South Meridian
Puyallup, WA 98372

Jo Ann Tomberlin, M.A., P.T.
Partner, Physical Therapy Services
Director, Department of Physical Therapy
Transitional Learning Community
Galveston, TX
and
Physical Therapy Services
1810 Tremont Street
Galveston, TX 77440

Linda C. Veldheer, D.P.A.
Department of Mental Health, Mental Rehabilitation
    and Substance Abuse Services
P.O. Box 1797
109 Governor Street
Richmond, VA 23214

Pamela Kaye Waaland, Ph.D.
Senior Neuropsychologist
Children's Neurological Services
Adjunct Faculty
Department of Rehabilitation Medicine
Medical College of Virginia
1825 Monument Avenue
Richmond, VA 23220

Paul Wehman, Ph.D.
Professor
Department of Rehabilitation Medicine
    and Special Education
Medical College of Virginia
Director
Rehabilitation Research and Training Center on
    Supported Employment for Persons with Severe
    Disabilities
Virginia Commonwealth University
Box 2011
Richmond, VA 23298-2011

Nathan D. Zasler, M.D.
Director, Brain Injury Rehabilitation Services
Assistant Professor
Department of Rehabilitation Medicine
Medical College of Virginia
Virginia Commonwealth University
Box 677, MCV Station
Richmond, VA 23298-0677

Foreword

The 1980s witnessed an exponential growth in the quantity and scope of facilities that serve the needs of those with traumatic brain injury and their families. The field has advanced beyond concerns of immediate survival to long-term issues relating to quality of life. Since the typical brain-injured person can often expect to enjoy a normal life span, rehabilitation professionals have been expected to confront an enormous challenge: How can the child or adult with brain injury successfully return to the community and live a meaningful and productive life? This book represents one of the best efforts to date to answer this perplexing question.

Why is community integration so difficult after traumatic brain injury? There are many reasons: Enduring neurocognitive and psychosocial problems, such as diminished capacity to attend, remember, and learn; and difficulties in reacting to stress, modulating emotion, and interacting appropriately with peers and significant others are but a few of the many problems that have an impact on community integration. The nature of brain injury—a sudden event that permanently alters brain function and consequently both physical and neuropsychological capacities—is such that the process of rehabilitation must extend beyond the basic functions of talking, walking, and caring for basic hygiene. Instead, the rehabilitation process must be concerned with capacities to engage in education, vocation, recreation, social interaction, and community activities. For this reason, the rehabilitation process for persons with brain injury extends beyond the intensive care unit and the inpatient rehabilitation unit into facilities and programs whose focus is on teaching the necessary skills to both the brain-injured survivor and his or her family in order to achieve optimal community integration.

Many critical issues in community integration are explored in this book by a multidisciplinary group of contributors representing the fields of rehabilitation medicine, neuropsychology, vocational rehabilitation, physical therapy, occupational therapy, speech/language pathology, and education. The interdisciplinary approach to community integration is absolutely an essential and defining characteristic of most respectable community integration programs. The importance of establishing a sound methodology in this area has been recognized by the Commission for the Accreditation of Rehabilitation Facilities, which adopted special standards for post–acute brain injury rehabilitation in 1988.

For the practitioner and researcher, community integration demands creativity and innovation. This book highlights the most current thinking in treatment strategies and models of service delivery. In practical terms, the contributors describe how cognitive rehabilitation can be employed successfully in the real world; which types of vocational rehabilitation practices, such as supported employment, hold promise for this group of individuals who have difficulty in finding and maintaining employment; the unique problems that confront children with brain injury and their teachers, in attempting to return to school; what strategies families can use to restore and maintain balance within the family system while aiding the brain-injured survivor in day-to-day functioning; and why attention to medical needs and physical capacities is a critical, but sometimes overlooked element in the community reentry equation.

Successful community integration is dependent on many sectors of our society—the health care community, consumers, regulatory agencies, and government. To meet the overwhelming demand of 50–75,000 severely head-injured persons per year, it is important that local and national governmental agencies recognize this need and create programs that foster the development and evaluation of new treatment techniques and models of cost-effective service delivery. This is particularly relevant in the field of community reintegration, where there is less uniformity in service delivery practices than in the acute stages of brain injury rehabilitation; treatment may extend for many months or years and costs of service provision are often of great magnitude.

For you, the reader, this book should serve as a guide that will enable you to critically evaluate your current methods of community integration and expand your knowledge base and treatment repertoire. This will surely assist you in improving the quality of life for those who are faced with the enormous challenge of rebuilding their lives after a traumatic brain injury.

Mitchell Rosenthal, Ph.D.
Rehabilitation Institute
Wayne State University School of Medicine
Detroit, Michigan

Preface

Initial efforts toward improving outcome following traumatic brain injury were focused on improving survival rates. Advances in medical care including neuroimaging techniques, surgical intervention, intensive care technology, and emergency transport contributed to substantial progress. As survival rates increased, clinicians and researchers began to focus their attention on acute medical treatment and rehabilitation within the hospital environment. Increased attention yielded significant progress as evidenced by standardization of treatment protocols, the proliferation of medical rehabilitation facilities, improved outcome measurement, and the increased availability of information for professionals and family members.

Unfortunately, despite the many recent advances in medical and rehabilitation interventions, substantial problems remain for many persons with traumatic brain injury. Many of those who participate in early rehabilitation face disappointment and frustration in their pursuit of independent living following discharge. Unemployment, inadequate academic resources, financial hardships, lack of transportation alternatives, intermittent medical problems, the unavailability of recreational opportunities, and difficulty maintaining interpersonal relationships are partly a consequence of underdeveloped community resources. We also know that family members often face daily crises and assume the long-term burden of care despite limited resources and training.

Our primary purpose in editing and writing this book was to facilitate efforts to extend the continuum of care for persons with traumatic brain injury. Necessarily, a diversity of topics are covered, including medical and pharmacological treatment, communication disorders, the role of neuropsychology and psychotherapy, physical therapy, transitional living, community networking, educational reintegration, family adjustment, and daily living skills. Given their special importance, individual sections of the book were allocated to rehabilitation of children and vocational rehabilitation.

Despite the diversity of topics covered by the book, the authors share two important philosophies. First, rehabilitation for many persons with traumatic brain injury is a long-term and, in some cases, a lifelong phenomenon. Second, rehabilitation is most efficacious using an interdisciplinary team that includes the client as well as the family. We have gathered work by a number of distinguished authors to help advance knowledge in the field, enhance existing services, stimulate additional research, and facilitate the development of new programs. It is hoped that, in the next few decades, advances in community program development will parallel those evident in early medical care and acute rehabilitation.

We are thankful to the authors of individual chapters for their important contribution to this text. Our gratitude is extended to J. Paul Thomas, Richard Melia, and Toby Lawrence at the National Institute on Disability and Rehabilitation Research. Their guidance and support were essential in the preparation of this book. Much of our own research, which is cited within this book, was funded by the National Institute on Disability and Rehabilitation Research as well as the Office of Special Education and Rehabilitative Services, within the United States Department of Education. Our heartfelt thanks are extended to our colleagues and staff at the Medical College of Virginia and Virginia Commonwealth University, including Stephen Ayres, Henry Stonnington, Guy Clifton, Schontel Abdulrazaaq, Paul Mazmanian, Mike West, Paul Sale, and Jan Smith. Their support, advice, and assistance were critical to the production of this book. Also, special thanks to Muriel Lezak and Harvey Levin: scientists, teachers, and relentless advocates who helped inspire the writing of this book. Additionally, we appreciate the efforts of Paul Brookes, Melissa Behm, and their colleagues at Brookes Publishing Company for their advice and assistance in the editing and production process. Most of all, we would like to thank our clients and their family members. We appreciate their sharing part of their lives with us and helping us understand their needs and the true value of intervention.

We dedicate this book to the memory of Mary Romano. Mary helped underscore the important role of patient advocacy and helped us understand the unique and valuable role of families in the process of rehabilitation.

SECTION I

Medical and Physical Aspects of Rehabilitation

CHAPTER 1

Medical Advances in the Treatment of Brain Injury

Catherine F. Bontke

INCIDENCE

It is estimated that between 500,000 and 1.5 million Americans sustain brain injuries of all severities each year. Of these, between 50,000 and 70,000 injuries are classified as moderate to severe; those persons will live the rest of their (normal life-span) lives with a combination of cognitive, physical, behavioral, and/or emotional deficits and require rehabilitation services. The peak incidence for traumatic brain injury is between the ages of 15 and 24 years and it is two to three times more common in males than females. Most persons with traumatic brain injury are single and are in lower socioeconomic groups. There is a significant number who have a history of alcohol use, drug use, and/or who have undergone psychiatric care prior to their head injuries (Kraus et al., 1983).

Motor vehicle accidents, and then falls, are the leading causes of traumatic brain injury. In most motor vehicle accidents where persons are screened for blood alcohol level, 72% had alcohol in their blood, and 52% were noted to have a blood alcohol level of 0.1% or higher (Rimel & Jane, 1983). The increased use of the automobile in the past century has lead to an increased risk of severe traumatic brain injury. The number of survivors has also increased dramatically since the introduction of helicopter evacuation and skilled emergency medical technicians, which enable quick transportation to specialized trauma centers as well as rapid prehospital stabilization. These developments are a direct result of similar techniques introduced during the wars in Korea and Vietnam.

In addition, there have been dramatic advances made in the diagnosis and neurosurgical treatment of persons with severe brain injury, and widespread application of these advances has markedly decreased the morbidity and mortality associated with traumatic brain injury. Reports of mortality in severe brain injury range from a low of 30% to a high of 70% (Eisenberg, Weiner, & Tabaddor, 1987).

PATHOPHYSIOLOGY

The brain destruction seen after traumatic brain injury occurs primarily at the moment of impact. Secondary damage results from complications arising from both intracranial and extracranial injuries. Only prevention of head injuries can lessen the primary brain damage. Secondary damage is lessened via advanced neurosurgical care.

Primary Brain Damage

As the soft but incompressible brain slides and strikes the rigid and rough skull, primary brain damage occurs—usually over the frontal lobe

This work was supported in part by Grant G0087C2016 awarded by the U.S. Department of Education, National Institute on Disability and Rehabilitation Research (NIDRR) to the Head Injury Rehabilitation Program at The Institute for Rehabilitation and Research, Catherine F. Bontke, M.D., principal investigator. The author thanks Betty C. Olson for expert help in the preparation of this manuscript.

and the anterior tip of the temporal lobes, as they glide over the rough falx cerebri and the wings of the sphenoid bones, respectively. Hemorrhagic contusions or bruises can vary in extent from small collections of blood on the surface of the brain to intracerebral hemorrhages throughout the whole depth of the cortex. Contusions are usually bilateral but asymmetric in their severity. In addition to the frontal and temporal contusions, localized contusions under areas of depressed skull fracture can also occur. In addition to the focal damage, movement between the different components of the brain as a result of rotational acceleration results in shear injury or diffuse axonal injury. The corpus callosum and the brain stem are the most commonly affected areas.

Secondary Brain Damage

As hematomas enlarge, brain edema causes intracranial pressure, which in turn causes tissue necrosis and obstruction of intracranial veins. This further increases the pressure, compromising the cerebral blood flow. With decrease in cerebral blood flow and increase in intracranial pressure, areas of infarction secondary to ischemia can occur. In addition, increased intracranial pressure, when uncontrolled, can cause herniation and thus compromise brain-stem function, lead to cranial nerve paralysis, and lead to contusion of the herniated parts of the brain.

In addition, traumatic brain injury is frequently accompanied by subarachnoid hemorrhage that can cause vasospasm and additional ischemia. Early hydrocephalus can occur secondary to cerebrospinal fluid malabsorption by arachnoid villi that have become blocked with blood or white blood cells.

Extracranial factors such as hypoxia secondary to respiratory failure and hypotension following significant blood loss may further compromise cerebral blood flow.

ACUTE NEUROSURGICAL INTERVENTION

Advances in the treatment of survivors of traumatic brain injury have evolved to include early identification of complications with the help of neuroradiological procedures such as computerized axial tomography (CT), ultrasound, and magnetic resonance imaging (MRI). Routine intracranial pressure monitoring, frequent neurological checks utilizing the Glasgow Coma Scale (GCS), as well as electrophysiological monitoring and enhanced measurement of metabolic and caloric needs have allowed neurosurgeons to monitor for subtle changes that may indicate a potential complication and therefore allow intervention before secondary damage occurs. Better monitoring and assessment techniques also permit prognostication (Eisenberg, Weiner, & Tabaddor, 1987).

In addition to assessment techniques, acute neurosurgical treatment has included routine management of increased intracranial pressure by techniques such as positioning, hyperventilation, sedation, osmotic diuretics, steroids, ventricular drainage, and paralyzation. Aggressive surgical decompression, early ventricular peritoneal shunting, and shunting of hygromas have resulted in marked decrease in secondary damage (Marshall & Marshall, 1987). The recent release of a nimodipine, a new calcium antagonist that reduces vasospasm after subarachnoid hemorrhage, has added to the neurosurgeon's armamentarium in the battle against secondary damage (Allen et al., 1983; Petruk et al., 1988; Scriabine & Van Den Kerckhoff, 1988).

Once the patient is in the intensive care unit the priority shifts from saving life to enabling life. The patient is evaluated for additional extracranial injuries such as vertebral instability or spinal cord injury. Definitive orthopedic management of fractures often can be delayed, but early surgical treatment of orthopedic injuries will frequently minimize disability later in the patient's course (Hanscom, 1987). Infections are guarded against, but if they occur are aggressively treated.

Rehabilitation efforts can start while the patient's medical and neurosurgical status is being stabilized. Patients are positioned in ways to prevent decubitus formation, edema, and contractures. It has been noted that patients who receive passive range of motion twice a day, unless orthopedically contraindicated, have fewer contractures (Kottke, 1982). Improved attention to nutritional needs and bowel and bladder management can prevent further disability. Further, family intervention with adequate information and support should be started as soon as the patient is under the care of the medical team (Sandel, 1989).

REHABILITATION

In the past decade there has been a tremendous increase in the number, types, and locations of acute rehabilitation programs in the United States. The National Head Injury Foundation noted fewer than 40 dedicated head injury programs in 1980. By 1988, they estimated over 700 such programs existed. Even with this tremendous growth, not all patients with moderate and severe injuries can be accommodated in acute rehabilitation programs due to shortages of beds, funding sources, location of programs, and because patients are simply not being properly referred by the hospital teams who saved their lives. In 1988, the National Head Injury Foundation estimated that less than 10% of patients with moderate and severe injuries get adequate rehabilitation services. The picture is changing, however. Better marketing efforts heighten awareness of the availability of services and the very presence of such a program in a community raises the standard of care for survivors of traumatic brain injury.

Cost-effective treatment and improved long-term outcome have become priorities for such rehabilitation programs, not only because of the support and encouragement from third-party payers (both private and governmental), but also because the traumatic brain injury rehabilitation professionals recognize the need for alternative rehabilitation programs that are not based on a medical model. The development of an integrated system of care with a common language and data system, shared technologies, fully trained rehabilitation professionals that function as a transdisciplinary team is being championed by the leaders in traumatic brain injury rehabilitation medicine and by the families of survivors (Dixon, 1989).

Most patients referred to acute rehabilitation programs, once they are medically stable, begin the long process of recovery and reintegration in one of the more than 700 acute dedicated head injury rehabilitation programs in the United States. The usual length of stay is 2–8 months. These programs are usually lead by a physiatrist, a physician trained in physical medicine and rehabilitation, and comprise a team of professionals that may include: neuropsychologists, social workers, case managers, occupational therapists, physical therapists, speech/language pathologists, therapeutic recreation specialists, audiologists, pharmacists, dieticians, rehabilitation nurses, orthotists, vocational counselors, respiratory therapists, and persons trained in pastoral care. Consultants in all branches of medicine may also be involved. Family members, and when appropriate, the patient, are considered integral members of the team. The team works together to assess the patient's strengths and deficits and then to plan incremental functional goals based on the patient's progress. Each program has its own criteria for admission; patients may still be comatose (coma management program) or the program may require that he or she be able to follow one-step or two-step commands (acute rehabilitation program). Some programs may not be able to care for patients with respiratory problems or patients who are ventilator dependent.

Coma Management Programs

Coma management or coma stimulation programs have increased in number in recent years. They are usually based in a skilled nursing facility or are a component of a hospital-based dedicated brain injury program. The goals of these programs are to bring the patients out of coma, to increase consistency of response to commands, to prevent complications related to immobility and malnutrition, and to educate families and involve them proactively (Whyte & Glenn, 1986). Multimodality sensory stimulation programs, although frequently used, have not been proven to be effective in enhancing patients' ability to respond. They are, however, an effective way to monitor patients for change over a period of time and, if taught, families can be involved proactively. Patients' medications that may be sedating are eliminated or changed to others having less cognitive effects.

In addition, patients may be tried on medications to increase arousal and enhance cortical functioning. The pharmacological classes include dopamine agonists (e.g., L-dopa, bromocriptine mesylate, amantadine hydrochloride), psychostimulants (e.g., methylphenidate hydrochloride, dextroamphetamine sulfate, pemoline), and antidepressants (e.g., protriptyline) (Sandel, 1989). The use of such drugs is based on animal studies. These studies indicate enhanced recovery when used with appropriate physical trials such as beam walking, in comparison to animals that were not medicated or were administered sedating medications and confined to small cages without physical trials (Sutton, Weaver, & Feeney, 1987).

Acute Rehabilitation Programs

Although there are increasing numbers of coma management programs, most patients are transferred to acute rehabilitation programs when their Glasgow Coma Scale (GCS) score is 8 or 9 and they have begun to follow one-step commands consistently. Here the focus is to increase orientation. Most patients are still confused and in a state of post-traumatic amnesia (PTA) with severely impaired short-term memory.

Unfortunately, it is not unusual for patients to experience a phase of acute agitation as they emerge from coma and are still in PTA. Agitated patients are often a danger to themselves and to others. They may thrash about; remove restraints, tubes, and catheters; fall out of bed; and/or wander away from the rehabilitation unit.

The etiology of this behavior is usually related to severe confusion and lack of ongoing memory. However, related contributing factors such as electrolyte imbalances, sleep disturbances, seizure activity, malnutrition, or vitamin deficiencies must first be ruled out. Any condition that may cause discomfort such as a traumatized extremity or an infection must be ruled out as well. Medications commonly used to control agitation, such as minor tranquilizers, neuroleptics, and other central nervous system de-

pressants can increase the patient's confusion and actually increase agitation (Cardenas, 1987).

Behavioral and environmental approaches are the usual first line of management. Utilization of quiet, safe, structured areas such as a floor bed; removal of as much noxious stimulation as possible, such as tubes, catheters, restraints, and traction set-ups; and gentle physical and verbal reassurance by trained personnel can help alleviate agitation.

Pharmacological intervention may be necessary when behavioral and environmental techniques do not succeed and the patient is still a danger to him or herself and to others. In recent years there has been a trend to move away from the use of sedating medications such as neuroleptics and minor tranquilizers. Neuroleptics, such as haloperidol and chlorpromazine, may contribute to the underlying confusional state, may have long-term side effects, and, theoretically, may impede recovery (Sutton et al., 1987). Minor tranquilizers such as benzodiazepines may decrease the patient's ability to learn, increase memory deficits, and may have paradoxical as well as enhanced side effects in patients with traumatic brain injury.

Physiatrists experienced in traumatic brain injury are more apt to try antidepressants, mood stabilizers such as lithium, and psychostimulants with agitated patients. The practice of eliminating sedating drugs and switching to medications with the least amount of cognitive side effects has led to the widespread use of carbamazepine for seizure prophylaxis as well as for behavioral control (Glenn & Wroblewski, 1986).

If agitation is ameliorated or was never a problem, the goals for the patient with PTA are to increase basic functions such as eating, communication, ambulation, and bowel and bladder continence; and to improve orientation.

Patients are evaluated frequently by each discipline in order to follow neurological and cognitive recovery, which is usually quite rapid and dramatic during this stage. Goals are upgraded and changed accordingly. Swallowing evaluations may be done at bedside by speech/ language pathologists and a videofluoroscopy may be done to confirm the absence of silent aspiration and adequate coordination and efficacy of swallowing before oral feeding is begun. Once the patient is aware of bodily functions, rehabilitation nurses begin bowel and bladder training programs, and occupational therapists usually begin basic activities of daily living (ADL) training. These usually include grooming, hygiene, dressing, and feeding, and advance to more complex tasks such as shopping, cooking, and checkbook balancing. Physical therapists assess the patient's motor and sensory functions and begin transfer training, wheelchair training, and progressive ambulation. Emergence from PTA is documented by the neuropsychologist through the use of standardized tests such as the Galveston Orientation and Amnesia Test (GOAT).

Once the patient emerges from PTA, more thorough neuropsychological evaluations can be performed, and more accurate prosnostication and long-term planning can occur. Discharge from the acute rehabilitation program ideally occurs when the patient is independent in activities of daily living and is behaviorally able to function at home. Discharge planning involves knowing the patient's physical, cognitive, and behavioral limitations; available resources within the community; financial resources; home environment; and family support system.

Patients may also go home with day care for respite if no further progress is anticipated, to day treatment to improve functioning, or to a skilled nursing home. Family members may need training in their new caregiving responsibilities, and the patient and family members may wish to have a therapeutic day or overnight pass to practice new skills.

ADVANCES IN THE TREATMENT OF COMPLICATIONS

Seizure Prophylaxis

It is estimated that approximately 5% of all persons with traumatic brain injury who are hospitalized will develop post-traumatic epilepsy (PTE). Patients who have depressed skull fractures, acute intracranial hematomas, or seizures during the first week have an increased risk of developing late PTE (Jennett, 1983). Other factors such as dural tearing, focal signs such as aphasia and hemiplegia, and post-traumatic amnesia present for longer than 24 hours are also considered as increased risk. However, determining the degree of each individual patient's risk is a bit more difficult. Feeney and Walker devised a mathematical model in 1979 to estimate seizure risk based on a combination of risk factors. Studies are underway to determine the efficacy of using such mathematical models in a clinical setting. In the interim, clinicians must often judge seizure risk on individual patients without the benefit of such models, and seizure prophylaxis is customarily continued for a period of 1–2 years.

Patients are often placed on seizure prophylaxis in the acute neurosurgical setting, where the usual medications chosen by neurosurgeons are phenytoin or phenobarbital because these medications can be administered parenterally and have been in use the longest (Epstein, Ward, & Becker, 1987; Jennett, 1979; Thompson & Trimble, 1982). Once the patient is transferred to the rehabilitation program, the physiatrist often reassesses the actual need for seizure prophylaxis medication, and if the risk is judged to be high, medications with the least behavioral and cognitive side effects are chosen. Currently, carbamazepine (Tegretol) is the drug of choice among physiatrists, although valproic acid (Depakote) is gaining favor among some clinicians. Therefore, it is not uncommon for patients with high risk of developing post-traumatic epilepsy to be switched from phenobarbital or phenytoin to carbamazepine or valproic acid in the acute rehabilitation setting (Glenn & Rosenthal, 1985).

In one study, switching patients to carbamazepine was shown to improve speed of mental processing, visual scanning, and memory (Trimble & Thompson, 1984). Furthermore, other studies show that phenytoin decreases attention, concentration, mental processing, and motor speed (e.g., Andrewes, Tomlinson, Elwes, & Reynolds, 1984; Reynolds & Trimble, 1985). Phenobarbital side effects include lethargy, sedation, and reversal hyperactivity (Reynolds & Trimble, 1985). Although valproic acid can have initially sedating effects, patients usually accommodate to them, and certainly do not have the persistent lethargy and other cognitive side effects noted in phenytoin and phenobarbital (Vining, 1987).

Most post-traumatic epilepsies are thought to be of the partial variety, either simple partial or complex partial, which secondarily generalize. Carbamazepine was shown to be as effective as phenytoin and phenobarbital for generalized tonic-clonic seizures and more effective in the control of partial seizures (Jennett, 1975; Mattson et al., 1985).

Carbamazepine is an easy-to-tolerate drug with few side effects (gastrointestinal distress, headaches, dizziness, and diplopia) that are usually ameliorated by starting with a low dose and gradually building up to therapeutic range. The most limiting side effect of carbamazepine is bone marrow suppression. However, transient leukopenia, primarily a relative neutropenia, can usually be monitored, and as long as the white blood cell count is above 4,000 cells/mm^3 with 50% of the white cells being neutrophils, there appears to be no reason to stop or change the drug (Pisciotta, 1982). The disadvantage of carbamazepine appears to be its relatively short half-life, which makes three times daily dosing mandatory. In patients with memory impairment this can significantly decrease compliance. However, memory aids such as beeping pill boxes or alarm watches seem to help with this problem.

Post-traumatic Hydrocephalus

True post-traumatic hydrocephalus (PTH) following severe brain injury is, fortunately, relatively uncommon. One study estimated the incidence at 1%–8% (Gudeman et al., 1981). However, the neurological symptoms can range from deep coma to the typical triad for normal pressure hydrocephalus (NPH) of dementia, ataxia, and incontinence. Atypical presentations can include emotional problems, seizures, and spasticity (Beyerl & Black, 1984). PTH is felt to be secondary to the impairment of flow and absorption of cerebrospinal fluid. This blockage may be around the cerebral convexities or may be, as some authors suggest, around the arach-

noid granulations by subarachnoid blood (Beyerl & Black, 1984). Patients with subarachnoid hemorrhage that may lead to adhesive arachnoiditis, as well as patients with meningitis and severe skull fractures, appear to be at greatest risk for the development of this complication (Beyerl & Black, 1984).

It was hoped that magnetic resonance imaging would reveal periventricular lucency more accurately, and that the diagnosis of post-traumatic hydrocephalus would be eased by this new radiographic modality (Zimmerman, Fleming, Lee, Saint-Louis, & Deck, 1986). Unfortunately this has not been the case, and clinicians must rely on computerized axial tomography criteria developed by Kishore in 1978, which includes enlarged ventricles, normal or absent sulci, and enlargement of the basil cisterns in the fourth ventricle; if suspicion is high, serial monthly CT scans for comparison may help make the diagnosis of PTH (Cope, Date, Mar, 1988; Kishore et al., 1978).

Improved methods of determining which patients will benefit from shunting include the use of an adapted version of the cerebrospinal fluid tap test (Wikkelso, Anderson, Bloomstrand, Lindqvist, & Svendsen, 1986). This test involves utilization of psychometric measures and gait pattern before and after lumbar puncture in which a quantity of fluid is removed. Improvement in test results after the removal of fluid implies a successful result will occur if the patient is shunted.

Injuries and Fractures

It is unusual for persons to sustain traumatic brain injury in isolation. Rimel and Jane (1983) have noted that 82% of patients with brain injuries admitted to the hospital sustained one or more extracranial injuries. There has been a movement toward early identification and management of these injuries in the acute neurosurgical phase of treatment in order to minimize long-term disability (Botte & Moore, 1987).

In the acute care setting a minimal series of radiographs is usually done, which includes the cervical spine, pelvis, hips, and knees as well as routine anterior-posterior radiographs of the extremities in order to minimize the chance of missing an injury. Some clinicians even recommend a bone scan 7–10 days after the injury occurred to detect occult fractures (Botte & Moore, 1987).

Orthopedic surgeons now recommend early fracture stabilization and espouse that treatment should always be based on the assumption that the patient will make a good recovery regardless of the prognostic indicators to the contrary (Hanscom, 1987). This is in marked contrast to the way patients with traumatic brain injury were treated in the late 1970s, when patients were first allowed to "wake up" before their fractures were repaired.

Heterotopic Ossification

It is noted that persons with brain injuries with spasticity, prolonged coma (greater than 2 weeks), and long bone fractures are at the highest risk for development of heterotopic ossification (HO) (Spielman, Gennarelli, & Rogers, 1983). The incidence of HO ranges from 11% to 76%, depending on the method of detection and the population studied (Garland, Blum, & Waters, 1981; Sazbon, Najenson, Tartakovsky, Becker, & Grosswasser, 1981). Major long-term disability from untreated HO can include limited range of motion and joint ankylosis, pain, spasticity, vascular and nerve compression, lymphedema, and loss of nerve length (Garland & Keenan, 1983). Various medications have been shown to halt the progression of HO including etidronate disodium (EHDP) as well as nonsteroidal anti-inflammatory drugs (NSAID) and salicylates (Gennarelli, 1988; Mital, Garber, & Stinson, 1987; Ritter & Gioe, 1982; Rogers, 1988; Spielman et al., 1983; Stover, Hahn, & Miller, 1976).

Although prophylaxis is not currently a routine practice in the United States, there are improved techniques for early detection and early treatment. Some of these improvements include triple-phase bone scan, which may pick up increased vascularity earlier than radiographs, and use of medications such as EHDP, NSAID, or salicylates following its detection. These medications coupled with progressive range of motion with adequate analgesia, control of spas-

ticity to maintain range of motion, and a functional positioning so that if ankylosis should occur the joint would fuse in the best possible position are current practices by most physiatrists in the United States (Bontke, 1988; Freed, Hahn, Menter, & Dillon, 1982). Forceful manipulation and/or surgical removal of mature HO with concomitant use of EHDP may allow some functional use of the involved extremity (Garland, Razza, & Waters, 1982).

Spasticity

Up until the early 1980s, spasticity following traumatic brain injury was often treated in the same way spasticity induced by spinal cord injury was treated—that is, with medications causing sedation, such as baclofen or diazepam. In reality, spasticity that results from traumatic brain injury is more heavily influenced by such factors as postural changes, body positioning, and labyrinthine and tonic neck reflexes. Spasticity can be a source of extreme discomfort and pain in persons with traumatic brain injury with intact sensation. Additionally, as volitional motor control returns, and as the brain heals, tone may normalize and medication is then no longer necessary.

Spasticity has some beneficial effects such as maintaining muscle bulk, preventing a deep vein thrombosis and osteoporosis, and allowing a patient with marginal motor strength to stand and transfer. It is only when spasticity interferes with function, causes pain, does not allow nursing care, or contributes to the formation of contractures that spasticity needs to be treated.

The current trend has drifted away from pharmacological intervention. Instead physical modalities are tried, such as: the application of cold or heat; stretching, splinting, and casting (including inhibitive casting); adequate positioning; functional electrical stimulation; vibration; relaxation techniques; motor reeducation; and biofeedback (Glenn & Rosenthal, 1985). In addition, modalities such as chemical neurolysis (nerve blocks and motor point blocks) may be tried before drug therapy is begun (Weintraub & Opat, 1989). When drug therapy is indicated, dantrolene sodium (Dantrium) is the preferred drug as it appears to have the least cognitive or sedating effects.

Respiratory Complications

Most patients with severe brain injuries require hyperventilation for the control of intracranial pressure. Therefore the development of respiratory complications is quite common. Most patients with severe injuries are subject to oral or nasal intubation and most will require tracheostomy. With tracheostomy comes a high percentage of patients who develop colonization of the tracheostomy site and pneumonia. Additionally, neurological deficits may impair patients' ability to cough or breathe. Recurrent regurgitation with aspiration as a consequence of dysphagia may further compromise their respiratory status.

Despite the fact that tracheostomy tubes appear to be a source of continual bacterial colonization, one recent study concludes that patients with lower cognitive levels should retain their tracheostomy tubes until they are more aware (Nowak, Cohn, & Guidice, 1987). There appears to be a high rate of morbidity and mortality associated with decannulation (Klingbeil, 1983; Nowak, Cohn, & Guidice, 1987).

Nutritional Status and Swallowing

Patients with acute brain injuries are known to be hypermetabolic and thus require increased calories and increased protein (Epstein et al., 1987). Most trauma centers now take into account the nutritional needs of the acutely injured patient, and patients are primarily being fed via enteral tube feedings. Patients who have suffered severe visceral trauma may have been supplemented by hyperalimentation. Subsequently, they are usually transferred to rehabilitation settings in positive nitrogen balance.

Recognition of swallowing problems in the acute care setting is improving as the use of videofluoroscopy (a radiographic procedure that allows clinicians to observe the swallowing reflex, oral-motor and tongue control, and pharyngeal peristalsis) increases. Increased awareness of silent aspiration had decreased the mortality and morbidity of severely injured patients and has contributed to the development of improved therapeutic interventions for delayed or absent swallowing mechanisms (Lazarus & Logemann, 1987).

Genito-urinary Problems

Patients in acute care settings are very often subjected to indwelling Foley catheterization to monitor urine output. Such instrumentation is often a source of chronic infection (Whyte & Glenn, 1986).

Neurogenic bladder following traumatic brain injury is quite rare, and if it does exist, it is usually an uninhibited detrusor hyperreflexia causing the patient to void small amounts frequently (Anderson, 1977). Awareness that patients can also have detrusor hyporeflexia as a result of bladder overdistension that can occur secondary to outlet obstruction or iatrogenically in the acute care setting has minimized problems in this realm. Patients can usually be adequately managed with external collection devices or diapers until they are aware enough of their surroundings and have sufficient ongoing memory to benefit from being offered the commode or bedpan on a regular basis (Johnson, 1980).

Endocrine Complications

The most frequently encountered endocrine complication seen in the acute care setting is the disturbance of antidiuretic hormone (ADH) secretions (Epstein et al., 1987). Inappropriate ADH syndrome resulting in oversecretion of ADH with a resultant decrease in sodium concentration occurs frequently during the acute neurosurgical phase. Treatment is usually by fluid restriction and usually resolves spontaneously. Less common is the disruption of ADH release, which results in central diabetes insipidus (DI). DI can usually be treated with vasopressant tannate and oil, or with internasal 1-desamino-8-D-arginine vasopressin (DDAVP) (Notman, Mortek, & Moses, 1980).

Recent studies by Horn (1988a,1988b) looking at patients' endocrine function in a screening protocol indicate that 20% of persons with severe brain injuries suffer from one or more disturbances of anterior pituitary hormone levels. However, the significance of these are not yet known; further studies are needed and are ongoing.

CONCLUSION

Advances in the medical treatment of patients with traumatic brain injury have permitted an increase in the number who survive and a decrease in secondary injuries and complications. The increasing number of survivors has fueled the recent explosion in the number of facilities providing rehabilitation services. Yet, despite the increase in the number of rehabilitation programs, not all patients are afforded the opportunity to enter comprehensive programs and fewer still are guided by experts in their attempts at community reentry.

The medical advances achieved within the past century have been dramatic—but there is much more that needs to be done with alternative and innovative rehabilitation programs, in terms of their effectiveness and accountability.

REFERENCES

Allen, G.S., Ahn, H.S., Preziosi, T.J., Battye, R., Boone, S.C., Chou, S.N., Kelly, D.L., Weir, B.K., Crabbe, R.A., Lavik, P.J., Rosenbloom, S.B., Dorsey, F.C., Ingram, C.R., Mellits, D.E., Bertsch, L.A., Boisvert, P.J., Hundley, M.B., Johnson, R.K., Strom, J.A., & Transou, C.R. (1983). Cerebral arterial spasm—a controlled trial of nimodipine in patients with subarachnoid hemorrhage. *New England Journal of Medicine, 308,* 691–624.

Anderson, J.T. (1977). Neuro-urological investigation in urinary bladder dysfunction. *International Urology and Nephrology, 9,* 133–143.

Andrewes, D.G., Tomlinson, L., Elwes, R.D.C., & Reynolds, E.H. (1984). The influence of carbamazepine and phenytoin on memory and other aspects of cognitive function in new referrals with epilepsy. *Acta Neurologica Scandinavica, 69* (Suppl. 99), 23–30.

Beyerl, B., & Black, P.M. (1984). Posttraumatic hydrocephalus. *Neurosurgery, 15,* 257–261.

Bontke, C.B. (1988). Update on pharmacology: Pharmacological treatment of heterotopic ossification. *Journal of Head Trauma Rehabilitation, 3,* 86–89.

Botte, M.J., & Moore, T.J. (1987). The orthopedic management of extremity injuries in head trauma. *Journal of Head Trauma Rehabilitation, 2,* 13–27.

Cardenas, D.D. (1987). Antipsychotics and their use after traumatic brain injury. *Journal of Head Trauma Rehabilitation, 2*(4), 43–49.

Cope, D.N., Date, E.S., & Mar, E.Y. (1988). Serial computerized tomographic evaluations in traumatic head injury. *Archives of Physical Medicine and Rehabilitation, 69,* 483–485.

Dixon, T.P. (1989). Systems of care for the head injured. In L.J. Horn & D.N. Cope (Eds.), *State of the art review: Traumatic brain injury* (Vol. 3, No. 1, pp. 169–181). Philadelphia: Hanley and Belfus.

Eisenberg, H.M., Weiner, R.L., & Tabaddor, K. (1987). Emergency care: Initial evaluation. In P. R. Cooper (Ed.), *Head injury* (2nd ed., pp. 20–33). Baltimore: Williams & Wilkins.

Epstein, F.M., Ward, J.D., & Becker, D.P. (1987). Medical complications of head injury. In P.R. Cooper (Ed.), *Head injury* (2nd ed., pp. 390–421). Baltimore: Williams & Wilkins.

Feeney, D.M., & Walker, A.E. (1979). The prediction of posttraumatic epilepsy. *Archives of Neurology, 36,* 8–12.

Freed, J.H., Hahn, H., Menter, R., & Dillon, T. (1982). The use of the three-phase bone scan in the early diagnosis of heterotopic ossification (HO) and in the evaluation of Didronel therapy. *Paraplegia, 20,* 208–216.

Garland, D.E., Blum, C.E., & Waters, R.L. (1981). Periarticular heterotopic ossification in head-injured adults. *Journal of Bone and Joint Surgery, 62-A,* 1143–1146.

Garland, D.E., & Keenan, M.A.E. (1983). Orthopedic strategies in the management of the adult head-injured patient. *Physical Therapy, 63*(12), 2004–2009.

Garland, D.E., Razza, B.E., & Waters, R.L. (1982). Forceful joint manipulation in head-injured adults with heterotopic ossification. *Clinical Orthopaedics and Related Research, 169,* 133–138.

Gennarelli, T.A. (1988). Subject review: Heterotopic ossification. *Brain Injury, 2,* 175–178.

Glenn, M. B., & Rosenthal, M. (1985). Rehabilitation following severe traumatic brain injury. *Seminars in Neurology, 5*(3), 233–246.

Glenn, M.B., & Wroblewski, B. (1986). Update of pharmacology: Anticonvulsants for prophylaxis of post-traumatic seizures. *Journal of Head Trauma Rehabilitation, 1,* 73–74.

Gudeman, S.K., Kishore, P.R.S., Becker, D.P., Lipper, M.H., Girevendulis, A.K., Jeffries, B.F., & Butterworth, J.F. (1981). Computed tomography in the evaluation of incidence and significance of post-traumatic hydrocephalus. *Neuroradiology, 141,* 397–402.

Hanscom, D.A. (1987). Acute management of the multiply injured head trauma patient. *Journal of Head Trauma Rehabilitation, 2,* 1–12.

Horn, L.J. (1988a). Update in pharmacology: Pharmacological interventions in neuroendocrine disorders following traumatic brain injury, Part I. *Journal of Head Trauma Rehabilitation, 3*(2), 87–90.

Horn, L.J. (1988b). Update in pharmacology: Pharmacological interventions in neuroendocrine disorders following traumatic brain injury, Part II. *Journal of Head Trauma Rehabilitation, 3*(3), 86–90.

Jennett, B. (1975). *Epilepsy after non-missile head injuries* (2nd ed.). Chicago: William Heinemann Medical Books.

Jennett, B. (1979). Posttraumatic epilepsy. In R. A. Thompson, J. R. Green et al. (Eds.), *Advances in neurology* (Vol. 22, pp. 137–147). New York: Raven Press.

Jennett, B. (1983). Posttraumatic epilepsy. In M. Rosenthal, E.R. Griffith, M.R. Bond, & J.D. Miller (Eds.), *Rehabilitation of the head injured adult.* Philadelphia: F.A. Davis.

Johnson, J.H. (1980). Rehabilitative aspects of neurologic bladder dysfunction. *Nursing Clinics of North America, 15*(2), 293–307.

Kishore, P.R.S., Lipper, M.H., Miller, J.D., Girevendulis, A.K., Becker, D.P., & Vines, F.S. (1978). Post-traumatic hydrocephalus in patients with severe head injury. *Neuroradiology, 16,* 261–265.

Klingbeil, G.E.G. (1988). Airway problems in patients with head injury. *Archives of Physical Medicine and Rehabilitation, 69,* 493–495.

Kottke, F.J. (1982). Therapeutic exercise to maintain mobility. In F.J. Kotke, G.K. Stillwell, & J. F. Lehrman (Eds.), *Krusen's handbook of physical medicine and rehabilitation* (3rd ed., pp. 389–402). Philadelphia: W.B. Saunders.

Kraus, J.F., Black, M.A., Hessol, N., Ley, P., Rokaw, W., Sullivan, C., Bowers, S., Knowlton, & Marshall, L. (1983). The incidence of acute brain injury and serious impairment in a defined population. *American Journal of Epidemiology, 119,* 186–201.

Lazarus, C., & Logemann, J.A. (1987). Swallowing disorders in closed head trauma patients. *Archives of Physical Medicine and Rehabilitation, 68,* 79–84.

Marshall, L.F., & Marshall, S.B. (1987). Medical management of intracranial pressure. In P.R. Cooper (Ed.), *Head injury* (pp. 177–196). Baltimore: Williams & Wilkins.

Mattson, R.H., Cramer, J.A. Collins, J.F., Smith, D.B., Delgado-Escueta, A.V., Browne, T.R., Williamson, P.D., Treiman, D.M., McNamara, J.O., McCutchen, C.B., Homan, R.W., Crill, W.E., Lubozynski, M.F., Rosenthal, N.P., & Mayersdorf, A. (1985). Comparison of carbamazepine, phenobarbital, phenytoin and primidone in partial and secondarily generalized tonic-clonic seizures.

New England Journal of Medicine, 313(3), 145–151.

Mital, M.A., Garber, J.E., & Stinson, J.T. (1987). Ectopic bone formation in children and adolescents with head injury: Its management. *Journal of Pediatric Orthopaedics, 7,* 83–90.

Notman, D.D., Mortek, M.A., & Moses, A.M. (1980). Permanent diabetes insipidus following head trauma: Observations on ten patients and an approach to diagnosis. *Journal of Trauma, 20,* 599–602.

Nowak, P., Cohn, A.M., & Guidice, M.A. (1987). Airway complications in patients with closed-head injuries. *American Journal of Otolaryngology, 8,* 91–96.

Petruk, K.C., West, M., Mohr, G., Weir, B.K.A., Benoit, B.G., Gentili, F., Disney, L.B., Khan, M.I., Grace, M., Holness, R.O., Karwon, M.S., Ford, R.M., Cameron, G.S., Tucker, W.S., Purves, G.B., Miller, J.D.R., Hunter, K.M., Richard, M.T., Durity, F.A., Chan, R., Clein, L.J., Maroun, F.B., & Godon, A. (1988). Nimodipine treatment in poor-grade aneurysm patients. *Journal of Neurosurgery, 68,* 505–517.

Pisciotta, A.V. (1982). Carbamazepine: Hematological toxicity. In D.M. Woodbury, J.K. Penry, & C.E. Pippenger (Eds.). *Antiepileptic drugs* (2nd ed., pp. 533–541). New York: Raven Press.

Reynolds, E.H., & Trimble, M.R. (1985). Adverse neuropsychiatric effects of anticonvulsant drugs. *Drugs, 29,* 570–581.

Rimel, R.W., & Jane, J.A. (1983). Characteristics of the head injured patient. In M. Rosenthal, E.R. Griffith, M.R. Bond, & J.D. Miller, (Eds.), *Rehabilitation of the head injured adult* (pp. 9–22). Philadelphia: F.A. Davis.

Ritter, M.A., & Gioe, T. (1982). The effect of indomethacin on para-articular ectopic ossification following total hip arthroplasty. *Clinical Orthopaedics and Related Research, 167,* 113–117.

Rogers, R.C. (1988). Program idea: Heterotopic calcification in severe head injury: A preventive program. *Brain Injury, 2,* 169–172.

Sandel, M.E. (1989). Rehabilitation management in the acute care setting. In L.J. Horn & D.N. Cope (Eds.), *State of the art review: Traumatic brain injury* (Vol. 3, No. 1, pp. 27–42). Philadelphia: Hanley and Belfus.

Sazbon, L., Najenson, T., Tartakovsky, M., Becker, E., & Grosswasser, Z. (1981). Widespread periarticular new-bone formation in long-term comatose patients. *Journal of Bone and Joint Surgery, 63-B* (1), 120–125.

Scriabine, A., & Van Den Kerckhoff, W. (1988, March). Pharmacology of nimodipine: A review. Calcium Antagonists Pharmacology. *Annals of the New York Academy of Science, 522.*

Spielman, G., Gennarelli, T.A., & Rogers, C.R.

(1983). Disodium etidronate: Its role in preventing heterotopic ossification in severe head injury. *Archives of Physical Medicine and Rehabilitation, 64,* 539–542.

Stover, S.L., Hahn, H.R., & Miller, J.M. (1976). Disodium etidronate in the prevention of heterotopic ossification following spinal cord injury. *Paraplegia, 14,* 146–156.

Sutton, R.L., Weaver, M.S., & Feeney, D.M. (1987). Drug-induced modifications of behavioral recovery following cortical trauma. *Journal of Head Trauma Rehabilitation, 2,* 50–58.

Thompson, P.J., & Trimble, M.R. (1982). Anticonvulsant drugs and cognitive functions. *Epilepsia, 23,* 531–544.

Trimble, M.R., & Thompson, P.J. (1984). Anticonvulsant drugs and cognitive function. *Archives of Physical Medicine and Rehabilitation, 65,* 618.

Vining, E.P. (1987). Cognitive dysfunction associated with antiepileptic drug therapy. *Epilepsy, 28,* (Suppl. 2), S18–S22.

Weintraub, A.H., & Opat, C.A. (1989). Motor and sensory dysfunction in the brain injured adult. In L.J. Horn & D.N. Cope (Eds.), *State of the art review: Traumatic brain injury* (Vol. 3, No. 1, pp. 59–84). Philadelphia: Hanley and Belfus.

Whyte, J., & Glenn, M.B. (1986). The care and rehabilitation of the patient in a persistent vegetative state. *Journal of Head Trauma Rehabilitation, 1,* 39–54.

Wikkelso, C., Andersson, H., Bloomstrand, C., Lindqvist, G., & Svendsen, P. (1986). Normal pressure hydrocephalus. *Acta Neurologica Scandinavica, 73,* 566–573.

Zimmerman, R.D., Fleming, C.A., Lee, B.C.P., Saint-Louis, L.A., & Deck, M.D.F. (1986). Periventricular hyperintensity as seen by magnetic resonance: Prevalence and significance. *American Journal of Neuroradiology, 7,* 13–20.

CHAPTER 2

Neuropsychopharmacological Approaches to Traumatic Brain Injury

Gregory J. O'Shanick and Nathan D. Zasler

Sustaining a traumatic brain injury alters the individual in multiple ways. In their most obvious forms, these changes appear as problems with speech, gait, movement, and perceptual disturbances. At the other end of the continuum, however, exist alterations in the individual's cognitive, coping, and self-regulatory capacities. These alterations frequently endure far beyond the recovery and stabilization of more obvious physical disabilities. These "hidden" deficits often subvert the individual in his or her attempts at community reentry and vocational or scholastic productivity.

Over the years, substantial direct and indirect evidence has been accumulated supporting the notion that the brain is the organ of the mind. This concept has been overlooked relative to traumatic brain injury behavioral disturbances and especially with regard to intervention strategies for these problems. Compelling information now exists indicating that underlying these behavioral disturbances are alterations in neurophysiological elements of the central nervous system (O'Shanick, 1988). While the majority of investigations correlating neurochemical alterations with behavioral abnormalities have been done in non–head-injured persons, the extrapolation of this research has led to exciting and innovative discoveries regarding the underpinnings of traumatic brain injury behavioral disturbances and their biological management.

Biological interventions have largely been focused upon the use of pharmacological agents that act upon the multiple types of neurotransmitters found in the central nervous system

(O'Shanick, 1987). Many of these agents have been used for decades in the management of primary psychiatric disturbances; however, their use in individuals with traumatic brain injury is a relatively new addition to the rehabilitation armamentarium. While these chemicals are used to counteract the alterations that occur secondary to the injury process, most possess not only their primary therapeutic action, but also other interactions with neurochemical systems that result in a constellation of side effects. These side effects can range from minor inconveniences to major annoyances and may have an adverse impact upon occupational performance. In toxic levels (unintentionally induced by various causes), the medications may also present fairly characteristic symptoms that again would adversely affect job performance. This chapter is designed to familiarize those individuals working with persons with traumatic brain injury with the major classes of pharmacological agents employed, their indications, actions, side effects and potential interactions on the job site.

ANTIDEPRESSANTS

Multiple types of antidepressants exist. The oldest of these agents are the monoamine oxidase inhibitors (MAOI) whose use requires careful dietary restriction of foods that contain high levels of tyramine (e.g., aged meats, aged cheese, wine, beer, sardines, sauerkraut) and other medications (meperidine, certain cold medications, certain antiparkinsonian agents) to prevent potentially life-threatening elevations in blood pressure. As such, they are rarely used in patients with traumatic brain injury. Another group of antidepressant agents are the tricyclic antidepressants (TCA), which include those listed in Table 2.1. These agents possess in addition to their antidepressant activities potent antihistaminic and anticholinergic activities that define their most commonly encountered side effects (Richelson & Nelson, 1984). Newer antidepressant agents are pharmacologically designed to be more specific in their therapeutic actions with fewer side effects.

In general, the actions of the antidepressants are designed to result in a net increase of the availability of the neurotransmitter to act from one neuron to another. This net increase may be achieved by: 1) preventing the reabsorption of the neurotransmitter into the discharging neuron, 2) by reducing the amount of the neurotransmitter that is metabolized and rendered inactive, or 3) by both mechanisms. The primary neurotransmitter systems affected by antidepressants are norepinephrine and serotonin.

The indications for antidepressants in individuals with traumatic brain injury are multiple (O'Shanick & Parmelee, 1989). These include the standard clinical target symptoms that are the neurovegetative symptoms of depression. These include disorders of sleep continuity, anorexia, diurnal variation in mood (worse in the morning, better in the evening), anhedonia, psychomotor retardation, and concentration impairment. These target symptoms may predate the occur-

rence of the injury and, certainly in some cases, the brain injury is secondary to some degree of self-destructive behavior due to significant depressive disease. Other focal lesions in the central nervous system may also respond to antidepressant therapy (Lipsey, Robinson, Pearlson et al., 1984). Included in this are pathological emotionality (the mood lability often present following injury); depression secondary to injuries at the dominant temporal lobe region; postconcussive symptoms (dizziness, irritability, headache, and anxiety) due to "mild" traumatic brain injury; and agitation/aggressive behavior due to injuries of the frontal cortex, which controls the modulating response to actions, anxiety disorders, and cyclic disturbances of sleep.

In general, antidepressant activity requires 2–4 weeks from initiation of treatment to recognize any consistent therapeutic impact (O'Shanick, 1984). During this initial phase, the individual may experience multiple side effects while acclimating to these agents. The side effects include initial sedation with fatigue and lassitude, tremor, increase in heart rate, blurred vision, dry mouth, and lightheadedness. While not all individuals experience all side effects, during the early phases of treatment it is imperative to recognize the potential limitations upon climbing ladders, performing fine motor work, strenuous manual activity, and bending or squatting. Controversy exists regarding the ability of these agents to lower seizure threshold; however, with adequate anticonvulsant coverage, problems with breakthrough seizures are rare.

In the work environment, these agents should have relatively little impact due to their once-a-day dosing. Primarily this is done in the evening prior to retiring to minimize the individual's awareness of the acute side effects. The initiation phase (the first 2–4 weeks of ingesting the antidepressant) may reduce the individual's productivity; however, the upward or downward adjustment of antidepressant may minimize the side effects and their disruption of the individual's life. Discontinuation of antidepressants can generally be accomplished in 1 or 2 days with no substantial tapering required. Toxic effects of these agents relate to their increased concentration in the blood stream resulting in

Table 2.1.   Antidepressants

Monoamine oxidase inhibitor (MAOI)
   Phenelzine (Nardil)
   Tranylcypramine (Parnate)

Tricyclic antidepressants (TCA)
   Amitriptyline (Elavil)
      Nortriptyline (Aventyl)
   Imipramine (Tofranil)
      Desipramine (Norpramin)
   Doxepin (Sinequan)
   Protriptyline (Vivactil)

Tetracyclic antidepressants
   Maprotilene (Ludiomil)

Other
   Trazodone (Desyrel)
   Fluoxitane (Prozac)

various cardiac rhythm disturbances, acute confusional episodes, and hypertension relating to postural changes (O'Shanick, 1987). As alcoholic beverages typically increase the sedating qualities of these antidepressants, their use is actively discouraged.

ANTIPSYCHOTICS

Antipsychotics (neuroleptics, major tranquilizers) were initially introduced as agents to control the severe symptoms of schizophrenia. Their success with treating the positive symptoms (e.g., auditory hallucinations, delusions) of schizophrenia resulted in a dramatic reduction in length of hospital stays for individuals with this disorder. Their ability to decrease agitation and irritability in individuals with schizophrenia was generalized for use in agitation and irritability secondary to persons with organic brain syndromes, including traumatic brain injury (O'Shanick & Parmelee, 1989). While multiple chemical structures exist under the larger rubric of antipsychotics, their net clinical effect appears to be mediated by their ability to block postsynaptic receptors of the neurotransmitter dopamine in the mesolimbic cortex. Clinical studies that compare the efficacy of agents thought to be antipsychotics consistently show the ability to bind (block) with postsynaptic dopamine receptors to be the governing variable in terms of potency (Peroutka & Snyder, 1980). Agents such as chlorpromazine (Thorazine) and thioridazine (Mellaril) are less potent antipsychotics than agents such as haloperidol (Haldol), fluphenazine (Prolixin) and thiothixene (Navane) for this reason (Table 2.2). While the major indications (target symptoms) for anti-

Table 2.2. Antipsychotics (and their relative potencies)

1 mg of fluphenazine (Prolixin)
    = 2 mg of haloperidol (Haldol)
    = 6 mg of thiothixene (Navane)
    = 8 mg of perphenazine (Trilafon)
    = 10 mg of trifluoperazine (Stelazine)
    = 15 mg of molindone (Moban)
    = 20 mg of loxapine (Loxitane)
    = 100 mg of thioridazine (Mellaril)
    = 100 mg of chlorpromazine (Thorazine)

psychotics have been the positive psychotic symptoms associated with schizophrenia, other uses for antipsychotics exist (O'Shanick & Parmelee, 1989). These include their use as antinausea or antiemetic agents due to their ability to block dopamine receptors in the medulla, their use as potentiators of narcotic analgesics such as morphine and meperidine (Demerol), their ability to decrease gastrointestinal activity, and their ability to provide a "chemical straitjacket" for individuals with extreme agitation or aggressive behavior.

In 1982, an experiment conducted by Feeney, Gonzalez, and Law revealed that rodents exposed to neuroleptics following traumatic brain injury had a much longer recovery curve than those not so exposed. It was hypothesized that the relearning necessary to recover motor function following this experimentally induced injury was inhibited by the neuroleptic's ability to block dopamine receptors. Later clinical studies have not shown any difference in ultimate outcome in humans exposed to neuroleptics following brain injury; however, there does appear to be a prolonged recovery phase for the exposed group versus the non-exposed group (Rao, Jellinek, & Woolston, 1985). For this reason, the use of agents that block dopamine receptors has largely been discouraged following traumatic brain injury.

In addition to the potential prolongation of recovery, other side effects are seen with antipsychotics, including extrapyramidal symptoms that relate to changes in the smoothness of voluntary muscle activities (O'Shanick, 1984). These are manifested by tremor, rigidity, difficulty initiating or stopping movements, profuse sweating, and mask-like facies. Other side effects from antipsychotics include a lowering of seizure threshold, drowsiness, potential for decrease in cognitive capacity, increase in pulse, and a potential for jaundice and photosensitivity (O'Shanick, 1987).

Perhaps the most dramatic side effect of antipsychotic use is tardive dyskinesia. This involuntary movement disorder occurs in up to 25% of persons on long-term neuroleptics and affects the mouth, lips, tongue, and occasionally the trunk and arms. This entity is, for all intents and purposes, irreversible once developed and markedly impairs the individual's ability to work productively (Gerlach, 1979).

The therapeutic effects of antipsychotics are countered by exposure to ethanol, with the exception of their sedative properties, which are increased. These agents generally are given in a once-a-day dose at bedtime. Some preparations are available for long-term intramuscular injection (Haldol Decanoate, Prolixin Decanoate). This permits once-a-month injections, providing the maintenance medication for the individual. During the initial phases of medication, the individual may have some difficulty with sedation, muscle rigidity, or irritability. With discontinuation, given the long half-lives (how long it takes for the blood level of the drug to drop to half its initial value) of these agents and their storage in fat cells, no tapering is required and no withdrawal syndromes are generally observed.

ANTIANXIETY AGENTS (ANXIOLYTICS)

Control of anxiety has been a longstanding quest. For centuries, agents such as ethanol were used to decrease muscle tension, produce mild euphoria, and create some level of sedation for its partakers. Until relatively recently, most antianxiety agents were generally variations on the ethanol theme but possessed somewhat larger therapeutic windows (i.e., the difference in the amount of drug necessary to achieve the desired therapeutic effect versus the amount of the drug required to demonstrate a toxic effect). In general, anxiolytic agents currently in use in the United States are more than likely benzodiazepines whose main chemical activity is to potentiate the neurotransmitter GABA (gamma aminobutyric acid), which inhibits the firing of other neurons (Ameer & Greenblatt, 1981). The multiple available benzodiazepines (Table 2.3) vary in their time of onset, duration of action, and number of active byproducts created by their breakdown by the liver. Other older antianxiety agents include barbiturates such a phenobarbital and pentobarbital, meprobamate, and methaqualone. Other agents that act as sedative hyp-

Table 2.3.   Antianxiety agents (and their relative potencies)

0.5 mg of alprazolam (Xanax)
= 1 mg of lorazepam (Ativan)
= 5 mg of diazepam (Valium)
= 10 mg of chlordiazepoxide (Librium)
= 10 mg of prazepam (Centrax)
= 15 mg of oxazepam (Serax)
= 15 mg of chlorazepate (Tranxene)
= 40 mg of halazepam (Paxipam)

notics such as ethchlorvynol and glutethimide, also are similar in their neurochemical function.

The main indications for anxiolytic use in persons with brain injury (O'Shanick & Parmelee, 1989) are for control of intractable seizures (status epilepticus), and to decrease preoperative anxiety, muscle spasms, certain types of tremor, and acute agitation. Controversy exists regarding the use of shorter acting anxiolytics in the management of initial insomnia (difficulty falling asleep) due to their high potential for addiction and abuse (O'Shanick, 1984).

Major side effects of antianxiety agents relate to their ability to create dependency on these agents with resulting withdrawal symptoms upon abrupt discontinuation. The development of withdrawal symptoms relates to factors such as the duration of use, the amount of medication used daily, and the agent's duration of effect. For agents with relatively short durations (short half-lives), these withdrawal symptoms may be misdiagnosed as worsening anxiety symptoms with the individual then being given escalating doses of the antianxiety agent. Recent evidence illustrates that even "therapeutic" use of these agents can result in substantial abstinence syndromes (Lader & Higgitt, 1986). Other difficulties with such agents relates to their interference with memory and learning (Healey, Pickens, Meisch, & McKenna, 1983). The phenomenon of "state-dependent learning" has been well described for such agents. State-dependent learning means that information acquired under the influence of an antianxiety agent is best recalled under the influence of that agent. For the head-injured individual, this suggests that skills acquired through cognitive remediation, behavioral shaping, or other therapeutic interventions that occur while the individual is under the influence of these agents will be less completely recalled or efficiently performed once the agent has been withdrawn.

A second concern with the use of shorter acting antianxiety agents relates to their ability to induce forgetfulness (transient global amnesia) in individuals resulting in blackouts for which no memory exists whatsoever; however, the individual may be functioning in an apparently "normal" manner. A third significant side effect of antianxiety agents relates to the enhancement of their sedative properties when combined with other similarly acting agents. This phenomenon (called potentiation) is best illustrated by the combination of ethanol and benzodiazepine, which can be an extremely lethal combination in relatively modest amounts whereas large quantities of either agent would need to be ingested before significant medical difficulties were encountered. Some evidence also exists that the use of antianxiety agents in individuals with traumatic brain injury may result in a disinhibition phenomenon that creates increasing agitation and belligerence.

During the initial phase of medication with these agents, there is a tendency for the individual to be drowsy and less coordinated than usual. This may be compounded if the individual is also using alcohol to any degree. Once the individual is adjusted to the dosage of medication, which is often given three or four times per day, no significant difficulties are usually encountered. Some concern regarding the operation of potentially injurious machinery, including automobiles, exists during the initial medication phase. Discontinuation of these antianxiety agents must be done in a slow, tapering fashion to prevent the evolution of withdrawal phenomena, which would be characterized by increasing anxiety, irritability, agitation, and insomnia; elevations in blood pressure, heart rate, and respiratory rate; and (perhaps) visual hallucinations (Lader & Higgitt, 1986).

A new class of antianxiety agents has recently been released for use in the United States. These agents are characterized by the chemical buspirone (Buspar) and are notable for their lack of interaction with GABA (Eison & Temple, 1986). Their mechanism of action appears to be through serotonergic mechanisms and they are currently used for the control of chronic rather than acute anxiety states. Similarly, no efficacy is noted with these agents in terms of muscle spasm, status epilepticus, or alcohol withdrawal syndromes. As their onset of action is at least 2 weeks following initiation of treatment, their utility for acute anxiety is negligible compared to other antianxiety agents that potentiate GABA. Their use, however, in longstanding anxiety states (which one could argue would accompany virtually every traumatic brain injury) is well documented. Usually given in three- or four-times-a-day divided dosages, no difficulties are noted with sedation. The individual may even complain of no therapeutic benefit of the agent if he or she is expecting an acute response to his or her anxiety. Not infrequently, family and colleagues are the first to notice the decrease in irritability and aggressiveness often manifested in chronic anxiety situations. The agent has little abuse potential, and has very little potentiation by alcohol or other antianxiety agents. No evidence exists of any negative cognitive consequences for this agent at this time.

MOOD STABILIZERS

In the United States, the primary agent used to stabilize mood and decrease hyperactive grandiose or manic-like behavior is lithium (Preskorn et al., 1981). The major indications for this monovalent cation in addition to recurrent mood disorders are mood disorders refractory to single therapy with an antidepressant, aggressive behavior especially in individuals with preexisting organic brain injury, and behavior disturbances that arise between seizure episodes (O'Shanick & Parmelee, 1989). The mechanism of action of lithium relates to its ability to enhance the neurotransmitter serotonin in the central nervous system while decreasing the activity of dopamine and norepinephrine (Preskorn et al., 1981). The onset of action typically is 2–3 weeks with the individual receiving either three or four divided doses of this medication per day. Blood levels are assessed, with a therapeutic range of 0.6–1.2 mEq/1 being desired for the remission of symptoms. Significant side effects of lithium relate to both acute and long-term factors (Schou, Baastrup, Gross, et al., 1970). Acutely, the individual may report increased thirst, increased urination, and mild tremor at rest. In addition, complaints of mild gastrointestinal distress (nausea, vomiting, diarrhea) are not unusual in the first week or 10 days of treatment. Chronic administration of lithium may be associated with thyroid abnormalities as well as renal abnormalities, which require at least annual monitoring.

From a vocational perspective, the most significant difficulties with lithium relate to its induction of a fine hand tremor that could interfere with fine motor activities and with the individual's being at risk for developing severe lithium toxicity if placed in a situation where he or she is sweating profusely. With perspiration, the individual will greatly increase his or her blood concentration of lithium to toxic levels that could result in dizziness, irritability, lethargy, seizures, and even death (Schou et al., 1970). For these reasons, individuals on lithium are counseled to minimize warm-weather activities unless adequate hydration and salt replacement are given. During the discontinuation phase with lithium carbonate, no tapering or abstinence symptoms are observed. Some indication exists that alcohol may in fact decrease the efficacy of lithium due to the ability of ethanol to increase the clearance rate of lithium through the kidneys and decrease its blood levels.

In addition to lithium, carbamazepine, the anticonvulsant, has also been employed as a mood-stabilizing agent. The reader is directed to the section on anticonvulsants for further discussion.

STIMULANTS

Agents that increase arousal through augmenting the activities of the catecholamine neurotransmitters dopamine and norepinephrine have been especially interesting to individuals involved in traumatic brain injury rehabilitation (O'Shanick & Parmelee, 1989). Several different categories exist, including amphetamines, methylphenidate, and pemeline, that fundamentally act in the same way to increase the release of these neuro-

transmitters from the neurons in the central nervous system. Their primary use has been for individuals who are lethargic and hypoarousable, individuals with impaired concentration and attention, individuals with excessive daytime drowsiness, and the short-term treatment of significant depressive episodes. These agents have significant generalized effects requiring very close cardiovascular monitoring. Short-term side effects include irritability, insomnia, and aggressive behavior; long-term side effects relate to the development of paranoid delusions, hypertension, and the potential for addiction (Angrist, 1978).

Individuals receiving stimulants require close medical supervision to prevent abuse or toxicity (O'Shanick, 1986). Discontinuation should not be abrupt but rather should have a slow tapering of the medication to prevent dramatic abstinence syndromes that might be mistaken for delusional psychosis. The intercurrent use of alcohol or any other illicit drugs is *absolutely* contraindicated with these agents. Most often they are given in a twice-daily dosing schedule prior to 2:00 P.M. to decrease their potential to create initial insomnia. Perhaps the major vocational effect of these agents relates to the abuse potential—especially once others learn that the individual has a supply of these at his or her disposal.

ANTICONVULSANT MEDICATIONS

Aside from the issues of psychopharmacological intervention for neurobehavioral disorders following traumatic brain injury, one of the biggest controversies that presently exists in the post–acute care of the person with traumatic brain injury is the prescription of anticonvulsant medications. These medications can be used to suppress post-traumatic epilepsy (PTE) and theoretically to prevent the future occurrence of epileptic fits even after the drug is withdrawn. There continues to be significant differences of opinion regarding which persons are at higher risk for PTE and the duration of anticonvulsant therapy that is necessary for those persons at high risk. Although most physicians who deal with post-traumatic epilepsy tend to utilize risk factors set forth by Jennett (1975) more recent studies (Guidice & Berchow, 1987) indicate that these may be somewhat inaccurate. In most European countries, a person who has incurred a traumatic brain injury generally does not receive prophylactic anticonvulsant therapy; medications are only started when and if an individual has a seizure. The present trend at most academic institutions in the United States has been to increase the threshold for beginning prophylactic anticonvulsant medications. Philosophies regarding discontinuation of anticonvulsant medication following seizure-free periods vary from as short as 3 months to as long as 2 years after the initial injury. It is important for physicians to realize that the risk factors for development of post-traumatic epilepsy vary depending upon whether seizures occur early or late. Additionally, one seizure after a traumatic brain injury does not imply a diagnosis of PTE.

At the present time, most neurosurgeons in the United States use either phenytoin (Dilantin) or phenobarbital for early management of seizures and/or seizure prophylaxis due to the fact that these medications can be administered parenterally (by intravenous route) in the acute care setting. However, there are significant data to indicate that the anticonvulsants of choice for either treatment of post-traumatic epilepsy or prophylaxis for post-traumatic epilepsy are carbamazepine (Tegretol) and valproic acid (Depakote). Scientific data indicate that both phenobarbital and Dilantin have significant negative effects on cognitive abilities whereas medications such as carbamazepine and valproic acid have been found to cause relatively little cognitive impairment (Reynolds & Trimble, 1985; Trimble & Thompson, 1983). Important concepts to remember when treating the brain-injured individual with anticonvulsant agents are to minimize the degree of cognitive impairment by choosing the least sedating medication; minimizing, as much as possible, the number of medications being used; and using the minimum effective dosage required to control the seizure disorder. Aside from the lack of significant cognitive side effects, the use of carbamazepine and valproic acid for treatment and prophylaxis of post-traumatic epilepsy following traumatic

brain injury is also supported by the fact that most individuals who suffer from PTE will either experience partial or generalized tonic-clonic seizures, respectively.

Although carbamazepine and valproic acid are the anticonvulsants of choice in traumatic brain injury, multiple other medications are available, including: barbiturates (such a phenobarbital and primidone), benzodiazepines (such as clonazepan), hydantoins (such as phenytoin), oxazolidinediones (such as trimethadione), and succinimides (such as ethosuximide). It is important to be aware of these various agents and their potential interactions with other medications (not only other anticonvulsants), as well as their individual side effects.

Adverse effects of anticonvulsant agents are numerous and range along a whole spectrum of severity from those that are benign and reversible to those that are fatal and irreversible (Dam, 1988). Central nervous system side effects are quite common with anticonvulsant agents. Some of the side effects that occur more commonly include irritability, headache, restlessness, dizziness, vertigo, ataxia, drowsiness, and dysarthria. The central nervous system side effects tend to be dose related, and also tend to be worse during the initial phases of treatment. It is important, therefore, to initiate treatment at low doses and titrate the dose upward in a careful manner to achieve the minimum effective dose required for control. All of the available antiepileptic drugs have a fairly narrow therapeutic ratio. Common dose-related adverse effects include: the triad of clinical signs (nystagmus, ataxia, and dysarthria) frequently seen with phenytoin toxicity, sedation due to phenobarbital and primidone, and dizziness/double vision with carbamazepine.

Chronic use of anticonvulsant agents can lead to a cornucopia of adverse side effects. Phenytoin can cause overgrowth of gum tissue (gingival hyperplasia), coarsening of features and hirsutism, and various dermatological reactions most commonly in the form of benign rashes. Phenobarbital, primidone, and phenytoin commonly cause behavioral disturbances and impaired learning ability; hyperactivity and paradoxical irritability have been reported in the pediatric age group with these medications. Carbamazepine, phenytoin, phenobarbital, and primidone have all been implicated in induction of liver enzymes, which results in changes in the rate and quality of metabolism of other medications including anticonvulsant drugs, which in turn generally results in lower plasma anticonvulsant levels. Hepatic induction also affects the metabolism of other medications such as oral anticoagulants, steroid medications, and birth control pills. Anticonvulsant medications can also adversely affect the levels of various substances that occur naturally in the body including folic acid, steroid hormones, and vitamin D.

Since carbamazepine and valproic acid are now felt to be the drugs of choice for treatment and prophylaxis of post-traumatic epilepsy (Glenn & Wroblewski, 1986; Pellock, 1989), it is essential to have a good working understanding of their pharmacological properties. Many of the side effects seen on initiating carbamazepine therapy can be minimized by starting the drug at relatively low doses (i.e., 200 mg every day or 200 mg twice a day). It is not uncommon for early side effects such as dizziness, headaches, drowsiness, and gastrointestinal upset to be seen even when the medication is started at relatively low doses; however, these tend to decrease with continued administration. It is important to remember that carbamazepine not only induces the metabolism of other medications by increasing the activity of liver enzymes but also induces its own metabolism (auto-induction). Generally, auto-induction occurs within the first month of therapy and has been found to be both time and dose dependent. From a practical standpoint, this means that the drug's half-life will be much greater at initiation of therapy compared to 1 month postinitiation. Therapeutic serum concentrations are between 4 and 12 micrograms per milliliter. Due to the fact that the drug's half-life (once auto-induction has been established) is approximately 15 hours, it is important to dose the medication three to four times a day to maintain a more steady concentration in the blood and ultimately better seizure control. It is important to remember that higher doses of the medication will be needed when other anticonvulsant medications are used concomitantly as these other medications may also induce liver enzyme function. Carbamazepine levels need to be monitored closely when other anticonvulsant medications are withdrawn, as the serum level will tend to rise; lower doses of the medication will be necessary with time to maintain the same serum drug level. There has been much concern over the hematological side effects of carbamazepine; however, the occurrence of aplastic anemia (a condition that is generally fatal) is very uncommon, with an incidence of approximately 1 or less in every 10,000 persons.

It is important that all persons being considered for carbamazepine treatment undergo baseline laboratory investigations including complete blood count, platelet count, and possibly reticulocyte count, as well as baseline liver function tests. Additionally, baseline ophthamological examinations including funduscopic, slit-lamp exam, and tonometry are generally recommended. Proper follow-up of carbamazepine levels as well as hematological, hepatic, and ophthamological parameters are critical in order to minimize potential adverse drug reactions.

The main side effect that requires monitoring with valproic acid treatment is that of hepatotoxicity. Anticonvulsant polypharmacy increases the risk of valproic acid induced hepatotoxicity. It is essential to keep in mind that numerous medications can actually induce epileptic seizures in head-injured persons with PTE who are well controlled on anticonvulsant medication as well as in those who have no history of PTE and are not presently receiving anticonvulsant treatment. Drugs possessing this action include the phenothiazines, tricyclic and tetracyclic antidepressants, aminophylline, and many antihistamines. The atypical antidepressant trazodone, the antispasticity agent baclofen, and certain antibiotics (penicillin) have also been reported to elicit seizure activity. It should also be remembered that anticonvulsant medication withdrawal can itself precipitate seizure activity due to one of two phenomena: either the medication has been withdrawn too rapidly (more of an issue with phenobarbital than dilantin, carbamazepine, or valproic acid) or the individual requires continued anticonvulsant treatment for suppression of epileptogenic foci.

ANTISPASTICITY MEDICATIONS

In general, the use of oral medications to control spasticity in persons with traumatic brain injury should be considered only when more conservative interventions such as various physical modalities including heat/cold modalities, stretching, proper positioning, and inhibitory casting have been attempted (Katz, 1988). Additionally, more invasive interventions such as motor point blocks and/or nerve blocks with substances such as phenol can be utilized to control spasticitiy, thereby avoiding the central side effects of oral medications and allowing for more selective blockade of spastic muscles on a peripheral basis (Glenn, 1986).

The oral medications most commonly used for management of spasticity in general neurologic rehabilitation include baclofen (Lioresal), diazepam (Valium), and dantrolene sodium (Dantrium). Baclofen and diazepam both work at a central level by affecting the GABA neurotransmitter system. Dantrolene sodium works at a more peripheral level, specifically by causing release of calcium into the muscle, which is critical for full muscle contractile force to be established. Baclofen and diazepam can truly be considered as antispasticity agents based upon their mechanism of action; dantrolene sodium, however, would be considered more a muscle weakener than an antispasticity agent. The main disadvantage to the use of these types of medications in individuals with traumatic brain injury is that drugs such as baclofen and diazepam have significant sedating properties that can adversely affect cognitive function and work performance. Additionally, they act in a nonselective manner so that even muscles that are not spastic may be weakened (Davidoff, 1985). This can have functional consequence since many individuals will compensate for some of their motoric deficits with their "good muscles" and/or utilize spastic musculature in a functional way. Therefore, it is imperative that the physician prescribing antispasticity agents have a good understanding of the functional consequences of such treatment in terms of both cognitive and motoric side effects. Dantrolene sodium is generally considered the antispasticity

agent of choice since its central sedating affect is minimal. Because it acts directly at the muscle level, dantrolene sodium can cause generalized weakness. Although there is presently no way to predict which individuals will respond positively to the effects of dantrolene sodium, a decrease in spasticity with ice therapy has been used as a predictor for good response to baclofen therapy.

Adverse effects of antispasticity drugs are numerous. Secondary to potential muscle weakness caused by dantrolene sodium, functional impairment may be seen in ambulation, speech, and bladder control. Other common adverse side effects are drowsiness, dizziness, malaise, and numerous gastrointestinal side effects including diarrhea, constipation, nausea, anorexia, and abdominal cramps. Toxic effects to the liver have been reported, thereby necessitating intermittent follow-up of liver function tests. Hepatitis has been reported with the use of this medication and may be fatal. In general though, the current consensus is that the hepatotoxicity of the drug may be much less common than originally thought. The risk of hepatitis does seem to be greater with longer use and in general hepatotoxicity is seen more commonly in females who are older than 35 years of age and who may be receiving other drugs, particularly estrogens, concomitantly.

Numerous side effects have also been reported with baclofen, the most common being drowsiness, which may adversely affect the head-injured individual's work capacity. Other adverse symptoms that may impede the individual's work performance include fatigue, dizziness, muscle weakness, mental depression, and headache. Psychiatric disturbances including confusion, anxiety, depression, hallucinations, and euphoria have been reported and these seem to be more common in persons who have had premorbid psychiatric disturbances or any type of brain disorder (including traumatic brain injury). Baclofen should never be withdrawn abruptly as this can precipitate hallucinations and/or seizures in some persons or acute exacerbation of spasticity. The drug also has numerous potential gastrointestinal side effects including constipation, vomiting, and positive tests for occult blood in the stool. Changes in electroencephalographic readings as well as deterioration in seizure control have also been reported with baclofen in persons with epilepsy; this may have implications for persons with traumatic brain injury who are being treated for post-traumatic epilepsy.

Due to the potentially significant sedating effects of orally administered baclofen and diazepam there is really little reason for their use in spasticity management in the individual with traumatic brain injury.

ANTIHYPERTENSIVE MEDICATION

It is not uncommon for individuals with traumatic brain injury to have a premorbid history of medical problems including hypertension, diabetes, and substance abuse. It is important to keep in mind that there are numerous medications that may be used for treatment of other medical conditions unrelated to the traumatic brain injury itself that might have deleterious effects upon cognitive status as well as vocational reintegration. Probably the agents that have the greatest potential for this are the antihypertensive agents.

Generally, it is advisable that persons who have had a traumatic brain injury not be treated with antihypertensives that have a central depressant effect. Certain beta-blockers, such as propranolol, that penetrate the central nervous system may be suboptimal in terms of the potential side effects that can be encountered such as cognitive impairment, affective disturbance, and sedation. Beta-blockers that do not penetrate the central nervous system, such as atenolol, may be more appropriate in the head-injured individual with hypertension (if a beta-blocker is desired). Recent studies have indicated that the cognitive side effects of lipid-soluble beta-blockers (i.e., those penetrating the central nervous system) may not be any more adverse than the side effects from water-soluble beta-blockers (i.e., those not penetrating the central nervous system). None of these studies has been done in persons with brain injury yet the implications for treatment are important and further work is required to elucidate the implications to the treatment of chronic hypertension in traumatic brain injury. Other antihypertensive medications that may adversely

affect vocational reintegration potential secondary to sedation, cognitive depression, and/or other central nervous system side effects include clonidine, hydralizine, reserpine, and methyldopa (Croog, Levine, Testa et al., 1986; Solomon, Hotchkiss, Saravay et al., 1983).

Three classes of drugs have particular utility in the treatment of hypertension in persons with traumatic brain injury: calcium channel blockers, angiotensin-converting enzyme inhibitors, and diuretics. These agents are preferable secondary to their lack of central nervous system side effects; however, one does need to be aware of associated non–central nervous system problems that may arise with the use of these medications. Generally, these side effects will not interfere with vocational pursuits. Of the three classes of aforementioned drugs, probably the greatest potential for side effects is with the diuretics; the occurrence of electrolyte imbalances, sexual dysfunction, irregularities in cardiac rhythms, and increased urinary frequency need to be monitored closely. If the hypertension is secondary to the traumatic brain injury itself and not essential in nature, there may not be a need for long-term continuation of antihypertensive therapy and this needs to be reevaluated intermittently by the individual's primary care physician.

MEDICATIONS FOR ULCER PROPHYLAXIS

It is not uncommon for persons with moderate to severe traumatic brain injury to be treated prophylacticly with medications to prevent the occurrence of gastric ulceration secondary to the stress they incur during the acute and subacute postinjury phases. There are no specific recommendations regarding the length of prophylaxis and many patients will be discharged from the hospital on continued treatment. The medications most commonly used for stress ulcer prophylaxis are the H_2-antagonists and sucralfate. The H_2-antagonists include cimetidine, ranitidine, and famotidine (listed in order of decreasing central nervous system side effects) (Berardi, Tankanow, & Nostrant, 1988). This class of medications works by actually decreasing release of hydrochloric acid from parietal cells in the stomach. Due to the potential for adverse central nervous system side effects with the H_2-antagonists, their use is generally avoided unless there is active ulcer disease necessitating concomitant therapy with sucralfate. Sucralfate is a mucopolysaccharide that works through a mechanism of cytoprotection to the gastric mucosa, inhibits certain enzymes present in the gastric juices, and absorbs bile salts. There have been no significant adverse central nervous system side effects reported that might be deleterious to job performance (Marks, 1987).

The continued use of H_2-antagonists for stress ulcer prophylaxis in the postacute period needs to be examined more carefully, considering the potential negative effects that some of these agents may possess—with regard not only to central nervous system side effects and interference with vocational performance, but also the cost and the potential for interaction with other medications.

PHARMACOLOGICAL MANAGEMENT OF HETEROTOPIC OSSIFICATION

It is not uncommon for persons with traumatic brain injury to develop ectopic bone around joints secondary to an as-yet-unclarified neurogenic process related to their brain injury. This phenomenon, neurogenic heterotopic ossification (NHO), has a varying incidence related to the severity of brain injury, with rates reported in the literature to be as low a 11% and as high as 76% (Garland, 1988). Neurogenic heterotopic ossification typically occurs around large joints such as the elbows, shoulders, hips, and knees. The greatest functional morbidity can be loss of range of motion, which may impair not only mobility and activities of daily living but also vocational pursuits.

The only pharmacological therapy presently available to minimize the extent of morbidity associated with neurogenic heterotopic ossification is etidronate disodium (Didronel) (Bontke, 1988). Didronel works by interfering with biological calcification of bone and thereby impeding further progression of ectopic bone formation. Nonsteroidal anti-inflammatory agents

such as indomethacin have been used during the acute (early) stage of neurogenic heterotopic ossification to decrease the suspected inflammatory component of this process. Generally, by the time the individual is working toward vocational reintegration the use of nonsteroidal anti-inflammatory agents is no longer indicated; however, the use of etidronate disodium will generally continue into this part of the rehabilitation continuum. The incidence of side effects is quite low with etidronate disodium. The main adverse side effect involves gastrointestinal complaints in the form of diarrhea and nausea, which occur in approximately 1 in every 15 patients. Although the drug can be taken as one daily dose, it can also be divided to decrease gastrointestinal side effects. There have been no reported adverse central nervous system side effects from the use of etidronate disodium.

If heterotopic ossification secondary to traumatic brain injury interferes with vocational reintegration, referral to an orthopedic surgeon for resection of the ectopic bone can be considered. Generally, resection is not considered until at least 12–18 months postinjury to assure that maturation of ectopic bone has occurred, thereby minimizing recurrence after resection.

CIGARETTE SMOKING AND TRAUMATIC BRAIN INJURY

There has been little attention paid to the potential contraindications and adverse side effects of cigarette smoking after traumatic brain injury. In general, it is felt that nicotine causes arousal and this is supported by electroencephalographic changes that occur after cigarette smoking and/or administration of nicotine (Knott & Venables, 1977). This may be contraindicated in persons who may already be hypervigilant secondary to their traumatic brain injury; additionally, it may have adverse effects on ability to suppress impulsive/violent behavior. However, other studies have shown that nicotine may actually improve attention, learning, reaction time, and problem solving in non–brain-injured persons (Wesnes & Warburton, 1983); the implications of this are as yet unknown as they apply to the individual with traumatic brain injury. It is still unclear whether the improvements in performance are due to improved central nervous system function or to relief of abstinence symptoms. Nicotine has also been reported to have various endocrinological, metabolic, and neuromuscular side effects (Benowitz, 1988), none of which should dramatically interfere with vocational pursuits.

A significant side effect seen with cigarette smoking is the acceleration of drug metabolism. Although there are numerous compounds in cigarette smoke that may be responsible for altering drug metabolism, the most likely group of chemicals is the polycyclic aromatic hydrocarbons that are theorized to work through the cytochrome P448 enzyme system in the liver. There are a number of drugs commonly used in persons with traumatic brain injury whose metabolism may be accelerated by cigarette smoking, including: imipramine (used for treatment of affective disturbances including post-traumatic stress disorder) and propranolol (used in the treatment of aggressive behavior).

It is important to realize that as with many other medications rapid cessation of cigarette smoking can lead to withdrawal symptoms. Theoretically, withdrawal symptoms may be somewhat different and/or heightened in a person with concomitant brain injury. Typically, withdrawal symptoms consist of restlessness, irritability, drowsiness, anxiety, decreased frustration tolerance, confusion, and impaired concentration—all of which may be seen as part of the symptom complex associated with traumatic brain injury. Therefore, it is important always to be aware of any radical changes in tobacco usage especially in the presence of new subjective/objective deficits that could easily interfere with the individual's job responsibilities.

CONCLUSION

As part of the comprehensive rehabilitation of individuals with traumatic brain injury, the use of pharmacological agents can enhance the ultimate outcome. Common sense, however, must prevail when using these with a person in the transitional phase of reentry to personal and vocational independence. In his or her desire to be accepted by peers, the person with a brain injury might be, and often is, tempted to engage in socially "normal" behaviors (e.g., using ethanol and cigarettes). Conversely, the use of medication, *no matter how beneficial,* might be discontinued in an attempt to remove the "reminder" of past injuries. Therefore, when behavioral or physical deterioration occurs, the first inquiries are directed toward *compliance* with prescribed and proscribed agents.

Toxic effects and side effects are not inevitable when these agents are employed. Most disturbing problems can be reduced by avoiding sudden changes in habits (sleep, eating, activity), always checking for potential interactions with new medications (including over-the-counter medicines), and maintaining close medical supervision. Vocational problems may evolve, but are commonly manageable by changing doses, strengths, or preparations. Education of the consumer is mandatory for optimizing the therapeutic response.

REFERENCES

Ameer, B., & Greenblatt, D.J. (1981). Lorazepam: A review of its clinical pharmacological properties and therapeutic uses. *Drugs, 21,* 161–200.

Angrist, B.M. (1978). Toxic manifestations of amphetamine: *Psychiatric Annals, 8,* 13–18.

Benowitz, N.L. (1988). Pharmacologic aspects of cigarette smoking and nicotine addiction. *New England Journal of Medicine, 319*(2), 1318–1330.

Berardi, R.R., Tankanow, R.M., & Nostrant, T.T. (1988). Comparison of famotidine with dimetidine and ranitidine. *Clinical Pharmacy, F,* 271–284.

Bontke, C.F. (1988). Pharmacological treatment of heterotopic ossification. *Journal of Head Trauma Rehabilitation, 3*(1), 86–89.

Croog, S.H., Levine, S., Testa, M.A., et al. (1986). The effects of antihypertensive therapy on the quality of life. *New England Journal of Medicine, 314,* 1657–1664.

Dam, M. (1988). Side effects of drug therapy in epilepsy. *Acta Neurologica Scandinavica, 78*(Suppl. 11F), 34–40.

Davidoff, R.A. (1985). Antispasticity drugs: Mechanism of action. *Annals of Neurology, 17,* 106–166.

Eison, A.S., & Temple, D.L. (1986). Buspirone: Review of its pharmacology and current perspectives on its mechanism of action. *American Journal of Medicine, 80*(3B), 1–9.

Feeney, D.M., Gonzalez, A., & Law, W.A. (1982). Amphetamine, haloperidol, and experience interact to affect rate of recovery after motor cortex injury. *Science, 217,* 855–857.

Garland, D.E. (1988). Clinical observations on fractures and heterotopic ossification in the spinal cord and traumatic brain injured populations. *Clinical Orthopedics and Related Research, 219,* 86–101.

Gerlach, J. (1979). Tardive dyskinesia. *Danish Medical Bulletin, 26,* 209–245.

Glenn, M.B. (1986). Nerve blocks in the treatment of spasticity. *Journal of Head Trauma Rehabilitation, 1*(3), 72–74.

Glenn, M.B., & Wroblewski, B. (1986). Anticonvulsants for prophylaxis of post-traumatic seizures. *Journal of Head Trauma Rehabilitation, 1*(1), 73–74.

Guidice, M.A., & Berchou, R.C. (1987). Post traumatic epilepsy following head injury. *Brain Injury, 1,* 61–64.

Healey, M., Pickens, R., Meisch, R., & McKenna, T. (1983). Effects of chlorazepate, diazepam, lorazepam, and placebo on human memory. *Journal of Clinical Psychiatry, 44,* 436–439.

Jennett, W.B. (1975). *Epilepsy after non-missile head injuries.* London: Hienemann.

Katz, R.T. (1988). Management of spasticity. *American Journal of Physical Medicine and Rehabilitation, 67*(3), 108–116.

Knott, V.J., & Venables, P.H. (1977). EEG alpha correlates of non-smokers, and smoking deprivation. *Psychopharmacology, 14,* 150–156.

Lader, M., & Higgitt, H.A. (1986). Management of withdrawal from benzodiazepines. *International Drug Therapy Newsletter, 21,* 21–23.

Lipsey, J.R., Robinson, R.G., Pearlson, G.D., et al., (1984). Nortriptyline treatment of post-stroke depression: A double-blind study. *Lancet, 1,* 297–300.

Marks, I.N. (1987). The efficacy, safety and dosage of sucralfate in ulcer therapy. *Scandinavian Journal of Gastroenterology, 140* (Suppl.), 33–38.

O'Shanick, G.J. (1984). Emergency psychopharmacology. *American Journal of Emergency Medicine, 2,* 164–170.

O'Shanick, G.J. (1986). Neuropsychiatric complications in head injury. *Advances in Psychosomatic Medicine, 16,* 84–92.

O'Shanick, G.J. (1987). Clinical aspects of psychopharmacologic treatment in head-injured patients. *Journal of Head Trauma Rehabilitation, 2,* 59–67.

O'Shanick, G.J. (1988). Psychotropic management of behavioral disorders after head trauma. *Psychiatric Medicine, 6*(3), 67–82.

O'Shanick, G.J., & Parmelee, D.X. (1989). Psychopharmacologic agents in the treatment of brain injury. In D. Ellis & A.L. Christensen (Eds.), *Neuropsychological treatment after brain injury* (pp. 91–104). Boston: Martinus-Nijhoff.

Pellock, J.M. (1989). Who should receive prophylactic antiepileptic drugs following head injury? *Brain Injury, 3,* 107–108.

Peroutka, S.J., & Snyder, S.H. (1980). Relationship of neuroleptic drug effects and brain dopamine, serotinin, adrenergic, and histamine receptors to clinical potency. *American Journal of Psychiatry, 137,* 1518–1522.

Preskorn, S.H., Irwin, G.H., Simpson, S., Friesen, D., Rinne, J., & Jerkovich, G. (1981). Medical therapies for mood disorders alter the blood-brain barrier. *Science, 213,* 469–471.

Rao, N., Jellinek, H.M., & Woolston, D.C. (1985). Agitation in closed head injury: Haloperidol effects on rehabilitation outcome. *Archives of Physical Medicine and Rehabilitation, 66,* 30–34.

Reynolds, E.H., & Trimble, M.R. (1985). Adverse neuropsychiatric effects on anticonvulsant drugs. *Drugs, 313,* 145–151.

Richelson, E., & Nelson, A. (1984). Antagonism by antidepressants of neurotransmitter receptors of normal human brain *in vitro. Journal of Pharmacology and Experimental Therapeutics, 230,* 94–102.

Schou, M., Baastrup, P.C., Gross, P., et al. (1970). Pharmacological and clinical problems of lithium prophylaxis. *British Journal of Psychiatry, 116,* 615–619.

Solomon, S., Hotchkiss, E., Saravay, S.M., et al. (1983). Impairment of memory function by antihypertensive medication. *Archives of General Psychiatry, 40,* 1109–1112.

Trimble, M.R., & Thompson, P.J. (1983). Anticonvulsant drugs, cognitive function and behavior. *Epilepsia, 24*(Suppl.1), 555–563.

Wesnes, K., & Warburton, D.M. (1983). Smoking, nicotine and human performance. *Pharmacologic Therapeutics, 21,* 189–208.

CHAPTER 3

Physical Therapy in Community Reentry

Assessment and Achievement of Physical Fitness

Jo Ann Tomberlin

Any community reentry program must embrace the philosophy that individuals with brain injury are capable of achievement of positive change in their specific level of functional independence (DeLoach, Wilkins, & Walker, 1983). During the acute phase of the individual's illness, the responsibility for decisions, actions, and consequences is not demanded of the client, creating a state of dependency. Unfortunately, the dependency is prolonged and spills over into the latter phases of rehabilitation. During the early phases of rehabilitation, the therapeutic programs are designed to minimize confusion and ambiguity so that the person with brain injury has a consistent daily routine. This process allows the person to function successfully even with reduced cognitive, emotional, and physical skills. This pattern of "setting the stage" to prevent failure has merit in the early stages of recovery. However, it is unacceptable to continue the plateau of stage setting simply because it is easier and less time consuming. Health care professionals must be willing to allow individuals the risk of failure in the supported environments so that problems can be corrected prior to discharge into the home and community (Smith, 1983).

Few data exist that identify the individuals with brain injury who become ideal candidates to pursue ongoing rehabilitation and ultimately noninstitutional community reentry (Talmage & Collins, 1983). The assessment of

outcome has been studied for over 10 years (Bond, 1979; Jennett & Bond, 1975; Jennett, Bond, & Brooks, 1981; Jennett et al., 1979). Use of the Glasgow Coma Scale the first week after onset of injury compared to the outcome scores at 6 months postinjury using the Glasgow Outcome Scale, revealed that, of the persons surviving the brain injury, approximately 30%–40% achieved moderate to good recovery (Jennett et al., 1979). Unfortunately, the operational definition of moderate to good recovery is seldom based upon an individual's ability to function acceptably in a real-life activity (Brown, Gordon, & Diller, 1986). Rappaport, Hall, Hopkins, Belleza, and Cope (1982) have suggested using a disability rating (DR) scale to follow progress from coma to return to the community. Findings suggest that the DR provides greater sensitivity in measuring clinical changes when compared to the Glasgow Outcome Scale. These data could assist to identify the most appropriate candidates for intensive rehabilitation services.

Obviously, if the individual is to gain the ability to perform activities that are not routine within environments that are unfamiliar, strategies to upgrade such skills as planning, initiating, monitoring, and decision making must be developed. Therefore, the overall outcome goals of the rehabilitation process for each individual becomes: to develop compensatory strategies

The author acknowledges Don Danell, B.S., Certified Orthotist, for the orthotic concepts discussed in this chapter.

that provide the opportunity for pursuit of performance of behaviors of increased complexity, to master survival in a greater variety of environments, and to achieve maximum acceptance as a valued member of a community.

In preparing for community reentry, the individual must accept that success is measured on a continuous scale, that responsibility must be assumed for one's actions, and that the individual must develop the ability to advocate for him or herself. The family and professionals associated with the survivor must also support the community reentry activities by providing nonjudgmental feedback and must willingly diminish control as self-advocacy is established. There must be acceptance by all involved of a philosophy that people are able, not disabled, and that disability is not synonymous with illness.

In viewing a discussion of community reentry, one must establish a predetermined set of premises for clarification. First, community reentry may have a wide array of meaning depending upon the focus of the health professional. For the purposes of this chapter, community reentry is operationally defined as the ability of the individual with brain injury to physically access the community for self-advocacy, leisure pursuits, and vocational/avocational activities to as normal a degree as possible.

Second, successful access of the community in which one resides may have a wide array of forms depending upon the individual's interest, abilities, and financial status. Although this chapter emphasizes the use of physical therapy, the process of community reentry requires transdisciplinary consideration of all the residual disabilities and consistent use of strategies if the individual is to achieve community reentry with lifelong success.

PROGRESSION OF PHYSICAL THERAPY MANAGEMENT IN REHABILITATION

During the early management from onset of injury to intensive care unit placement, the individual's rehabilitation potential is determined by ongoing medical and neurological status as indi-

cated by traditional neurological examination, computed axial tomography, brain-evoked potentials, and various other neurological and radiological studies. Survival and motor response status of the individual are top medical priorities. However, motor response status does not define any characteristic that speaks to the quality of life for the survivor. Once medical stability is achieved the physical therapist can begin to provide ongoing evaluation and therapeutic management of neuromuscular sequelae. The selection of the treatment is dependent upon the level of consciousness of the individual. Although comprehensive care is provided by a cohesive interdisciplinary team, the following sections only address physical therapy intervention. It is beyond the scope of this chapter to cover total utilization of other services.

Physical Therapy in the Acute Phase

For persons in coma, but displaying medical stability, physical therapy, in cooperation with other personnel, has five major goals: 1) prevention of secondary physical problems due to immobility (e.g., pulmonary congestion, loss of skin integrity, and adaptive shortening of soft tissue); 2) monitoring of changes in neurological status with emphasis on emergence of or decrease in hypertonicity, reflex behavior, and movement disorders; 3) recommendation, application, and monitoring of external devices to retain neutral limb, trunk, and neck positions and lessen abnormal patterns or posturing; 4) sensory stimulation to elicit motor responses through manual guidance of normal movement patterns; and 5) evaluation for use of a neuromuscular electrical stimulation program (Boughton & Ciesla, 1986).

Physical Therapy in the Early Postacute Phase

As the emergence from coma occurs, the individual displays general and specific responses that allow the physical therapy management to be expanded. The type, frequency, and intensity of treatment is dependent upon the level of consciousness and duration of the alert state.

Provision of an intensive program includes: 1) intraoral stimulation to support normal tongue and jaw function; 2) tactile stimulation of the face, head, and neck to enhance neck and upper trunk movement; 3) visual and auditory cues to stimulate alertness and improve attention; and 4) kinesthetic stimulation to assist body part location and orientation, and to elicit normal gross motor patterns in the limbs, neck, and trunk. Such a program must be applied intermittently throughout the day.

Major objectives for the physical therapy program during this phase include but are not limited to: 1) continuation of objectives from the acute phase; 2) documentation of the cycle of alertness; 3) expansion and extension of the periods of alertness; 4) assessment and documentation of the increased number of appropriate responses, by category, during each intervention; and 5) establishment of specific methods for documentation of progress during each physical therapy session.

Mills (1985) reported on the performance of 24 persons with brain injury rated on the Rancho Los Amigos Levels of Cognitive Functioning to identify the numbers and types of physical therapy treatments tolerated and to determine the relationship between tolerated treatment and cognitive levels of function. The individuals rated on the lower cognitive levels of three and four were able to tolerate fewer specific physical therapy treatments in any session compared to those persons rated at the higher levels of cognition. Those with higher cognitive ratings were able to tolerate more tasks of greater complexity requiring attention, sequencing, and voluntary cooperation. The data suggest that intervention strategies for cognitive levels three and four should include activities that allow a more passive participation not requiring levels of cognition of which the individual is incapable. Activities recommended were supervised ambulation, use of a tilt table, joint range of motion, and mat activities providing limited use of gross body movements. The use of complex verbal cues or directions tended to diminish success.

Data obtained from such a study assists in the formation of guidelines for care. Further, early intervention by physical therapy may identify the appropriate type, level, and intensity of physical intervention with the medically stable person emerging from coma. Use of this information could: 1) educate family or personnel responsible for the daily ongoing care and decrease the inconsistency in physical management of the person, which often gives rise to inappropriate behaviors; and 2) provide opportunity for informal evaluation of changing motor responses and cognition, which will allow continuous feedback to family and personnel so the management plan is congruent with the individual's physical and cognitive needs.

Physical therapists must recognize the need to supply the family with ongoing information regarding changes in the client's status, to provide education to encourage family involvement, and to provide emotional support during all phases of recovery. A major responsibility of physical therapists is to create a continuum of care by developing a program that allows family interaction with the survivor on a day-to-day basis. Unfortunately, too often families report that health care professionals do not provide adequate information (Panting & Merry, 1972). It is possible that ongoing communication to relatives could provide needed emotional support and thus lessen the potential for psychosocial problems.

Since no objective data exist, evaluation of the relatives' ability to cope with the emotional burden through long-term survival has not been measured. Through experience, health care providers have found that utilization of family members as alternate care providers can assist in decreasing the family's feeling of helplessness and provide a more complete understanding of the recovery process as it occurs.

Also, because ongoing long-term care is dependent upon the availability of programs and resources, family members involved in the rehabilitation process from the early postacute phase could expand otherwise limited services for the survivor. Since some survivors have access to only a few services for short periods, special training for the family coupled with ongoing professional monitoring could provide care that might favorably influence the outcome of independence and thus lessen the burden on families.

Physical Therapy in the Late Postacute Phase

During the late postacute phase, which occurs as the individual appears to be less confused, more oriented to the daily routine, and to some degree able to demonstrate carryover in learning, physical therapy management should become more intense and complex. At this stage, physical achievement becomes one motivational factor for cooperation and positive emotional behavior by the individual.

Major goals of physical therapy become: 1) restoration of advanced weight-bearing skills and bimanual activities; 2) sensorimotor organization and integration for efficient coordinated movement of the limbs, head, neck, and trunk; 3) specific intervention for definable neurological or musculoskeletal deficiencies; 4) introduction to environments external to the institution that increase the complexity of incoming stimuli, to evaluate physical and cognitive responses; and 5) continuation of predetermined rating scales to identify changes in performance for the individual, the family, and other personnel interacting with the individual.

Physical Therapy in the Transitional Phase

There is a paucity of objective information on current physical therapy program development occurring during the transitional rehabilitation phase for individuals with brain injury. The ability of a survivor of brain trauma to seek and receive intensive transdisciplinary services is primarily dependent upon two factors: available space within a program and money to finance such a program. The relative success of physical intervention has yet to be determined. Because of wide differences in program outcome objectives and the heterogeneity of the client population in various programs, it is difficult to make comparisons of physical achievement among different programs, measured in outcome terms.

Traditionally, management of the individual's problems during the acute and early postacute phases is highly structured, aimed toward individual needs, and generally best provided in an interdisciplinary inpatient setting. By contrast, the late postacute and transitional rehabilitation programs require a transdisciplinary, holistic approach to create the final step forward into the mainstream of the community.

RATIONALE FOR PHYSICAL THERAPY INTERVENTION

Deficiencies that have been reported to block community reentry include maladaptive behavior, inability to self-initiate or direct attention, and residual deficits of orientation, memory, judgment, and problem solving (Garland, 1983; Hamish & Knight, 1988; Levin, Goldstein, High, & Williams, 1988). Brooks, McKinlay, Symington, Beattie, and Campsie (1987) studied rate and prediction of return to work. They reported cognitive, behavioral, and personality changes were significantly related to failure to return to work, while physical deficits were not. Jacobs (1988) randomly selected 142 families with a head-injured survivor to participate in the Los Angeles Head Injury Survey. Results indicated that physical deficits or secondary problems resulting from inactivity did have an impact on the survivor's ability to perform independently in the home and community. Lack of stamina significantly reduced community excursions in 46.5% of the survivors who reportedly were limited in ability to walk for long periods of time. Only 63% reported independence in personal safety, health care maintenance, and personal shopping. Problems of dependence in basic self-care skills were related to physical limitations in 21% of the group.

Despite the fact that in studies of adults with brain injury, cognitive and behavioral sequelae have been reported as of greater consequence than physical deficits, one must not underestimate the integrated effect of sensorimotor deficiencies on the long-term outcome of these individuals (Gilchrist & Wilkinson, 1979). Physical problems, coupled with cognitive, behavioral, and social deficits, change the individual's goals and curtail activity level (Ylvisaker, 1985). Any person who cannot perform daily routines in an automatic manner greatly increases the energy costs to complete the activities. Applied to the environments of work, school, or community, the person experiences fatigue, slowness of performance, and lack of attention—which may lead to risk of task error or injury. Further, the individual's ability to use strategies to inhibit inappropriate behavior is jeopardized by fatigue-related stress. Wood (1980) described stress as a discord between one's individual performance and one's expectations. Also, disorders of sensorimotor processing resulting from brain injury adversely affect the ability to perform meaningful, appropriate motor responses, and have an effect on the person's ability to become independent in community living skills, vocational/avocational endeavors, and use of leisure time (Panikoff, 1983).

PHYSICAL THERAPY MODEL FOR TRANSITIONAL REHABILITATION

The objective of this section is to discuss a specific physical therapy program model appropriate for the transitional rehabilitation phase. The section includes preadmission screening, postadmission evaluation, and components of the physical therapy program.

Preadmission Screening Process

Starting in 1985, observations and physical assessments have been collected by the physical therapist on adults with brain injury applying to the author's residential transitional rehabilitation program. The specific physical therapy screening form is provided in Form 3.1. The screening time available for physical therapy is 30–45 minutes. The provision of a structured treatment plan is routinely requested by the financing agency or individual prior to the decision to fund the applicant. The screening process in physical therapy must be based upon actual performance rather than projected by interview or past performance reports.

The first objective of the screening process is to sample those areas that may need to be included in a physical therapy program plan in the event the applicant elects to enter the program. The example presented in Form 3.2 represents only three physical areas that consistently deter ambulatory applicants from having access to the community with a high degree of independence. If an applicant needs to utilize mobility equipment such as wheelchairs, walkers, or canes, the treatment plan would reflect objectives leading to community independence with use of equipment. Recommendations for upgrading, repair, or replacement of equipment necessary throughout the residential period would be documented with the approximate cost and rationale for the request. Information necessary for decision making by the funding source includes identified problems, treatment goals with regard to each problem, therapeutic strategies, time frames of expected achievement, and methods of ongoing assessment of change. In addition, types and frequency of interventions must be recommended to enable a sound financial plan to be prepared.

The second objective of the screening process is to provide recommendations for home and community services in the event admission does not occur or the admission waiting period is prolonged. Physical therapy recommendations most frequently endorse basic activities that could provide maintained or improved flexibility through daily performance of body and limb movement, and increased endurance through walking or wheelchair manipulation outside the home, performed daily for a specified time and distance. Utilization of local resources such as the YMCA or YWCA, community college adult fitness programs, and fitness centers is consistently recommended. The follow-through of any recommendations made during the preadmission screening process becomes the responsibility of the individual and the family working directly with their local referring agency. Any specific recommendations given the applicant are sent to the referral source as well.

Postadmission Evaluation

The postadmission physical therapy evaluation occurs within the 2-week program evaluation phase after admission orientation. The evaluation battery was designed to establish the initial baseline in the areas of flexibility, muscle performance, sensation, balance, coordination, and

FORM 3.1

TRANSITIONAL LEARNING COMMUNITY
DEPARTMENT OF PHYSICAL THERAPY
SCREENING ASSESSMENT

NAME: _____ DATE OF BIRTH: _____ DATE OF SCREENING: _____

SCREENER: _____

SUMMARY OF RESULTS AND RECOMMENDATIONS

Recommended therapy: ____ group/s, ____ individual sessions for each week:

_____
_____
_____
_____
_____
_____
_____
_____

ORIENTATION	
Time, place, person	
KNOWLEDGE OF INJURY	
Where treated?	
How long?	
SELF-DIRECTION	
What are your goals?	
What are your major strengths?	
weaknesses?	
KNOWLEDGE OF TLC PROGRAM	
CURRENT MEDICATIONS	

AREA EVALUATED	NORMAL LIMIT	NOT TESTED	IDENTIFIED PROBLEMS AND COMMENTS
VISUAL INSPECTIONS			
Postural asymmetries			
Condition of skin			
scars			
temperature			
Peripheral pulses			
Limb length Discrepancies			
JOINT RANGE OF MOTION			
Upper limbs			
Lower limbs			

AREA EVALUATED	NORMAL LIMIT	NOT TESTED	IDENTIFIED PROBLEMS AND COMMENTS
SENSATION			
Gross touch			
Sharp/dull			
TONE/MOTOR CONTROL			
Upper limbs			
Lower limbs			
Neck			
Trunk			
GROSS PSYCHOMOTOR SPEEDS			
Upper limbs			
Lower limbs			
STRENGTH			
Upper limbs			
Lower limbs			
WEIGHT-BEARING SKILLS			
Level ambulation			
Tandem walking			
One-leg balance			
right			
left			
Stair climbing			
Hopping			
bilateral			
right foot			
left foot			
FITNESS SCREEN			
Stationary bicycle 80 rpm			
Treadmill (indicate speed)			
Stairmaster 40–60 spm			
Kinetron II 30 car/sec			

ADDITIONAL COMMENTS: _____

_____

_____

_____

_____

_____

Physical Therapist
Department of Physical Therapy

FORM 3.2

PHYSICAL THERAPY PREADMISSION TREATMENT PLAN

Name: Date screened:

Examiner: Admission status:

Individual = I   Group = G

Projected no. of hours, type and frequency of therapeutic plan
1. **2** Hours progressive exercise tests (I)
2. **5** Hours group physical therapy (G)
3. **2** Hours activity tolerance (G)

Problems identified	Objectives of therapy	Therapeutic strategies	Time	Objective assessment
1. Decreased aerobic capacity	1a. Establish physical workload level.	1a. Progressive exercise test (PET).	2 wks.	Repeat PET 3 mos., exit
	b. Increase aerobic capacity sufficient for 8–10 hours of activity necessary for community, avo-cational/vocational, or leisure pursuits.	b. Training on electric treadmill, bicycle, ergometer, and mechanical stairs 20 min. daily. Timed walking bouts in community: (4–8 blocks increased to 9–16 blocks). Planned walking or cycling trip in community.	3 mos.	Comparison of baseline perfor-mance with monthly scores on time, dis-tance, and speed.
2. Decreased balance in presence of activities requiring changes in ambulation	2. Establish ability to: a. Perform out-door ambulation with minimum ac-ceptable speed of 2 ft./sec. b. Perform street crossing at con-trolled intersections in 21 seconds or less.	2a. and b. Perfor-mance of walking with varying velocities in controlled and outdoor environments with monitoring, visual observation, and independent performance.	3–6 mos.	Comparison of initial and sub-sequent tests. Calculation of no. of safety er-rors.
3. Decreased ability to self-protect during weight bearing.	3. Establish to protect self when falling to decrease risk of injury in work, community, or leisure environ-ments.	3. Falling practice using protective mat and head gear. Progress to self-protection without head gear in con-trolled environ-ments. Falling and recovery in external environments.	1 mo.	Visual observa-tion of trials in all learning phases. Cal-culation of no. of errors.

endurance. Within the 2 weeks there are 4 hours each week for formal evaluation plus observation of behavior during 8–10 group exercise sessions. During the evaluative group sessions, participation is encouraged but not mandatory since the major objective is to record the behavior as the individual observes and interacts in the group. The group rules are punctuality, attendance, documentation of body weight one time weekly, observation of the group exercise process, and voluntary initiation to request a signature of the group monitor at the end of the class. Participation is mandatory after the evaluation period. A sample monitoring form is provided in Form 3.3.

During formal evaluation, definitive data on joint range of motion, muscle performance, and sensation including sharp/dull, temperature, sterognosis, and proprioception are recorded. Balance and coordination are evaluated through timed dynamic activities for upper limbs, lower limbs, and movement of upper and lower limbs used simultaneously (Nelson, 1983b). Cardiorespiratory status is evaluated by use of a progressive exercise test (PET). Following the evaluation phase, an individualized physical therapy program is developed based upon the evaluation results, the program mission to foster achievement of the reentry process to as independent a degree as possible, and the specific goals set by each client together with the family and clinical staff.

Components of a Physical Therapy Program

The overall goal of the physical therapy service is to assist clients to gain the knowledge and skills to develop the level of physical health necessary for independence. The program components are:

1. Muscle performance
2. Flexibility acquisition/maintenance
3. Balance development/refinement
4. Gait performance/refinement
5. Reaction time performance
6. Physical conditioning
7. Gross mobility performance

Program components for individualized physical therapy management plans are selected to support the transdisciplinary goals of the client. All clients are assigned to group and individual sessions or group sessions only. Assignment is dependent upon physical ability and underlying deficits. The process moves from simple to complex with a gradual decrease in structure and increase in stress and complexity. Examples of increasing stress and complexity are additions of environmental distractions and upgrading the number of sensory systems stimulated. The amount and type of cuing, monitored during physical therapy activities, allows evaluation of the degree of autonomy displayed by each client. These evaluations provide ongoing objective data for progression toward independence.

Muscle Performance: Upper Limbs
Muscle performance training in the upper limbs has as its outcome objectives to enable the client to lift, reach, push, or pull objects encountered in community shopping or travel. Initial training occurs using hydraulic exercise equipment coupled with activities combining lifting loads to selected heights, pushing weighted carts specified distances in external environments, and ambulating while carrying a specified load. Emphasis is on the ability to perform multijoint movements between waist and shoulders, waist and 150 degrees above horizontal, and from waist to floor during sitting, supported standing, or independent standing.

Muscle Performance: Lower Limbs
Training of the lower limbs occurs to assure ability to support the body for time periods that allow achievement of community, vocational, and leisure pursuits. Activities include non–weight-bearing training using hydraulic exercises machines for hips and knees, weight-bearing training using an electric treadmill, mechanical stairs, and timed walking in external environments (1–8 blocks) in combination with upper-limb training.

Flexibility
Decreased flexibility is defined as any adaptive shortening of soft tissue that could limit body movement and increase the risk of injury during physical activity. The concept of pre- and postactivity stretching is empha-

FORM 3.3

MONITORING FORM
DEPARTMENT OF PHYSICAL THERAPY

Name: _____   Initial evaluation: _____   Initial treatment: _____

Date of birth: _____   Current body weight: _____

Target fitness index: _____   Current fitness index: _____

Program for: _____   Target heart rate: _____ to _____

Legend

0—Not attempted	5—Needs only intermittent verbal cues
1—Step-by-step prompting	6—Needs only intermittent manual cues
2—Requires manual arousal	7—Needs only initial verbal prompting
3—Needs frequent verbal cues	8—Independent
4—Needs frequent manual cues	

Place legend number in date column for each item performed.

DATES

ITEM #

WEEKLY TOTAL ALL ITEMS: _____   BEST POSSIBLE WEEKLY SCORE: _____

% OF ACHIEVEMENT BY WEEK: ____ ____ ____ ____ ____

OPERATIONAL DEFINITIONS

1. Step-by-step prompting: Requires one-on-one verbal directions (more than 10 times) at all times during performance of the task.
2. Requires manual arousal: one-on-one manual touching during performance of the task to direct attention and ensure safety.
3. Needs frequent verbal cues: Verbal directions (four or less times a period).
4. Needs frequent manual cues: Assisting person to continue to stay on equipment or continue to use equipment. Assisting person onto the equipment.
(3 and 4: Safety, attention to task, and completion of task are emphases here.)
5. Needs only intermittent verbal cues: Verbal support to move smoothly from one activity to another without distraction (more than three times per period).
6. Needs only intermittent manual cues: Assistance to mount/start equipment when task is new to the person.
7. Needs only initial verbal prompting: Person can carry out the task with one set of directions.
8. Independent: Needs no verbal or physical cues to start and complete task following known treatment protocols for self-documentation of progress.

sized. A general stretching program is developed by the individual for any special needs and is carried out on a daily basis. As physical activities are pursued with ongoing independence, the flexibility program becomes self-monitored. In cases of persistent loss of soft tissue flexibility, neuromuscular electrical stimulation is used as an alternative or in combination with custom orthoses.

Balance Given that the client is independently ambulatory on level surfaces, emphasis is centered on achieving balance stability necessary for advanced physical endeavors. Motor tasks of unloading one limb, body pivoting, and moving with increasing and varied velocities are basic to physical accomplishments of shopping, moving in the worksite, maintaining a household, and participation in leisure pursuits such as group or individual sports. Tasks that challenge the individual include use of multidirectional beam walking, timed obstacle courses on uneven surfaces, and use of equilibrium boards. Activities that combine standing on stools while loading objects from a cart to shelves offer an integrated task that requires body control, balance, and multilimb activity.

Gait Refinement The program component of gait refinement has the outcome goal to enable the individual to perform weight-bearing activities, with or without equipment, on level or elevated surfaces in any environment necessary to pursue activities in the community.

Activities used for gait refinement with or without equipment include: 1) electric treadmill, with use of grade, speed, distance, and time as parameters of change in ability; 2) mechanical stairs, using stepping speed, number of floors climbed, and time as parameters of change in ability; and 3) timed ambulation trips of 1–8 blocks, encountering curbs of various heights and uneven concrete and dirt surfaces, with time, distance, and level of difficulty as parameters of change in ability.

Equipment Use for Ambulation Alternative Some individuals are able to ambulate for controlled distances but need other equipment for complete access to community resources. The philosophy emphasized is the use of judgment in selecting equipment that best suits the client's abilities and the activity. The discarding of a crutch for a cane because the change is thought to denote improvement would be an example of poor judgment if the client actually needed the crutch. The decision to use the crutch for mall shopping and practices with the cane during household activities would denote a degree of independent prioritizing and self-monitoring ability. A similar rule is used for assisting the client to select clothing for various occasions and changes in weather.

Orthotic Alternative Persons with equinovarus in one or both ankles present with a problem of decreased stability and mobility when walking in the community. Not only is the person at risk for injury due to poor foot position, but the likelihood of developing the ability to vary walking speeds is remote. Instability and slowness impede the development of advanced skills of weight bearing. During 1986–1988, 15 clients admitted to the author's transitional residential program presented with varying degrees of spasticity sufficient to limit improvement in weight-bearing activities. Each was fitted with the custom, dynamic ankle-foot orthosis (AFO) pictured in Figure 3.1. The objectives for use of the orthosis were to get the foot on the floor, to control genu recurvatum, and to prevent toe drag, thus increasing the velocity of swing in the limb with the AFO and decreasing the stance time of the limb without the AFO. The foot plate used to fabricate the AFO is pictured in Figure 3.2. The advantage gained during use of the orthosis are: foot control through reduction of the equinovarus position; maintenance of muscle length of plantar flexors, toe flexors, and tibialis posterior; and enhancement of balanced ankle dorsiflexion through the moveable, adjustable ankle joint. The reduction of spasticity through use of the molded foot plate has yet to be evaluated. In all cases, the use of the custom, dynamic AFO enabled the client to participate in an advanced weight-bearing program including use of an apparatus for endurance and ambulation velocity training. The improvement noted was translated into functional significance through the ability to walk increased numbers of blocks in less time judged by timed outings for banking and shopping.

Neuromuscular Electrical Stimulation (NMES) This technique is used to activate muscle groups to counteract the predominant pattern of spasticity commonly found in the lower limb. Parameters for use have been documented in the literature (Baker, Parker, & Sand-

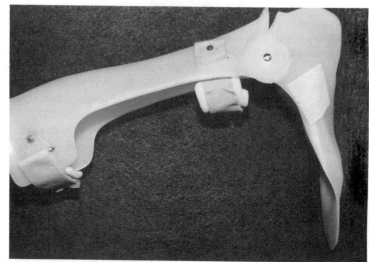

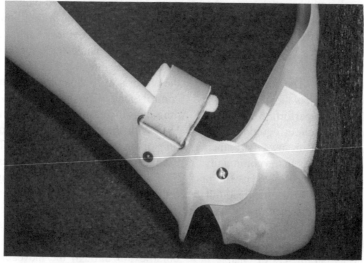

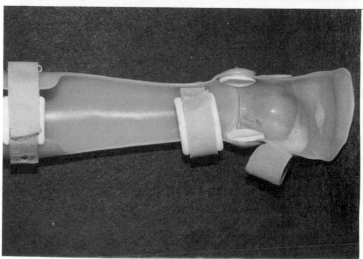

Figure 3.1. Front and side views of a custom, dynamic ankle-foot orthosis (AFO). Maximum allowable position of plantar flexion is controlled by approximation of posterior borders of shank and foot sections. Dorsiflexion is unlimited.

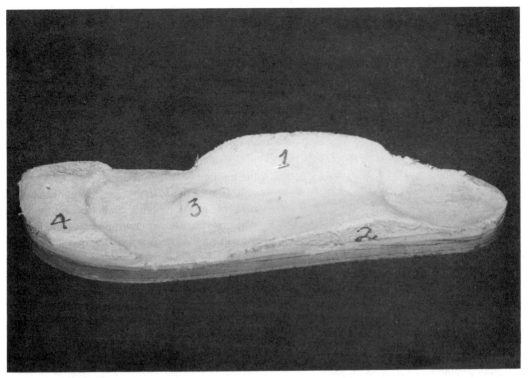

Figure 3.2. Foot plate. A plaster mold is used to fabricate the foot section of the custom AFO. Reliefs include: 1) medial longitudinal arch, 2) peroneal arch, 3) metatarsal arch, 4) toe raise.

erson, 1983; Zablotney, 1987). The primary use is to counteract the equinovarus position of the foot and ankle assumed during the ambulation activities of the client. The client's ability to apply, remove, and monitor the system indicates sufficient cognitive skills to use NMES effectively without risk. NMES in combination with orthotic application presents an effective method to establish a stable walking base and to provide consistent training in timing the muscle activity of dorsiflexors during weight-bearing activities.

Reaction Time Performance The major objective of this program component is to enable the client to respond rapidly to the need for body position changes in lying, sitting, standing, walking, or running with no loss of balance. Activities include: initial practice of moving on command through a planned sequence from chair to floor, floor to standing, and standing to lying in a time frame of 5 seconds for each move; moving through a random motor sequence; and practice in car or van en-

try, engaging the seatbelt and door locks in 60 seconds or less. An example of the random sequence is provided in Form 3.4. Community activities include entering or exiting a community building elevator in 5 seconds or less, and boarding or exiting a bus in 10 seconds or less. Task-specific activities are practiced to assist the client to increase efficiency. Examples include timed trials for sacking groceries, restocking items on shelves, and unloading supplies from large boxes. Fine motor activities such as adhering price tags, mailing labels, or stamps to items can also be used. All activities should be timed and percentage of production per unit of time calculated. The objective feedback assists the client to plot performance and provides motivation for improved production.

Physical Conditioning The client's inability to sustain activity levels throughout any time period set aside for daily routines, community involvement, work, and leisure activities creates unnecessary limitations. The implication

FORM 3.4

PHYSICAL THERAPY
RANDOM MOTOR SEQUENCE FORM

Preactivity stretch

Mat work: Start standing. All activities are performed as quickly as possible.

1. Down on right knee
2. Stand up
3. Down on left knee
4. Stand up
5. Down on both knees
6. Lie face down
7. Turn over on back
8. Turn face down
9. Spin body one full circle
10. Stand up
11. Lie face down
12. Turn over on back
13. Turn face down
14. Perform five push-ups
15. Stand up
16. Take 30-second rest period
17. Lie face down
18. Up on both knees
19. Lie face down
20. Turn over on back
21. Spin around one full circle on back
22. Stand up
23. Rest 30 seconds

Weight-bearing sequence

1. Forward walking 40 feet
2. Backward walking 40 feet
3. Forward walking 20 feet
4. Backward walking 20 feet
5. Lateral walking to the right 10 feet
6. Lateral walking to the left 10 feet
7. Lateral walking to the right 5 feet
8. Lateral walking to the left 5 feet
9. Forward walking 10 feet
10. Backward walking 10 feet
11. Lateral walking to the right 3 feet
12. Lateral walking to the left 3 feet
13. Forward walking 40 feet, stop

Repeat mat sequence

Cool down and stretch for 10 minutes

perceived by family and friends may be that the person with brain injury is dependent and cannot cope with the stress of day-to-day responsibilities. Although proper rest, nutrition, and schedule planning are factors to consider in this problem, the level of deconditioning occurring as a result of prolonged immobility must be explored. The outcome goal of physical conditioning is to enable the client to sustain activity levels necessary to achieve any desired community, work, or leisure endeavors. Activities include: bicycle riding (stationary or moving); electric treadmill; mechanical stairs; bilateral, reciprocal, isokinetic exercise (Nelson, 1983a); and rapid walking of 1 mile (in 24 minutes, gradually decreasing the time to 20 minutes). The progression of the exercise is based on increases in time and maintaining a steady work load once the training heart rate is achieved.

Gross Mobility The program component of gross mobility includes walking or wheeling in external environments, and use of available public transportation. The outcome objective is to enable the client to gain access to the community by walking, wheeling, or using the transportation systems available. Activities within the component include: planning an outing, gathering necessary information, carrying out the plan under visual supervision, and receiving feedback on performance. The number of outings requiring error-free performance is set so that the client understands the criteria for independence. Judgment in selecting the mode of transportation to meet the requirements of the planned activity is emphasized.

Use of Two- and Three-Wheel Bicycles Cycling may be a transportation alternative for selected clients. The choice of three-wheel or two-wheel cycles depends upon the physical and cognitive capacities of the client. Bicycle helmets are required regardless of the cycle type. Evaluations of street performance are made to destinations that sample the prevailing traffic patterns. The number of evaluations is dependent on the knowledge of road rules demonstrated through the street performance. In situations where the client demonstrates sufficient physical ability but insufficient cognitive abilities to be evaluated as a safe, independent bicycle user, recommendations for companion riding or limited-access riding are made.

Use of Walking Walking is evaluated by knowledge of pedestrian safety demonstrated during monitored planned outings. Maximum walking distances vary, depending upon the efficiency with which the client walks. The maximum acceptable time to negotiate a city block (330 feet) is 3 minutes, with ideal time set at 1½ minutes. In this case, a client is utilizing approximately 15–30 minutes to walk ½ mile (8 blocks). Time includes street crossings. Depending upon the activity at the destination, it might be more efficient to use public transportation, complete the planned task, and walk the return trip without time stress. Planning the utilization of time and energy output is vital to the ongoing success of community access.

In all gross mobility tasks, monitoring with written feedback is provided. Each activity has specific key indicators that have been identified as priorities for successful completion. Working from a checklist offers the client an opportunity to self-monitor the performance.

METHOD OF ASSESSMENT OF PHYSICAL FITNESS

Little data exist to substantiate physical therapy intervention as it relates to the outcome of im-

proved exercise performance in persons with brain injury. Becker, Bar-Or, Mendelson, and Najenson (1978) exercised healthy subjects and subjects with acute and chronic brain injury on a bicycle ergometer. The findings indicated decreased exercise tolerance in the subjects with brain injury. In order to examine the exercise performance of persons with brain injury and to establish the possible effectiveness of physical conditioning as a program component, clients in the author's transitional residential program were tested initially and again after participation in a 3-month physical therapy program. The component of the physical therapy program included preactivity stretching, activities for muscle performance, aerobics, and postactivity stretching. The frequency and duration of the program was 5 days a week, for 50 minutes.

Progressive test protocols are presented in Figure 3.3. The results are shown in Figures 3.4 and 3.5. Conclusions that may be drawn are that comparable results were achieved in progressive exercise testing using treadmill, bicycle, and

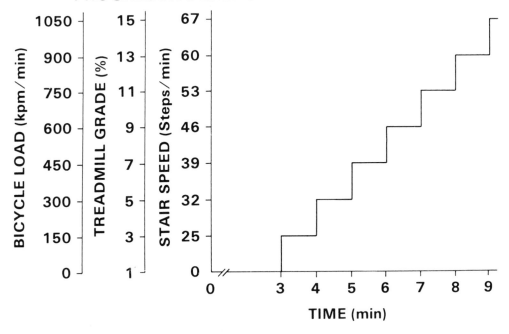

Figure 3.3. Progressive exercise test protocols. Bicycle: cycling speed 60 revolutions per minute; power output, increasing 150 kilopond meters per minute. Treadmill: speed fixed at 1.8, 2.5, or 3.5 miles per hour; grade progression from 1% to 25%, increasing 2% each minute. Stairs: initial stepping speed of 25 steps per minute; progressive speeds of 6–8 steps per minute. (Stepping speed dependent upon body weight.)

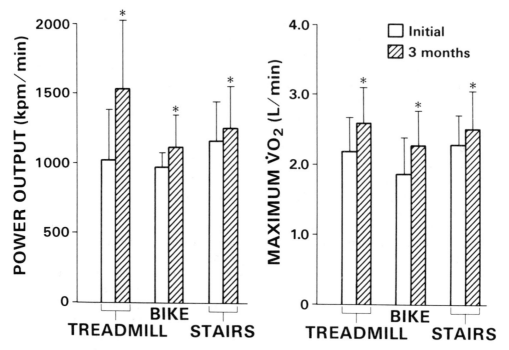

Figure 3.4.   Comparison of initial test and 3-month test on treadmill, bicycle and stairs. Mean $(+/-)$ standard deviation of maximum power output and maximum $\dot{V}O_2$ (maximum oxygen consumption) initially and at 3 months for all subjects. * = $p < 0.05$.

mechanical stairs, and as a result of the physical therapy program, improvement in exercise performance was demonstrated by the PET repeated at 3 months. These results suggest that when the clients entered the residential program they were deconditioned. After the 3-month training program, improved cardiac performance was noted. Possible changes in the exercises' efficiency are currently under investigation.

FITNESS BEYOND THERAPY

After the first 6 months, the physical therapy program lessens in intensity if the client is ready to assume less structure. To that end, clients are encouraged to explore local fitness centers or adult fitness classes to generalize their activities into the community. The department of leisure services in the author's program works directly with the client to plan a well-rounded, independent activity calendar to include participatory rather than simply spectator activities. Long-term physical health maintenance is a vital need

for clients with brain injury. The true success of any physical therapy intervention during the transitional rehabilitation phase is the client's use of activities within the community that maintain the level of physical health achieved through the intensive transitional program.

SUMMARY AND CONCLUSION

This chapter has defined community reentry in a framework of outcome goals or objectives. Physical therapy evaluation and therapeutic intervention for persons surviving brain injury has been compared along a continuum from acute care to transitional rehabilitation. Methods of assessment of community reentry outcome for the survivors of brain injury have been suggested. Results of therapeutic planning and implementation of a fitness program were presented.

The need for ongoing health maintenance for all individuals in this phase of community

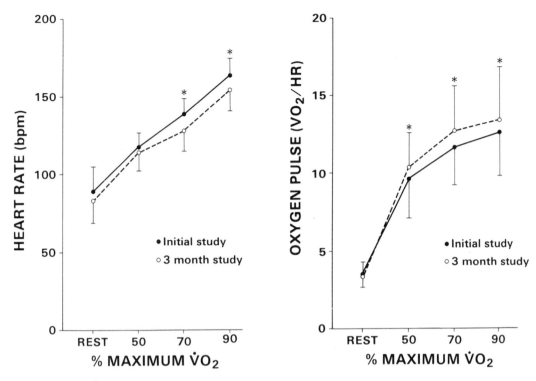

Figure 3.5.   Comparison of heart rate and oxygen pulse at selected levels of $\dot{V}O_2$ (maximum oxygen consumption). Left: Mean $(+/-)$ standard deviation of heart rate for all subjects at rest and given levels of maximum $\dot{V}O_2$ on initial and 3-month testing on stairs indicate a statistically significant decrease in heart rate at 3 months at the two highest levels of $\dot{V}O_2$. Right: mean $(+/-)$ standard deviation of oxygen pulse for all subjects at rest and given levels of maximum $\dot{V}O_2$ on stairs indicate a statistically significant increase in oxygen pulse at 3 months at the three highest levels of $\dot{V}O_2$. $^* = p < 0.05$.

reentry is vital. Obviously persons with brain injury are subject to the entire range of acquired disorders that can affect any individual. Secondary health issues arising out of decreased ability to sustain an appropriate activity level afflicts the person with brain injury with loss of lean body mass; decreased flexibility of trunk, neck, and limbs; increased obesity; increased risk of cardiac disease and stroke; and diminished respiratory status (Hacker & Tobis, 1983; Patterson, Pearson, & Fisher, 1985; Talmage & Collins, 1983). Monitoring and self-management of ongoing health must be taught and practiced, other-

wise the level of independence will be greatly reduced (DeVillis & Sauter, 1985).

Persons with brain injury should be afforded the same opportunities as their non–brain-injured counterparts to pursue, achieve, and maintain the highest degree of physical health possible. To this end the attitudes of individuals, communities, and societies must reflect a positive change toward persons who are physically challenged—to see them not as disabled persons in a community, but as productive citizens of the community (Crosby, 1980; Olson, 1985).

REFERENCES

Baker, L.L., Parker, K., & Sanderson, D. (1983). Neuromuscular electrical stimulation for the head-injury patient. *Physical Therapy, 63*(12), 1967–1974.

Becker, E., Bar-Or, O., Mendelson, L., & Najenson,

T. (1978). Pulmonary functions and responses to exercise of patients following craniocerebral injury. *Scandinavian Journal of Rehabilitation Medicine, 10,* 47–50.

Bond, M.R. (1979). Stages of recovery from severe

head injury with special reference to late outcome. *International Rehabilitation Medicine, 1,* 155–159.

Boughton, A., & Ciesla, N. (1986). Physical therapy management of the head-injured patient in the intensive care unit. *Topics in Acute Care and Trauma Rehabilitation, 1*(1), 1–18.

Brooks, D.N., McKinlay, W., Symington, C., Beattie A., & Campsie, L. (1987). Return to work within the first seven years of severe head injury. *Brain Injury, 1*(1), 5–19.

Brown, M., Gordon, W.A., & Diller, L. (1986). Functional assessment and outcome measurement: An integrative review. *Annual Review of Rehabilitation,* 93–120.

Crosby, K.G. (1980). Implementing the developmental model. In J.F. Gardner, L. Long, R. Nichols, & D. Iagulli (Eds.), *Program issues in developmental disabilities* (pp. 63–85). Baltimore: Paul H. Brookes Publishing Co.

DeLoach, C.P., Wilkins, R.D., & Walker, G.W. (1983). *Philosophy, process and services* (pp. 27–53, 95–112). Baltimore: University Park Press.

DeVillis, R.F., & Sauter, S.V.H. (1985). Recognizing the challenges of prevention in rehabilitation. *Archives of Physical Medicine and Rehabilitation, 66,* 52–54.

Garland, D.E. (1983). Rehabilitation of adults with head injuries. In H.S. Goldsmith, *Practice of surgery* (pp. 1–16). Philadelphia: Harper & Row.

Gilchrist, E., & Wilkinson, M. (1979). Some factors determining prognosis in young people with severe head injuries. *Archives of Neurology, 36,* 356–359.

Hackler, E., & Tobis, J.S. (1983). Reintegration into the community. In M. Rosenthal, E. Griffith, M. Bond, & J.D. Miller (Eds.), *Rehabilitation of the head injured adult* (pp. 421–434). Philadelphia: F.A. Davis.

Hamish, P.D., & Knight, R.G. (1988). Memory training and behavioral rehabilitation of a severely head-injured adult. *Archives of Physical Medicine and Rehabilitation, 69,* 458–460.

Jacobs, H.E. (1988). The Los Angeles head injury survey: Procedures and initial findings. *Archives of Physical Medicine and Rehabilitation, 69,* 425–431.

Jennett, B., & Bond, M.R. (1975). Assessment of outcome after severe brain damage: A practical scale. *Lancet, 3,* 1–12.

Jennett, B., Bond, M., & Brooks, W. (1981). Disability after severe head injury: Observations on the use of the Glasgow Outcome Scale. *Journal of Neurology, Neurosurgery and Psychiatry, 44,* 285–293.

Jennett, B., Teasdale, G., Brackman, R., Minderhoud, J., Heiden, J., & Kurze, T. (1979). Prognosis of patients with severe head injury. *Neurosurgery, 4,* 283.

Levin, H.S., Goldstein, F.C., High, Jr., W.M., & Williams, D. (1988). Automatic and effortful processing after severe closed head injury. *Brain and Cognition, 7,* 283–297.

Mills, V. (1985). Physical therapy and cognitive impairment in traumatically head injured patients: A clinical report. *Neurology Report, 9,* 51–54.

Najenson, T., Groswasser, Z., Mendelson, L., & Hackett, P. (1980). Rehabilitation outcome of brain damaged patients after severe head injury. *International Rehabilitation Medicine, 2,* 17–22.

Nelson, A.J. (1983a). Motor assessment. In M. Rosenthal, E. Griffith, M. Bond, & J.D. Miller (Eds.), *Rehabilitation of the head injured adult* (pp. 241–269). Philadelphia: F.A. Davis.

Nelson, A.J. (1983b). Strategies for improving motor control. In M. Rosenthal, E. Griffith, M. Bond, & J.D. Miller (Eds.), *Rehabilitation of the head injured adult* (pp. 313–334). Philadelphia: F.A. Davis.

Olson, R.S. (1985, November/December). Normalization: A concept in analysis. *Rehabilitation Nursing,* pp. 22–23.

Panikoff, L.B. (1983). Recovery trends of functional skills in the head injured adult. *The American Journal of Occupational Therapy, 37*(11), 735–743.

Panting, A., & Merry, P.H. (1972). The long term rehabilitation of severe head injuries with particular reference to the need for social and medical support for the patient's family. *Rehabilitation, 38,* 33–37.

Patterson, R.P., Pearson, J., & Fisher, S.V. (1985). Work-rest periods: Their effect on normal physiologic response to isometric and dynamic work. *Archives of Physical Medicine and Rehabilitation, 66,* 348–352.

Rappaport, M., Hall, K.M., Hopkins, K., Belleza, T., & Cope, D.N. (1982). Disability rating scale for severe head trauma: Coma to community. *Archives of Physical Medicine and Rehabilitation, 63,* 118–123.

Smith, R.K. (1983). Prevocational programming in the rehabilitation of the head-injured patient. *Physical Therapy, 63,* 2026–2029.

Talmage, E.W., & Collins G.A. (1983). Physical abilities after head injury: A retrospective study. *Physical Therapy, 63*(12), 2010–2017.

Wood, P.H. (1980). The language of disablement: A glossary relating to disease and its consequences. *International Rehabilitation Medicine, 2,* 86–92.

Ylvisaker, M. (Ed.). (1985). *Head injury rehabilitation: Children and adolescents.* San Diego: College-Hill Press.

Zablotney, C. (1987). Using neuromuscular electrical stimulation to facilitate limb control in the head injured patient. *The Journal of Head Trauma Rehabilitation, 2*(2), 28–33.

SECTION II

Cognitive and Neuropsychological Rehabilitation

CHAPTER 4

The Evolving Role of Neuropsychology in Community Integration

Jeffrey S. Kreutzer, Bruce E. Leininger, and Jennifer A. Harris

Especially during the 1980s, researchers and clinicians have developed an improved understanding of traumatic brain injury. We know with greater certainty that brain injury results in a variety of adverse, enduring alterations in cognitive ability, intellectual functioning, personality, emotional functioning, and behavior (Levin, Benton, & Grossman, 1982; Levin, Grossman, Rose, & Teasdale, 1979). These alterations affect complex abilities related to community integration including academic ability, interpersonal skills, and vocational functioning (Lezak, 1978; Lezak, 1987). Furthermore, independent living skills such as using transportation, managing personal finances, housekeeping, cooking, and managing emergency situations are frequently compromised by brain injury.

The adverse effects of brain injury often persist for many years. For example, Brooks and colleagues thoroughly documented long-term problems including high rates of unemployment, criminal behavior, assault on family members, family psychiatric disturbance, behavioral disorders, and cognitive impairment (Brooks, Campsie, Symington, Beattie, & McKinlay, 1986; Brooks, McKinlay, Symington, Beattie, & Campsie, 1987). Furthermore, Thomsen's (1984) survey of severely injured persons at 10 or more years postinjury revealed that the majority of individuals demonstrated personality change, poor concentration, loss of social contact, slowness, and fatigue.

Only recently have rehabilitation programs become available that are specifically designed for persons with traumatic brain injury. In the past, head injury survivors were treated within programs developed for persons with acquired physical disabilities caused by stroke, neuromuscular disease, and spinal cord injury. With improvements in neurosurgical management, physiatry, pharmacology, diagnostic evaluation, and other medical intervention techniques, an increased number of persons with brain injury began to survive. Increased survival rates and the unique sequelae of persons with head injury necessitated the development of specialized brain injury rehabilitation programs. Rehabilitation program development initially occurred within inpatient hospital facilities as neurosurgical teams required an appropriate treatment setting to accommodate the needs of patients with combinations of medical, cognitive, and behavioral problems. Many hospital systems now have coordinated medical and rehabilitation treatment systems whereby patients are admitted to intensive care, treated in an acute care medical unit, and transferred to and treated in an inpatient rehabilitation unit before being discharged (Thomas, 1988).

Progress in program development for community rehabilitation programs has proceeded

This work was partly supported by Grants #H133B80029 and #G0087C0219 from the National Institute on Disability and Rehabilitation Research, United States Department of Education.

slowly relative to inpatient programs for numerous reasons.

1. Persons discharged from inpatient rehabilitation facilities rarely develop life-threatening medical problems.
2. The problems of discharged rehabilitation patients are relatively subtle in comparison to the early medical and independent living problems that are obvious in the inpatient rehabilitation facility.
3. Discharged patients are often able to walk, comprehend language, speak, maintain personal hygiene, and eat independently.
4. The relative subtlety of problems and the absence of data indicating program cost-effectiveness contributes to problems obtaining funds needed for program development and implementation.
5. There are few cost-effective community service delivery models developed for persons with other types of disability that could be adapted for persons with brain injury.

Many individuals are discharged to their homes after maximum progress has been realized in inpatient rehabilitation settings. Research by Jacobs (1988) has indicated that family members subsequently assume the long-term burden of care. Unfortunately, helping the person with head injury return to maximum independence in the community is an extremely difficult task for family members. Relative to the inpatient setting, the quality and availability of community rehabilitation services is usually lacking and some families cannot afford these services. Where services are provided by several agencies, interagency communication problems contribute to confusion, resulting in fragmented or redundant service delivery. Furthermore, family members lack professional training, and so the combination of interpersonal, behavioral, and cognitive problems displayed by the client are likely to appear insurmountable. In addition, family members' ability to support the client may be compromised by prolonged stress. Inability to meet personal needs, assumption of additional household and work responsibilities, and the responsibility of caring for uninjured family members often proves overwhelming.

Community rehabilitation efforts ideally should be provided by a group of professionals working closely as a team. A team approach is required because of the multiplicity and interaction of problems arising from head injury. The team should comprise all persons involved in the rehabilitation process. The client, family members, and friends involved in caregiving are integral parts of the team. Disciplines commonly represented in such team approaches include physiatry, physical therapy, occupational therapy, social work, speech pathology, vocational rehabilitation, and neuropsychology.

Initially, the community rehabilitation team works with the head-injured individual to facilitate transition from the inpatient setting to the home setting. Following discharge, new treatment goals are established that focus on independent community living. To ensure retention of treatment gains, follow-up should not be time limited. Rather, follow-up services should be available throughout the client's lifetime. Every effort should be made to work proactively by anticipating problems and preventing their occurrence (Wehman, Kreutzer, Wood, Morton, & Sherron, 1988; Wehman et al., 1989).

Clinical neuropsychologists are likely to serve in a variety of roles as members of the community rehabilitation team. The exact nature of these roles is dependent on the client's needs and the availability of other professional services in the community. The more limited the availability of adjunct services, the greater the likelihood that the neuropsychologist will be called upon to fulfill a diversity of roles. Roles of the clinical neuropsychologist in community integration may include the following: 1) neuropsychological assessor; 2) individual, group, and family psychotherapist; 3) consultant to other professionals providing rehabilitation services to the client (e.g., vocational rehabilitation); 4) expert witness in litigation; 5) advocate; 6) cognitive remediation therapist; and 7) substance abuse evaluator and therapist. Several of these roles are discussed in greater detail in Chapters 2, 12, and 16 in this book. Consequently, to avoid redundancy, this chapter focuses on: the evolution of clinical neuropsychology as a professional entity, neuropsychological assessment, professional consultation, substance abuse, litigation, and advocacy.

EVOLUTION OF CLINICAL NEUROPSYCHOLOGY

Clinical neuropsychologists possess special knowledge of brain-behavior relationships and descriptive and prescriptive (i.e., treatment-directed) assessment and psychotherapy procedures for use with traumatically brain-injured and other neurologically impaired persons. Involvement of these specially trained professionals is critical if community integration efforts for persons with traumatic brain injury are to succeed.

Clinical neuropsychology is a discipline in evolution that recently entered its third developmental phase (Costa, 1983; Rourke, 1982). Linked with each phase has been a particular focus and application of assessment. The initial developmental phase of clinical neuropsychology originated during World War II and lasted until the mid-1960s. During this time, Ward Halstead (e.g., Halstead, 1947; Halstead & Wepman, 1959) pioneered efforts to develop a group of tests that were sensitive to the effects of brain injury and could reliably discriminate between brain-injured, psychiatrically disturbed, and normal individuals. As a consequence of systematic research and clinical experience, relationships were established between patterns of test performance, specific sites of brain lesions, and types of neurological disorders. On the basis of assessment results, clinicians were able to establish diagnoses, discriminate between static and progressive conditions, and provide relatively accurate indications of brain lesion sites. Halstead's procedures were later adapted by Reitan in the formation of the now commonly used Halstead-Reitan Neuropsychological Test Battery (Reitan & Davison, 1974). During this initial developmental period, neuropsychological assessment became a highly prized adjunct to the neurological examination by offering unparalleled information about functional capabilities and the integrity of higher cortical centers.

The role of neuropsychological tests for diagnostic purposes began to diminish in the late 1960s. This shift was in part precipitated by the rapid development of sophisticated and relatively inexpensive computer technology. Noninvasive neuroradiological tests including computerized axial tomography (CT), positron emission tomography (PET), and magnetic resonance imaging (MRI) were more accurate and efficient than neuropsychological tests for establishing diagnoses and lesion localization. Previously, the more valued medical diagnostic tests (e.g., angiography) were painful, potentially dangerous, and sometimes associated with mortality. With technological advances, neuropsychologists focused their evaluations on assessment of discrete abilities. Testing began to be used for elucidating relative strengths and weaknesses across various cognitive and psychomotor domains. Referring physicians more frequently asked clinical neuropsychologists to describe the behavioral, cognitive, and psychomotor consequences of neurological disorders rather than to establish diagnoses.

The focus of the newly emerging third phase in the development of clinical neuropsychology places a greater emphasis on treatment and the practical value of testing. Delineation of relative strengths and weaknesses is still requested by referral sources. However, practical statements about everyday behavioral competencies are often the primary goal of assessments (Chelune & Moehle, 1986; Heaton & Pendleton, 1981). Referring professionals typically ask questions about employability, academic potential, ability to live independently, and treatment needs. Clinical neuropsychologists increasingly provide recommendations to enhance treatment efficacy, consultation, and treatment implementation. These professionals also are devoting greater attention to psychotherapy, cognitive remediation, behavior management programs, and community education.

Some professionals have suggested that diagnosis is no longer a useful endeavor for clinical neuropsychologists (Mapou, 1988). In fact, one author of a recent chapter pertaining to neuropsychological assessment did not include diagnosis as a common use for test results (Acker, 1986). However, neuropsychological assessment retains an important role in brain damage detection and diagnosis particularly in the most difficult clinical cases (such as minor head injury; Leininger, Gramling, Farrell, Kreutzer, & Peck, in press) where neurological and neuroradiological procedures fail to provide objective evidence of brain damage (Kane, Goldstein, & Parsons, 1989).

Despite their sophistication, present-day neuroradiographic diagnostic procedures are associated with numerous shortcomings. Positron emission tomography provides important information about brain structure and function, but this procedure is expensive and unavailable to most clients. In contrast, CT and MRI have limited resolution, only provide information about brain structure, and are best suited to the detection of focal lesions. Microscopic damage, such as diffuse axonal injury, is typically not evident on CT or MRI scans. Scanning also has limited utility given the sometimes uncertain relationship between brain structure and function. For example, relatively large lesions may yield few functional impairments. Conversely, small lesions in combination with diffuse axonal injury may yield severe dysfunction. Imaging is undoubtedly useful for neurosurgical intervention. Nevertheless, from a rehabilitation perspective, clinicians are trained to rehabilitate by enhancing functional abilities rather than by "shrinking" lesions. Given the situations outlined above, neuropsychological evaluation is sometimes the most objective means of detecting brain injury and lends the greatest information regarding rehabilitation needs and treatment directions.

A growing number of psychologists who work with head-injured persons have training in both clinical neuropsychology and rehabilitation psychology. Those with rehabilitation psychology backgrounds possess knowledge of the psychological aspects of chronic disability, psychological assessment, and psychotherapy. These professionals can enhance the emotional adjustment of brain-injured persons who frequently experience depression, diminished self-esteem, and grieving following injury, and in addition, are the unfortunate victims of rude comments and insensitive behavior motivated by public stereotypes concerning disability. Rehabilitation

psychologists also are usually knowledgeable about vocational issues and may become involved in job placement, in training interview techniques, in job maintenance skills, and as a liaison between the employee and employer.

NEUROPSYCHOLOGICAL ASSESSMENT

An overview of issues pertaining to neuropsychological assessment of persons with traumatic brain injury who are facing community integration is provided in this section. The concerns addressed by the clinical neuropsychologist in this role are different from those relevant to other populations and inpatient settings. The reader is referred to other sources (e.g., Levin et al., 1982; Lezak, 1983) for a comprehensive discussion of neuropathology, functional neuroanatomy, and assessment techniques.

Most clients are referred for neuropsychological evaluation by physicians. In other cases, allied health professionals, insurance companies, attorneys, vocational rehabilitation counselors, or others, including the client and his or her family members, provide the referral. Primary goals for the neuropsychological evaluation usually include description of the client's intellectual, cognitive, sensory, and psychomotor skills; description of the client's emotional and behavioral status; and description of family support systems and their value to the client. The descriptive information in the report is intended to facilitate treatment planning. Clinical neuropsychologists rarely are asked specific referral questions. Nevertheless, specific referral questions can enhance the value of the examination by guiding the assessment process. Persons with head injury certainly constitute a heterogeneous group; as each client is an individual, the examination process should not be identical for all persons evaluated. Discussion with referral sources is often essential to ensure that the lengthy examination process meets the unique needs of the client and answers the questions most important to treating professionals. The evaluation and descriptive report may address any of the referral questions pertaining to the client's cognitive, intellectual, sensory, and psychomotor skills listed in Table 4.1. Additionally, because clinical neuropsychology is a relatively new field and because practitioners vary widely in terms of training and philosophy, referral sources can often benefit from a discussion of the

Table 4.1. Referral questions pertaining to clients' cognitive, intellectual, sensory, and psychomotor skills

Describe the client's preinjury vocational and educational history.

Within each area of cognitive, intellectual, and psychomotor functioning, compare the client's performance to the normal population. Which areas would you consider to be relative strengths and which areas would you consider to be weaknesses?

Describe levels of functioning in each area, relative to preinjury and relative to the client's last evaluation. Which skills have improved, declined, and remained the same? Identify factors that may have contributed to or limited change.

Can the client live independently? If not, can the client be left alone and for what period of time? Identify emotional, behavioral, and cognitive factors that primarily contribute to dependence. To what extent will the client benefit from behavioral, psychotherapeutic, and pharmacological treatment strategies?

Is the client competent to: manage his or her own financial affairs? drive? judge right from wrong? take medications on schedule and respond appropriately if dangerous side effects arise?

Based on the client's strengths and limitations, expectations, and interests, which vocations or vocational environments would be most suitable?

Which factors will affect the client's ability to benefit from physical and vocational rehabilitation? Which techniques (e.g., pharmacological, compensatory) might be useful to minimize limiting factors?

To what extent are the client's neurological deficits a function of his or her most recent injury and preinjury factors (e.g., learning disability, prior head trauma)?

When will it be helpful to evaluate the client again? For what purposes?

Will the client's level of self-awareness influence his or her ability to benefit from therapy and live independently?

How responsive is the client to feedback? What techniques can be utilized to increase responsiveness to feedback?

examination process. Information about test content, procedures, and goals of the examination should be conveyed.

As noted previously, traumatic brain injury can cause a wide variety of functional impairments. For this reason it is often important to evaluate the client using diverse tests that are indicative of a wide variety of abilities. There are many tests available and clinicians occasionally have difficulty selecting the "best" test. Factors that guide test selection include evidence of reliability and validity. For example, some tests such as the Paced Auditory Serial Addition Test and the Wechsler Memory Scale Logical Memory subtest have demonstrated criterion-related validity and are useful in predicting head-injured persons' capacity to return to work (Brooks et al., 1987). Tests that have been used extensively with head-injured persons, as evident in the research literature, usually possess greater clinical utility than tests used infrequently. Additionally, preference is given to selecting tests that have been used extensively with non-injured persons. Normative data for persons varying in age, education, race, and sex are helpful in establishing comparisons to peers.

Clinical neuropsychologists are also encouraged to use tests that have the greatest relevance to real-life functioning. For this reason, standardized measures of spelling, reading accuracy, reading comprehension, and arithmetic reasoning are useful. A listing of neuropsychological functions (abilities) and corresponding tests that apparently measure those abilities is presented in Table 4.2. Clinically, the authors have found these tests to be useful and they meet many of the selection criteria just stated. Notably, neuropsychological tests do not reflect singular neuropsychological abilities. Rather, most tests appear to reflect a myriad of interrelated abilities, some to a greater extent than others.

Clinical neuropsychologists are typically asked to make three important judgments for each skill area tested. A checklist has been developed to summarize and cogently present the results of these judgments (see Form 4.1). First, the client's ability in a given domain is determined by comparing his or her performance to the normal population. This comparison allows

Table 4.2.   Tests and corresponding neuropsychological functions

Neuropsychological function	Test
Old learning, verbal skills	
Oral fluency and speech quality	Controlled Oral Word Association Test; Boston Diagnostic Aphasia Examination; Clinical Interview
Oral reading	Gray Oral Reading Test–Revised; Reading subtest (Wide Range Achievement Test–Revised; WRAT-R)
Spelling	Spelling subtest (WRAT-R)
Writing	Spelling subtest (WRAT-R)
Fund of information	Information subtest (Wechsler Adult Intelligence Scale–Revised; WAIS-R); Vocabulary subtest (WAIS-R)
Reasoning and judgment	
Concept formation	Similarities subtest (WAIS-R); Comprehension subtest (WAIS-R); Wisconsin Card Sorting Test; Category Test; Picture Arrangement subtest (WAIS-R)
Reading comprehension	Gray Oral Reading Test–Revised
Judgment of safety	Comprehension subtest (WAIS-R)
Self-awareness	Clinical Interview
Logical-deductive reasoning	Luria-Nebraska Receptive Speech Scale (selected items)
Verbal memory	
Immediate	Babcock Story Recall; Rey Auditory Verbal Learning Test (Trial I); Logical Memory (Wechsler Memory Scale)
Delayed	Babcock Story Recall; Logical Memory (Wechsler Memory Scale)
Remote	Information subtest (WAIS-R); Personal and Current Information (Wechsler Memory Scale)
Learning	Rey Auditory Verbal Learning Test
Arithmetic	
Calculation	Arithmetic subtest (WRAT-R)
Reasoning	Arithmetic subtest (WAIS-R)
Attention and concentration	
Immediate	Digit Span Forward (WAIS-R)
Sustained	Paced Auditory Serial Addition Test; Symbol Digit Modalities Test; Digit Symbol subtest (WAIS-R); Mental Control (Wechsler Memory Scale); Digit Span Backward (WAIS-R)
Visual-based skills	
Perception	Motor Free Visual Perception Test; Line Orientation Test; Line Bisection Test; Symbol-Digit Modalities Test (Oral); Visual Form Discrimination Test
Reasoning	Hooper Visual Organization Test; Object Assembly subtest (WAIS-R); Picture Arrangement subtest (WAIS-R); Block Design subtest (WAIS-R)
Construction	Rey-Osterrieth Complex Figure Test; Block Design subtest (WAIS-R); Hooper Visual Organization Test; Object Assembly subtest (WAIS-R)
Nonverbal memory	
Immediate	Visual Reproduction (Wechsler Memory Scale); Benton Visual Retention Test; Motor Free Visual Perception Test; Corsi Block Test
Delayed	Rey-Osterrieth Complex Figure Test; Tactual Performance Test (Recall, Location); Recognition Memory Test
Learning	Symbol Digit Modalities Test; Digit Symbol subtest (WAIS-R)

(continued)

Table 4.2.   (*continued*)

Neuropsychological function	Test
Motor functions	
Dexterity (R/L)	Grooved Pegboard
Speed	Finger Tapping Test; Grooved Pegboard
Grip strength	Hand Dynamometer
Coordinated bilateral movement	Luria Motor Tests
Hand-eye coordination	Luria Motor Tests; Grooved Pegboard; Symbol Digit Modalities Test (written); Digit Symbol subtest (WAIS-R); Trail Making

For further information on the tests cited here, the reader is advised to consult Lezak (1983).

the clinician to estimate how the client performed relative to persons of similar age, education, and sex. Second, a judgment is made of how the client's performance has been affected by the injury. Reported sequelae, review of academic and vocational records, estimation of preinjury level of ability, and knowledge of common consequences of injury can help the clinician determine which skills are impaired relative to preinjury status. Third, clinical neuropsychologists estimate whether a client's functioning in each area has improved, remained the same, or declined relative to previous testing. Direct comparisons with prior test scores can help establish whether therapy, subsequent injury or disease, recovery, or medication has affected client status over time.

Careful observation during the course of the evaluation can provide useful qualitative information about how clients solve problems. This information can be used by therapists and vocational rehabilitation professionals to structure environments and provide feedback. Examiners observe whether the client is able to recognize errors and whether the client demonstrates initiative to correct errors that were recognized. Information is also obtained about executive skills including planning and organization. Rate of information processing and mental flexibility can also be assessed both formally and informally during the examination process.

To prevent possible accidents and for educational purposes, clinicians have the responsibility of commenting on the client's ability to engage in potentially dangerous activities. The client and his or her family members frequently have questions regarding the client's ability to drive, operate mechanical/electrical equipment, manage finances, and take medication as prescribed. Interview information pertaining to the client's current responsibilities is integrated with test information to estimate levels of competence in these skill areas. When possible, the opinions of other professionals should be solicited before reaching final determinations. For example, based on a neuropsychological evaluation that reveals visuoperceptual problems, the clinical neuropsychologist may suggest that the client submit to a formal driving evaluation before resuming driving.

Assessment of the client's emotional and behavioral status is another important area included in the neuropsychological evaluation. Questions to consider in the evaluation of emotional and behavioral status are listed in Table 4.3. In addition to behavioral observation during the course of examination, several other types of data are useful in describing the client's reaction to the injury. The interview with the client provides useful data in that his or her perception of emotional changes, present coping ability, and level of pessimism are assessed. Since depression often follows injury, clinicians are encouraged to be sensitive to reports of suicidal ideation, sleep disturbance, appetite change, weight fluctuations, and lack of initiative. Medical examination can help distinguish between pathophysiological changes arising from injury and psychological changes. Interview with family members provides another important perspective on the client's emotional and behavioral status.

FORM 4.1

NAME: _____   DATE: ____-____-____

NEUROPSYCHOLOGICAL PROFILE

Performance and Impairment Levels

Functional skills	High average (>75th percentile)	Average or normal (26th–75th percentile)	Low average (11th–25th percentile)	Borderline defective (6th–10th percentile)	Defective (<6th percentile)	Impaired relative to premorbid status[a]	Relative to prior testing[b]
I. Arithmetic (written, oral)							
A. Computation							
B. Reasoning							
II. Attention and concentration							
A. Immediate							
B. Sustained							
III. Language							
A. Word finding							
B. Oral fluency							
C. Auditory comprehension							
D. Handwriting accuracy							
E. Spelling							
F. Reading accuracy							
G. Reading comprehension							
IV. Learning and memory							
A. Auditory memory (1) Immediate							
(2) Delayed							
B. Visual memory (1) Immediate							
(2) Delayed							
C. Remote/fund of information							
D. Learning (1) Auditory							
(2) Visuomotor							
V. Motor							
A. Right hand (1) Speed/dexterity							
(2) Strength							
B. Left hand (1) Speed/dexterity							
(2) Strength							
C. Bilateral coordination (1) Sequencing/speed							

(continued)

Performance and Impairment Levels

Functional skills	High average (>75th percentile)	Average or normal (26th–75th percentile)	Low average (11th–25th percentile)	Borderline defective (6th–10th percentile)	Defective (<6th percentile)	Impaired relative to premorbid status[a]	Relative to prior testing[b]
VI. Reasoning A. Common sense, judgment of safety							
B. Logical deductive							
C. Hypothesis testing							
VII. Visual skills A. Perception							
B. Construction							

Performance levels are considered relative to the normal population, whereas impairment is considered relative to preinjury or premorbid status.

[a]"*" denotes impairment.

[b]"+" denotes improved; "=" denotes same; "−" denotes worse.

Qualitative Aspects of Performance

Cognitive skill areas	Good	Adequate	Poor or defective
Error recognition			
Error correction			
Mental flexibility			
Organization			
Planning			
Rate of information processing			

"Good" denotes a functional skill that is an asset and contributes to performance.

"Adequate" indicates that a skill is functional and does not prohibit performance of interdependent skills.

"Poor or defective" denotes an impaired, nonfunctional skill that adversely affects performance of interdependent skills.

Competencies

Competencies	Yes	?	No
Dangerous machinery and electrical appliances: operation			
Driving			
Financial management			
Medication management			

In appropriate cases, questionable ("?") competencies will be assessed by referral to relevant medical professionals.

Formal psychological assessment of emotional status and personality may have limited value because most tests have been standardized on psychiatric populations. However, some tests can yield useful insights when interpreted cautiously. Information from these tests should be

Table 4.3. Referral questions pertaining to clients' emotional and behavioral status

What was the client's level of preinjury psychosocial functioning? Address issues related to previous emotional disturbance and interpersonal relationships.

What is the client's present emotional status? Is there evidence of suicidal ideation, diminished self-esteem, and feelings of hopelessness?

To what extent are the client's behavioral and emotional problems a function of neuropathology versus psychological factors?

Will increased self-awareness cause or contribute to depression?

Does the client demonstrate any behavioral problems (e.g., aggressive, socially inappropriate) in the testing, home, or other environments? Which factors appear to influence the frequency and maintenance of behaviors?

How is the client coping with his or her disability? How does the client respond to stress? Identify adaptive and maladaptive coping mechanisms.

Is the client a suicidal risk?

Is there evidence of pre- or postinjury substance abuse?

compared with the client's self-report, the report of family members, and the clinician's knowledge regarding the common effects of injury. For example, the Beck Depression Inventory can provide useful information regarding self-esteem, levels of pessimism, appetite disturbance, and libido (Beck, 1967; Beck, Ward, Mendelson, Mock, & Erbaugh, 1961). However, this instrument is highly susceptible to a social desirability response style. The Minnesota Multiphasic Personality Inventory (MMPI) provides some indication of test-taking attitudes and social desirability through examination of this test's validity scales. Additional valuable information about depressive symptoms, family disturbance, somatic discomforts, and social isolation can be obtained via use of the MMPI (Dahlstrom, Welsh, & Dahlstrom, 1972; Graham, 1987). However, standard clinical interpretation of scale elevations for brain-injured persons should be avoided considering that certain clinical scales are frequently elevated over a T score of 70 for this population (scales #1, #2, #3, #7, #8; Leininger, Kreutzer, & Hill, 1989; Novack, Daniel, & Long, 1984). Clinicians who

use the MMPI may derive the most valid conclusions about the emotional and personality functioning of head-injured persons through examining responses to individual test items, including those designated as "Critical Items."

As family members can facilitate or impede rehabilitation efforts, two important intervention goals for clinical neuropsychologists are to maximize family support for the client's rehabilitation and to enhance family coping. To help meet these goals, immediate family members should be interviewed during the course of the evaluation. Perceptions of the client prior to the injury, how the client's present status compares to preinjury, and family members' goals for the client should be discussed. Additionally, clinicians should obtain an understanding of the emotional status of family members and evaluate their coping abilities. Information relevant to the family situation that may be included in the neuropsychological report is presented in Table 4.4. More

Table 4.4. Referral questions pertaining to clients' family situation

How aware is the family of the client's current level of abilities?

To what extent is the family educated regarding the typical effects of brain injury?

Is the family a good support system? How are family members helping the client or contributing to present difficulties?

Describe the emotional status of immediate family members, including siblings and children. Are family members using adaptive or maladaptive coping mechanisms?

How have family roles and relationships changed as a consequence of the client's injury?

How do outside family members and friends understand the client's problems and how are they reacting?

To what extent are extended family members and friends supportive? Are these individuals willing and able to offer respite? Is the client's family willing to request and take advantage of offers to provide respite?

Are family members reinforcing inappropriate behaviors and dependency?

Do family members feel guilty about the client's initial injury and limited recovery?

What are the family's expectations regarding recovery and the client's ability to return to previous activities (e.g., work, school)?

complete information regarding family assessment and intervention for families of children and adults with head injury is presented in Chapters 14 through 18 of this book.

To summarize, the neuropsychological evaluation begins with a clarification of the reasons for the examination. The clinical neuropsychologist then carefully reviews medical records to ascertain neurological consequences of injury and treatment history. The client and his or her family are interviewed to obtain historical information and to elicit their perceptions about client status and changes. Valid and reliable tests are selected to provide an overview of strengths and limitations in functional areas, and in some instances, to provide diagnostic information. Behavioral observations are collected to help understand problem-solving strategies and levels of executive functioning. The primary challenge to the clinical neuropsychologist is to integrate information from these diverse sources and help prepare a treatment plan that incorporates the client's strengths and acknowledges his or her uniqueness.

CONSULTATION TO REHABILITATION PROFESSIONALS AND COMMUNITY AGENCIES

Many clinical neuropsychologists involved in head injury rehabilitation serve as consultants. During inpatient rehabilitation, clinical neuropsychologists often work with physicians and members of allied health professionals. Results of the neuropsychological evaluation are shared with team members to help them gain a more complete understanding of the client's strengths and limitations as well as the emotional consequences of the injury that can interfere with ongoing therapies. Clinical neuropsychologists are called upon to facilitate adaptive coping and to help manage the client's behavior in the context of therapy to assure maximum therapeutic effectiveness. Allied health therapists are taught basic principles of reinforcement, target behavior identification, and extinction procedures. With an understanding of basic behavioral principles, therapists representing other disciplines can learn to reduce the frequency of behaviors that

interfere with therapy and increase the frequency of appropriate behaviors.

The role of the clinical neuropsychologist as consultant is similar during both the person's inpatient hospitalization and the process of community integration. Educating other rehabilitation professionals about the manifestations of brain injury and their implications for independent living remains an important activity. Teaching behavior management strategies also continues to be important. Neuropsychological evaluations are repeated as needed and, as before, the evaluation results are communicated to other members of the rehabilitation team.

Clinical neuropsychologists also work with community service organizations to help them better meet the needs of persons with head injury and their families. For example, clinical neuropsychologists work with chapters of the National Head Injury Foundation in many communities. Roles fulfilled by these professionals include gathering of educational materials for local libraries, establishing and facilitating support groups, educating families and clients through organized lectures and discussions, and lobbying with local governments and third-party payers to develop and fund services.

The supported employment program for persons with traumatic brain injury developed by Wehman and associates (e.g., Wehman et al., 1988; Wehman et al., 1989) provides an excellent example of the consulting role that clinical neuropsychology has played in vocational rehabilitation. Supported employment is a vocational program that helps persons with disabilities who are unable to gain or maintain competitive employment. Persons with head injury are helped by specially trained employment specialists to secure competitive employment. Employers and co-workers are educated about the effects of head injury. Compensatory strategies, social skills, and behavior management techniques are used in the workplace to help clients complete their job activities. Employment specialists provide intensive on-site intervention. After the job is mastered, a fading process begins, during which the employment specialist significantly reduces time spent at the work site. Continuing follow-along is provided indefinitely. Employment specialists regularly check with clients and employers to help prevent and eliminate problems that may arise.

Following referral for supported employment, clients are referred for neuropsychological evaluation and screened for substance abuse problems. The neuropsychological evaluation provides an understanding of clients' strengths and weaknesses and is used to select jobs congruent with abilities. Clients found to possess significant emotional or personality problems are seen by the clinical neuropsychologist for treatment. Additionally, compensatory strategies are developed for each client for use in the workplace. Strategies are designed on the basis of client ability levels and consultation with the employment specialist. The clinical neuropsychologist provides regular consultation to the employment specialist as part of a proactive approach. Every effort is made to prevent problems and to solve those that arise at the earliest feasible time. Biweekly support groups are provided to clients, and independently to family members, to help them cope with the stresses of injury and employment. As part of a substance abuse prevention program, clients and family members participate in an alcohol and drug education program developed and implemented by a clinical neuropsychologist in conjunction with employment specialists. Furthermore, clients with possible substance abuse problems are referred for evaluation and treatment by an experienced substance abuse counselor.

SUBSTANCE ABUSE

An increasing number of clinical neuropsychologists are becoming involved in the identification, treatment, and referral for treatment of substance abuse problems. The problems of dependency, co-dependency, denial, and rationalization are extremely complex and challenging, and result in high rates of ineffective treatment and recidivism. Clinical neuropsychologists may have training in substance abuse assessment but often lack formal training in treatment techniques. Treatment should ideally be provided by persons with specialized training and experience in substance abuse issues. These persons primarily identify themselves as substance abuse or alcohol counselors. Unfortunately, many persons with this specialized training are unaware of how the unique problems of head injury can adversely affect the efficacy of traditional treatment techniques. Cognitive problems such as impaired self-awareness, memory loss, and reasoning deficits contribute to difficulties in responding to techniques that have proven effective for persons without brain injury. Clinical neuropsychologists increasingly are working with substance abuse counselors and sharing knowledge in an effort to maximize treatment effectiveness.

Clinical neuropsychologists and other professional caregivers are increasingly concerned about substance use in persons with traumatic brain injury. Research suggests that alcohol is present in the bloodstream of at least two thirds of all persons who sustain serious head injury, and at least one fourth of these individuals have alcohol abuse histories (Kreutzer, 1989; Rimel, Giordani, Barth, & Jane, 1982; Sparadeo & Gill, 1989). Furthermore, one study reported that nearly one third of head-injured persons used illicit drugs preinjury (Kreutzer, Harris, & Doherty, 1989). Intoxication at the time of injury has been linked with greater mortality, lengthier duration of agitation, and greater cognitive impairment upon discharge (Sparadeo & Gill, 1989). Also, it has been recently noted that substance abuse problems negatively affect community integration efforts (Burke, Weselowski, & Guth, 1988). Unfortunately, a number of clients continue their patterns of substance abuse postinjury, with a negative influence on rehabilitation efforts.

Langley, Lindsey, Lam, and Priddy (in press) and Kreutzer and Harris (1990) have described model systems of care for persons with traumatic brain injury who have substance abuse problems. These model systems of rehabilitation focus on prevention. Prevention begins with an educational program that informs family members and clients of the negative effects of substance abuse. Assertiveness training is provided to help clients say "No!" to alcohol and drugs. Information is provided in a format that is understandable to laypersons, and is adapted for effectiveness in acknowledgment of the clients' unique nature of cognitive impairments. Educational efforts are shared with staff and family members since limiting substance abuse problems is most efficacious when clients, family, and staff possess similar attitudes and ideas. Disagreements pertaining to substance use, especially among staff and family members, only contribute to client confusion. Prevention efforts can be enhanced by facilitating and encouraging the clients' participation in social and recreational activities that do not include the use of alcohol and illicit drugs.

Several instruments can assist in the identification of substance use and abuse. The Michigan Alcoholism Screening Test (Selzer, 1971; Zung, 1970) and the Quantity-Frequency-Variability Index (Cahalan & Cisin, 1968) are self-report measures that assess drinking patterns. The Michigan Alcoholism Screening Test provides important information about correlates of alcohol dependence and helps clinicians in establishing a diagnosis of alcohol dependence. Information is collected regarding guilt associated with drinking as well as alcohol's negative influence on work and interpersonal relationships. The Quantity-Frequency-Variability Index provides information regarding how much and how often the individual typically drinks. This information is utilized to assign clients to one of five categories of drinker: abstinent, infrequent, light, moderate, or heavy.

The General Health and History Questionnaire (Kreutzer, Leininger, Doherty, & Waaland, 1987; see Appendix A, chap. 16, this volume) has proven useful for assessment of both alcohol and drug use patterns. This instrument can be administered to both clients and family members for purpose of comparison. Information is gathered regarding preinjury and postinjury alcohol and illicit drug use and perceptions of whether the client has a substance abuse problem. This form, along with a thorough history-taking interview, can assist in the determination of whether substance use problems exist.

Additional evidence of preinjury substance abuse can be derived from multiple sources such as blood alcohol level upon hospital admission (especially if above the legal limit), and driving or criminal records indicating arrest for alcohol-related offenses, including driving under the influence of alcohol. Employment records may provide other clues of substance abuse as suggested by irregular work performance, frequent tardiness, and high rates of absenteeism.

Ironically, community integration may contribute to the availability of addictive substances. The availability of drugs and alcohol increases the likelihood of abuse for most clients with substance abuse histories. The successful vocational rehabilitation client earns income, which enables an independent or less supervised living situation and increased mobility. Transportation and spendable income allows increased opportunities for socialization, and unfortunately, "normality" for most young adults includes alcohol and/or drug use. Nevertheless, abstinence from alcohol and drugs is recommended for all persons with traumatic brain injury, especially those involved in rehabilitation programs. Rehabilitation staff should be sensitive to the fact that this newly established abstinence can result in rejection and ostracism from former "friends." The authors, therefore, encourage professionals to use written contracts with their clients to make expectations explicit. Many clients have poor memory and forget verbal instructions. Some professionals may consider abstinence to be unreasonable and allow clients to use their own judgment. However, persons with head injury have problems with judgment and self-awareness, which often lead to poor decisions. Clinicians should acknowledge that substance use has a negative effect on both client safety and head injury recovery. Clinicians also are encouraged to acknowledge that assessment and prevention of substance abuse must continue throughout the rehabilitation and follow-up process. Community integration presents a new series of choices and challenges for the client. Continued support and education can help ensure that the client makes wise choices and that the benefits of rehabilitation are not lost.

In summary, clients with identified substance abuse problems should be referred for treatment to experienced substance abuse counselors where available. Clinical neuropsychologists can facilitate treatment by helping counselors to understand the diverse consequences of head injury. Community integration efforts need not cease during substance abuse treatment. In fact, substance abuse counselors should become part of the rehabilitation team, participate in treatment planning, and communicate means of reinforcing positive changes with other team members.

LITIGATION

Clients frequently use litigation to obtain compensation for emotional distress and disability arising from head trauma. The role of the clinical neuropsychologist includes providing emotional support and education to injured litigants and their families, and serving as an expert witness.

In many cases, clients' injuries are attributable to negligence on the part of another party. However, during the first year postinjury, clients and their families are usually immersed in various crises related to medical problems and recovery. Every effort is made to ensure that maximum gains arise from therapy and that the client is able to return to former levels of functioning. As recovery runs its course and evidence mounts that many impairments may be permanent, attention becomes more focused on litigation issues. Following discharge, family members usually begin to encounter difficulties obtaining additional funds to help meet the growing costs of medical treatment and rehabilitation. Unfortunately, funds for treatment contributed by the defendant most often become available only after settlement, and there is a delay of 2–3 years before most cases go to trial. Financial hardships contribute to blame and anger directed at the defendant and at the legal system in general.

For many persons with brain injury, intensive preparation for litigation occurs during the process of attempted community integration. The client may be a participant in day rehabilitation, transitional living, or vocational rehabilitation therapies. During this period, many clients feel they are in a "double-bind." Those who rarely complain and work diligently to maximize their recovery may feel they are ultimately hurting their chances to receive a substantial, appro-

priate settlement. Family members and friends also can indirectly "sabotage" therapeutic efforts by discussing cases they "heard about" in which other brain-injured persons were awarded large settlements. This may suggest how clients should "act" to achieve the greatest settlement possible. Frank discussion with the client will help the clinician develop an understanding of pressures and conflicts related to litigation. Ultimately, clients should be helped to understand that maximum participation in rehabilitation, rather than concerted demonstrations of disability, will yield the greatest benefits to their long-term outcome.

The process of litigation is stressful for nearly all persons with traumatic brain injury and a variety of interventions can prove beneficial. During the initial evaluation process, clinical neuropsychologists should ascertain whether a case involves litigation. Expectations regarding the outcome of litigation and the client's beliefs regarding degree of participation should be assessed. Clients may be unaware of the stresses of litigation and may require greater emotional support during the process. Meetings involving family members also may be helpful to assess their reactions and develop mutual support among family members during the litigation process.

Other aspects of the litigation process also may be upsetting. Clients participate in a series of meetings and depositions, and are asked questions regarding the circumstances of the accident and the effects of the injury. The process of questioning and review is frequently counterproductive to the client's attempts to cope with the life changes brought about by the accident. In many cases, psychotherapy has assisted the client to focus less on the past and more on constructive problem solving, as well as on future goals. Elaborate descriptions of the emotional distress and disabilities resulting from the accident contribute to pessimism and diminished self-esteem. Expert witness testimony about the severity and permanence of the injury and eyewitness recounts of the accident can increase clients' anxieties to dangerous levels. During the trial the clinical neuropsychologist should help the client and attorney remain sensitive to this possibility. It may be preferable at times to have the client wait outside the courtroom during testimony and questioning.

Insensitive and ignorant defense attorneys can also contribute to clients' emotional distress. For example, the attorney who is ignorant about head injury may attribute the client's poor motivation to greed and ignore the fact that depression and neuropathological changes contribute to present difficulties. Unfortunately, the legal system in the United States places the defense attorney in an adversarial position. Inevitably, the client's comments about his or her disability and need for treatment are more likely to be met with skepticism and disbelief than with acceptance and understanding. Furthermore, some attorneys may accuse clients of exaggerating their complaints in order to gain larger settlements, although research has not supported this claim (Binder, 1986). In turn, clients occasionally report feeling that they, rather than the defendant, are on trial.

Serving as an expert witness is an additional function of the clinical neuropsychologist in litigation. Attorneys often require assistance in collecting information, understanding medical records, and documenting the emotional, cognitive, and psychomotor consequences of the injury. The clinical neuropsychologist may be asked to provide an independent evaluation and address the effects of the injury, projected degree of permanence, need for treatment, and expected costs. Clinical neuropsychologists usually feel most comfortable working with the plaintiff's attorney, helping to demonstrate the long-term negative impact of the injury. Professionals who agree to help attorneys representing the defense may feel they face a complicated ethical dilemma. The adversarial role of the defense attorney may appear to be directly in conflict with the clinical neuropsychologist's role to advocate for and serve the client. However, the clinical neuropsychologist's only choice is to provide an objective opinion, regardless of which side he or she represents.

ADVOCACY

Clinical neuropsychologists may serve as client advocates in a variety of contexts. They may work with community agencies to establish a rationale for the development of new services as well as to modify and extend existing services to meet the unique needs of persons with brain injury (Rosenthal & Young, 1988). Lobbying with legislators and private agencies to obtain funding and other forms of support may be necessary. In this role, the clinical neuropsychologist carries out research to assess the need for services. Written or oral reports are prepared that discuss issues of need, alternative mechanisms of service delivery, costs and efficacy of each alternative, timelines for development and implementation, and staffing needs.

In addition to lobbying and working with community agencies, clinical neuropsychologists fulfill the role of advocate in dealings with families, employers and co-workers, and school systems. Advocacy efforts begin when intervention is requested by either the brain-injured person or the other party. The clinical neuropsychologist initially intervenes by assessing the situation. Points of view are obtained from both sides. The clinical neuropsychologist also provides information about the consequences of the injury and any implications for the client's adjustment and behavior. In addition, the clinician serves as mediator. Mediation efforts are directed at helping each party avoid blaming, incorrect assumptions of intentionality, denial, and defensiveness. Each party is encouraged to discuss his or her perspective, goals, and willingness to contribute to problem resolution. Once agreement is reached, the clinical neuropsychologist monitors the situation to help assure that both parties are working to attain mutual goals as promised. If the agreed-upon solution is not successful, alternatives are discussed and the most promising alternative is selected for implementation. Newly emerging conflicts are dealt with proactively.

As an advocate in educational settings, clinical neuropsychologists intervene by teaching education professionals about the unique problems faced by students with head injury. Relationships between students with head injury, families, and school systems are often strained because school personnel typically lack experience in dealing with the problems of head-injured students. Furthermore, school systems have limited financial resources and may be unable to provide needed assistance. As a result, students with head injury may inappropriately receive services developed for persons with attention deficit disorder, mental retardation, congenital neurological disorders, and learning disabilities. Students with head injury may benefit from flexible classroom approaches such as extended deadlines for papers and exams. Because of slowness and handwriting problems they may do best by recording their test responses on audiotape and having these transcribed. Additionally, these students typically benefit more from classroom instruction when they are not hindered by note-taking, but rather are supplied with notes and outlines provided by the teacher.

Clinical neuropsychologists also are advocates in family issues. Characterological changes arising from traumatic brain injury frequently alienate immediate and extended family members (Lezak, 1978). Family members sometimes perceive clients as "difficult strangers." Relationships are especially strained by behavioral problems including aggression, substance abuse, and lack of empathy for others. Crises often occur during which communication between the client and others is either nonexistent or characterized by aggression. The clinical neuropsychologist's initial role as client advocate involves helping the family understand the consequences of the injury and their personal reactions to the injury. The clinical neuropsychologist must also act as an advocate for the family by helping the client understand how the family has been burdened by the injury. Advocacy for the client and family members is an essential, ongoing part of the family therapy process, which is described in greater detail in Chapter 16 in this book.

As noted previously, behavioral and intellectual problems also contribute to difficulty finding and maintaining employment. Employers and co-workers may perceive the client as unmotivated and incompetent. Ignorance and misperceptions about the effects of the injury as well as negative stereotypes about persons with disabilities also contribute to conflicts in the work setting. As with other types of advocacy, intervention begins with education regarding the effects of head injury and the establishment of a commitment on the part of the client, employer, and co-workers to work toward mutual goals. Through education, expressed motivation by the client, and negotiation, employers and co-workers usually develop greater empathy and demonstrate willingness to provide appropriate assistance to their colleague with brain injury.

SUMMARY AND CONCLUSIONS

Clinical neuropsychology is an evolving subspecialty of psychology and one of many disciplines providing services to persons with traumatic brain injury. Before the development of sophisticated radiographic assessment procedures, clinical neuropsychologists primarily served a diagnostic function. The neuropsychological evaluation became a valuable adjunct to the neurological examination for its ability to lateralize lesions, distinguish between static and progressive conditions, and differentially diagnose neurological and psychiatric conditions.

Increased survival rates for persons with brain injury also has influenced the practice of clinical neuropsychology. Traumatically brain-injured persons incur a variety of personality, behavioral, intellectual, cognitive, and psychomotor problems. Because of their specialized training, clinical neuropsychologists are frequently called upon to provide assessment, behavior management, and psychotherapy. Assessment has a special role in the context of community integration as the clinical neuropsychologist helps treatment team members understand the client's strengths and limitations, and any implications for daily living. Practical recommendations and treatment needs are of primary importance. Additionally, clinical neuropsychologists are often asked to help facilitate academic adjustment, enhance employability, and improve cognitive functioning.

To a great extent, clinical neuropsychologists in community rehabilitation settings recognize the value of involving families in treatment. Programs of family education and advocacy are often developed, along with family support groups. Assessment of family members' emotional status and coping abilities is often necessary given the prolonged stress of client disability. Family assessment skills, family therapy skills, and knowledge of family systems theory often prove invaluable.

The problems of community integration for persons with traumatic brain injury are serious and the number of those in need has increased significantly, but many communities still lack the diversity of necessary services. In response, clinical neuropsychologists now sometimes provide substance abuse assessment and counseling, advocacy, and case management to help alleviate gaps in the service delivery system. Given the relative scarcity of community rehabilitation services, clinical neuropsychologists who are flexible, adaptive, and sensitive to

the changing needs of clients and their families are likely to be most effective.

Presently, the implementation of community neuropsychological services is guided primarily by common sense and lessons learned in the process of limited experience. As time passes, experienced rehabilitation professionals representing other disciplines will become more available, adding to the number and diversity of rehabilitation services offered. As a consequence, neuropsychologists will become more specialized members of the rehabilitation team. Additionally, community services will become more efficacious as a greater knowledge base develops through research and accumulated experience.

REFERENCES

Acker, M.B. (1986). Relationships between test scores and everyday life functioning. In B.P. Uzzell & Y. Gross (Eds.), *Clinical neuropsychology of intervention* (pp. 85–118). Boston: Martinus Nijoff.

Beck, A.T. (1967). *Depression: Clinical, experimental, and theoretical aspects.* New York: Harper & Row.

Beck, A.T., Ward, C., Mendelson, M., Mock, J., & Erbaugh, J. (1961). An inventory for measuring depression. *Archives of General Psychiatry, 4,* 561–571.

Binder, L.M. (1986). Persisting symptoms after mild head injury: A review of the postconcussive syndrome. *Journal of Clinical and Experimental Neuropsychology, 8*(4), 323–346.

Brooks, N., Campsie, L., Symington, C., Beattie, A., & McKinlay, W. (1986). The five year outcome of severe blunt head injury: A relative's view. *Journal of Neurology, Neurosurgery, & Psychiatry, 49,* 764–770.

Brooks, N., McKinlay, W., Symington, C., Beattie, A., & Campsie, L. (1987). Return to work within the first seven years of severe head injury. *Brain Injury, 1*(1), 5–19.

Burke, W.H., Weselowski, M.D., & Guth, W.L. (1988). Comprehensive head injury rehabilitation: An outcome evaluation. *Brain Injury, 2,* 313–322.

Cahalan, D., & Cisin, I. (1968). American drinking practices: Summary of findings from a national probability sample: Extent of drinking by population subgroups. *Quarterly Journal of Studies on Alcohol, 29,* 130–151.

Chelune, G.J., & Moehle, K.A. (1986). Neuropsychological assessment and everyday functioning. In D. Wedding & A.M. Horton (Eds.), *The neuropsy-*

chology handbook: Behavioral and clinical perspectives (pp. 489–525). New York: Springer.

Costa, L. (1983). Clinical neuropsychology: A discipline in evolution. *Journal of Clinical Neuropsychology, 5,* 1–11.

Dahlstrom, W.G., Welsh, G.S., & Dahlstrom, L.E. (1972). *An MMPI handbook* (Vol. 1). Minneapolis: University of Minnesota Press.

Graham, J.R. (1987). *The MMPI: A practical guide* (2nd ed.). New York: Oxford University Press.

Halstead, W.C. (1947). *Brain and intelligence.* Chicago: University of Chicago Press.

Halstead, W.C., & Wepman, J.M. (1959). The Halstead-Wepman Aphasia Screening Test. *Journal of Speech and Hearing Disorders, 14,* 9–15.

Heaton, R.K., & Pendleton, M.G. (1981). Use of neuropsychological tests to predict adult patients' everyday functioning. *Journal of Consulting and Clinical Psychology, 49,* 807–821.

Jacobs, H.E. (1988). The Los Angeles Head Injury Survey: Procedures and initial findings. *Archives of Physical Medicine and Rehabilitation, 69,* 425–431.

Kane, R.L., Goldstein, G., & Parsons, O. (1989). A response to Mapou. *Journal of Clinical and Experimental Neuropsychology, 11,* 589–595.

Kreutzer, J.S. (1989, June). *Alcohol and drug use among TBI survivors.* Lecture presented at the 13th Annual Postgraduate Course on the Rehabilitation of the Brain Injured Adult and Child, Williamsburg, VA.

Kreutzer, J. S., & Harris, J. (1990). Model systems of treatment for alcohol abuse following traumatic brain injury. *Brain Injury, 4*(1), 1–5.

Kreutzer, J., Harris, J., & Doherty, K. (1989, August). *Substance abuse patterns before and after traumatic brain injury.* Paper presented at the 97th Annual Convention of the American Psychological Association, New Orleans, LA.

Kreutzer, J., Leininger, B., Doherty, K., & Waaland, P. (1987). *General Health and History Questionnaire.* Richmond, VA: Rehabilitation Research and Training Center on Severe Traumatic Brain Injury, Medical College of Virginia.

Langley, M.J., Lindsay, W.P., Lam, C.S., & Priddy, D.A. (in press). A comprehensive alcohol abuse treatment program for persons with traumatic brain injury. *Brain Injury.*

Leininger, B., Gramling, S., Farrell, A., Kreutzer, J., & Peck, E. (in press). Neuropsychological deficits in symptomatic minor head injury patients after concussion and mild concussion. *Journal of Neurology, Neurosurgery, and Psychiatry.*

Leininger, B., Kreutzer, J., & Hill, M. (1989, August). *Emotional functioning after minor and severe head injury.* Paper presented at the 97th Annual Convention of the American Psychological Association, New Orleans, LA.

Levin, H.S., Benton, A.L., & Grossman, R.G. (1982). *Neurobehavioral consequences of closed head injury.* New York: Oxford University Press.

Levin, H.S., Grossman, R.G., Rose, J.E., & Teasdale, G. (1979). Long-term neuropsychological outcome of closed head injury. *Journal of Neurosurgery, 50,* 412–422.

Lezak, M.D. (1978). Living with the characterologically altered brain-injured patient. *Journal of Clinical Psychiatry, 39,* 592–598.

Lezak, M.D. (1983). *Neuropsychological assessment* (2nd ed.). New York: Oxford University Press.

Lezak, M.D. (1987). Relationships between personality disorders, social disorders, social disturbances, and physical disability following traumatic brain injury. *Journal of Head Trauma Rehabilitation, 2*(1), 57–69.

Mapou, R.L. (1988). Testing to detect brain damage: An alternative to what may no longer be useful. *Journal of Clinical and Experimental Neuropsychology, 10,* 271–278.

Novack, T.A., Daniel, M.S., & Long, C.J. (1984).

Factors related to emotional adjustment following head injury. *International Journal of Clinical Neuropsychology, 6,* 139–142.

Reitan, R.M., & Davison, L.A. (1974). *Clinical neuropsychology: Current status and applications.* New York: Hemisphere.

Rimel, R., Giordani, B., Barth, J., & Jane, J. (1982). Moderate head injury: Completing the clinical spectrum of brain trauma. *Neurosurgery, 11*(3), 344–351.

Rosenthal, M., & Young, T. (1988). Effective family intervention after traumatic brain injury: Theory and practice. *Journal of Head Trauma Rehabilitation, 3*(4), 42–50.

Rourke, B.P. (1982). Central processing deficiencies in children: Toward a developmental neuropsychological model. *Journal of Clinical Neuropsychology, 4,* 1–18.

Selzer, M.L. (1971). The Michigan Alcohol Screening Test: The quest for a new diagnostic instrument. *American Journal of Psychiatry, 127,* 1653–1658.

Sparadeo, F.R., & Gill, D. (1989). Effects of prior alcohol use on head injury recovery. *Journal of Head Trauma Rehabilitation, 4*(1), 75–82.

Thomas, J.P. (1988). The evolution of model systems of care in traumatic brain injury. *Journal of Head Trauma Rehabilitation, 3*(4), 1–5.

Thomsen, I.V. (1984). Late outcome of severe blunt head trauma: A 10–15 year follow-up. *Journal of Neurology, Neurosurgery, and Psychiatry, 47,* 260–268.

Wehman, P., Kreutzer, J., Wood, W., Morton, M., & Sherron, P. (1988). Supported work model of competitive employment for persons with traumatic brain injury. *Rehabilitation Counseling Bulletin, 31,* 298–312.

Wehman, P., Kreutzer, J., West, M., Sherron, P., Diambra, J., Fry, R., Groah, C., Sale, P., & Killam, S. (1989). Employment outcomes of persons following traumatic brain injury: Preinjury, postinjury, and supported employment. *Brain Injury, 4*(3), 397–412.

Zung, B. (1970). Psychometric properties of the MAST and two briefer versions. *Journal of Studies on Alcohol, 40,* 845–850.

CHAPTER 5

Evaluation and Treatment of Communicative Skills

McKay Moore Sohlberg and Catherine A. Mateer

Individuals who survive head trauma with damage to the areas of the brain directly involved in speech and language function will exhibit the typical problems associated with the corresponding site of lesion. Particularly in the early stages following a head trauma, many persons will demonstrate marked disruption in speech and language abilities. There is not good agreement, however, regarding the incidence of specific speech and language disorders. As discussed by Schwartz-Cowley and Stephanik (1989), the reason for the confusion in the literature is twofold. First, many of the early studies examining communication disorders in persons with head injury failed to identify the time postinjury when communication data were gathered. The nature of impairment varies dependent upon the stage in the recovery process; thus, time postonset can be a confounding variable (see Groher, 1983, for a review of this problem). Second, confusion arises from inconsistencies and imprecision in the use of terminology. The nomenclature for communication deficits that are linguistic in nature (e.g., aphasia) as opposed to being a by-product of impaired cognitive processes (e.g., confused language secondary to attention or orientation deficits) has not been established.

In this chapter, studies pertaining to the incidence of aphasia in persons with head trauma are reviewed briefly. Aphasia is distinguished from communication impairments that appear to be more cognitively based. Given that extensive reviews of aphasia and dysarthria are available elsewhere, management of specific language

and motor speech deficits is not reviewed. The primary focus of this chapter is on the less understood and often overlooked impairment of communication so prevalent in persons with head injury, namely poor pragmatics or deficient use of language in a social context. A review of pragmatics is provided, as well as a discussion of current assessment and treatment techniques.

THE INCIDENCE OF APHASIA IN CLOSED HEAD INJURY

There is much discrepancy in the literature concerning the incidence of aphasia in closed head injury. A study by Heilman, Safran, and Geschwind (1971) examined the relationship between closed head injury and the presence of aphasia. The authors suggested aphasia to be a rare sequela of head injury and reported that only 13 of the 750 head-injured patients (1.7%) admitted to a city hospital over a 10-month period exhibited aphasia. A similar study (Constantinovici, Areni, Iliesciu, Debrota, & Gorgea, 1970) found only 34 closed head injury cases out of 1,544 (2.2%) to demonstrate aphasia. In contrast to the aforementioned two studies, an investigation by Levin, Grossman, and Kelly (1976) reported that nearly half of 50 patients studied had aphasic disturbances. Thompson (1975) conducted a long-term observation of closed head injury and, as did the Levin et al. study, reported that nearly half of 26 patients who had sustained closed head trauma exhibited symptoms of aphasia. Sarno (1980) found that

Portions of this chapter were adapted with permission from: Sohlberg, M.M., & Mateer, C.A. (1989). Language remediation. In *Introduction to cognitive rehabilitation: Theory and practice*. New York: Guilford Publications.

32% of patients admitted to a rehabilitation hospital with closed head injury over a 7-year period had frank aphasic disturbance.

Although the reported incidence of aphasia in closed head injury varies greatly, in general, it might be said that aphasia can be a sequela of closed head injury, but it is not nearly as prevalent as other cognitive disturbances such as memory and attention. It is difficult to compare available studies because of the differences in subject-selection criteria, as well as in the measures and definitions used to evaluate the presence of aphasia.

More interesting and relevant than the frequency of aphasia is a review of the types of aphasic disturbance that are most common following head injury. The most common type of language disturbance is anomic aphasia characterized by impairment in confrontation naming and specific word-retrieval processes (Heilman et al., 1971; Levin et al., 1976; Sarno, 1980; Thompson, 1975); these studies all cited the vulnerability of visual naming and word association in closed head injury.

Sarno (1980) identified a subgroup of persons with closed head injury that she labeled as having subclinical aphasia. These were persons without signs of aphasia in their conversational speech but who exhibited linguistic disturbances upon evaluation. The identification of aphasia depends heavily upon an examiner's particular definition of aphasia and his or her method of evaluating the disorder. Sarno reminds clinicians of the importance of understanding and treating the subclinical as well as clinical manifestations of verbal impairment. In order to accomplish this, however, it is important to investigate the underlying pathology and to discern what represents linguistic deficits of an aphasic nature and what might be manifestations of other contributing cognitive problems.

COGNITIVE VERSUS
LINGUISTIC IMPAIRMENT

Some researchers encourage the testing of "higher language functions" as a means of delineating the nature of verbal impairment after closed head injury. Such researchers warn clinicians that the administration of an aphasia battery is not sufficient for diagnosing and describing potential language impairments associated with closed head injury (e.g., Levin et al., 1976; Sarno, 1980; Thompson, 1975). Typical measures of high-level language include tests sensitive to abstract language such as descriptions of thematic pictures, synonyms, antonyms, and metaphors, as well as assessments of verbal power and speed such as word fluency. Language, however, cannot be easily separated from the gestalt of cognitive processing. One cannot separate perceptual processes from symbolic processes. Symbols or words have meaning beyond their linguistic function; they have meaning because of the way they subserve patterns of social interaction.

Halpern, Darley, and Brown (1973) indicated that an individual's language capabilities after closed head trauma may often be described as confused. Also, in a study looking at the major language and memory deficits in closed head injury, Groher (1977) administered the *Porch Index of Communicative Ability* (Porch, 1967) and the *Wechsler Memory Scale* (Wechsler, 1945) to persons with closed head injury at 1-month intervals for a duration of 4 months. Results suggested that clients initially suffered a reduction of both memory and language skills; after 4 months, expressive and receptive language abilities improved, although language remained confused (Groher, 1977).

Both Halpern et al. (1973) and Groher (1977) contend that there is a dichotomy between confused language skills and those that deserve the term aphasia. Aphasia is considered a reduced capacity to interpret and formulate language symbols, whereas confused language skills involve faulty short-term memory, mistaken reasoning, inappropriate behavior, poor understanding of the environment, and disorientation. Groher (1977) further contends that most persons with closed head injury initially manifest both aphasia and confused language skills and then gradually become less aphasic while still remaining confused. Groher's (1977) theory may be important in that it could account for some of the variability found in the literature. The nature of language impairments would depend upon when the individual was evaluated with respect to his or her injury. Many of the studies cited did not control for time post-trauma. Weinstein and Keller (1963) also support the theory that persons with head injury initially demonstrate aphasic disorders, but that these gradually resolve to a more confused-language profile.

Confusion produces a disorientation with regard to language as well as to time, place, and person. This suggests that assessment of orientation, memory, judgment, and reasoning will be important facets of a thorough language evaluation, as these are components that relate closely to confused language. In terms of remediation, communication disorders that are secondary to cognitive impairment will best be addressed by cognitive rehabilitation techniques focusing on the impaired processes (see Sohlberg & Mateer, 1989, for a review of cognitive rehabilitation principles).

A review of the literature specific to language and closed head injury establishes the notion that the language abilities of persons with closed head injury must be viewed in a broad context, beyond the purely linguistic realm (e.g., Milton, Prutting, & Binder, 1984; Prigatano, 1986). This chapter now turns to a discussion of pragmatics, which allows consideration of language in a much more comprehensive and holistic framework.

PRAGMATICS

Holland (1977) notes that most persons with certain classic types of aphasia communicate better than they talk. The converse might be said of individuals who have sustained head injury; these persons often appear to talk better than they communicate. The relatively spared verbal skills in the midst of decreased cognitive abilities and compromised psychosocial functioning frequently afford persons with head trauma with a poor ability to use language effectively in interpersonal situations. Prigatano (1986) described three nonaphasic language disturbances observed following significant craniocerebral trauma: problems of talkativeness, tangential verbalizations, and the use of peculiar phraseology.

Additionally, he reported that these disturbances greatly compromise the individual's ability to communicate effectively in both social and vocational settings and may result in significant social isolation or unemployment.

Many of the nonaphasic and high-level language disturbances are captured by a branch of speech/language pathology termed "pragmatics." Pragmatics might be considered the manner in which language is used within a social context. Some communication specialists view pragmatics as a distinct component of language, along with syntax and semantics (e.g., Bloom & Lahey, 1978). Others view pragmatics as an umbrella function comprising all other aspects of language behavior including phonology, syntax, and semantics (Bates, 1979). Despite one's particular definition or theoretical orientation, the issue of how language is used in naturalistic situations has received increasing attention (Milton, Prutting, & Binder, 1984; Prutting & Kirchner, 1983). In the authors' experience, pragmatic deficits are perhaps the most pervasive communication problems present in adults with acquired brain injury.

In this chapter, pragmatic behaviors refer to those behaviors that, if used inappropriately, or in some cases, if absent, would penalize the speaker in a conversational exchange. Milton, Prutting, and Binder (1984) described pragmatics as that component of communication that transcends language in terms of its isolated word meanings and grammatical structures. This crucial aspect of interaction, the ability to manage one's communication, needs to be an important part of every language assessment and, if appropriate, targeted in a treatment program.

ASSESSING PRAGMATIC FUNCTION

As noted earlier, Groher (1977) administered the *Porch Index of Communicative Ability* (Porch, 1967) to a series of persons with head injury to assess their communication deficits. He suggested that although this measurement might offer good indication of aphasic characteristics, it did not provide information about the presence of high-level language deficits or pragmatic problems. Similarly, Halpern et al. (1973) used the Minnesota Test for the Differential Diagnosis of Aphasia (Schuell, 1965) to examine the speech and language patterns in a group of persons with head injury, again concluding that the use of an aphasia battery is an incomplete measure of communication function. Aphasia batteries do not measure cognitive factors or pragmatic skills. A comprehensive evaluation of communication function in persons with head injury needs to consider the following three areas: speech/language abilities, cognitive capacity, and pragmatic functions.

Assessment Protocols

Pragmatics is a very young area of speech/language pathology and has only been addressed clinically since 1983. As such, assessment and treatment instruments are not yet well established. However, there are some pragmatic assessment protocols available that may be easily adapted to persons with head injury. Regardless of the specific tool used to gather information on pragmatic functioning, the following ingredients need to be present for assessment of communication ability:

1. The clinician must observe the individual with head injury in a natural communication situation in which he or she is conversing with a discourse partner.
2. The clinician needs to have a list or taxonomy of pragmatic behaviors upon which to judge performance.
3. A method for translating information gleaned via observation into treatment goals and objectives should be established.

Pragmatic Protocol

Prutting and Kirchner (1983) developed an assessment protocol to evaluate pragmatics in school age and adult clients. The Pragmatic Protocol provides an extensive taxonomy of pragmatic abilities (see Appendix A at the end of this chapter for a list and description of the taxonomy of pragmatic behaviors). There are 32 pragmatic behaviors assessed that cut across the spectrum of our communication system (phonology, syn-

tax, semantics, and pragmatics). The behaviors are organized according to the "speech act" theoretical framework (Austin, 1962; Searle, 1969), which includes four speech act categories: the utterance act, the propositional act, the perlocutionary act, and the illocutionary act. The utterance act includes verbal, nonverbal, and paralinguistic behaviors related to how a message is presented. There are 13 behaviors within this category. The second area, the propositional act, refers to the linguistic meaning of the sentence. The illocutionary act refers to the speaker's intention, whereas the perlocutionary act relates to the effects of the speaker on the listener. These last two areas regulate the discourse between speaker and listener and contain 15 pragmatic items.

The Pragmatic Protocol is designed to be sensitive to aspects of discourse and to facilitate a clinician's understanding of how an individual uses language. The clinician's task is to observe the client in a conversation and to judge the appropriateness or inappropriateness of each pragmatic behavior that the client exhibits. When judging the appropriateness of communication, the clinician is to decide whether the behavior would be socially maladaptive. The Pragmatic Protocol is used for screening purposes to identify problem areas. A more in-depth analysis of the topography of various behaviors may be performed when designing treatment programs.

Milton, Prutting, and Binder (1984) administered a standard aphasia battery as well as the Pragmatic Protocol to assess pragmatic skills in five adults with head injury and five noninjured adults matched for age, sex, and education level. Each of the subjects with head injury had suffered acceleration/deceleration closed head injuries and all were greater than 6 months postinjury (range, 6–112 months; mean, 34 months). The Pragmatic Protocol was employed while observing the subjects engaged in 15 minutes of videotaped spontaneous conversation. The subjects were videotaped in unstructured discourse with a familiar conversation partner. Results suggested that although all the subjects with head injury scored above the aphasia cut-off criteria, they differed from the control group on the Pragmatic

Protocol, which assessed a range of behaviors present in normal discourse. The pattern of distribution for percentage of inappropriate pragmatic behaviors for each speech act category was obtained. The highest proportion of inappropriate pragmatic behaviors exhibited by the adults with head injury was in the illocutionary and perlocutionary acts. Milton et al. suggested that communication breakdown occurs most frequently in the ability of persons with head injury to regulate discourse. The types of behaviors that were observed to be the most problematic included: prosody, topic selection (e.g., restricted range of topics), topic maintenance (e.g., topic change occurred following minimal speaking turns), turn-taking initiation, turn-taking pause time, turn-taking contingency (e.g., awkward phrasing of new information added to the ongoing exchange), and quantity/conciseness (e.g., redundant information or excess detail). The control group was judged appropriate in almost all pragmatic behaviors with the exception of one speaker who showed inappropriate fluency and was judged as speaking too rapidly, and a second subject who was marked down for topic initiation. Milton et al. concluded that the Pragmatic Protocol was useful in identifying strengths and weaknesses in conversational competence in adults with head injury. They also suggested that it provided a focus of treatment for pragmatic deficits.

Communication Performance Scale

Ehrlich and Sipes (1985) developed a behavioral rating scale, the Communication Performance Scale, to assess pragmatic skills in clients with head injury. The scale was adapted from the Pragmatic Protocol just described. As shown in Appendix B at the end of this chapter, it contains 13 pragmatic behaviors, each of which is rated on a one-to-five interval scale. Ehrlich and Sipes included those behaviors most commonly disrupted in persons with head injury. The scale was intended to assist in the clinical judgment of clients' progress following communication intervention and to provide empirical documentation of change. Clinical implementation of the scale is described in the following section.

TREATMENT OF PRAGMATIC DEFICITS

Despite being at a rather exploratory phase in the implementation of pragmatic remediation techniques, it is important for clinicians to adopt the pioneer spirit and to implement trial remediation programs. The inability to communicate effectively may be the barrier that prevents an individual from being hired for a job or from fully reintegrating into society.

Intervention Utilizing a Group Context

Therapeutic treatment of pragmatics can be implemented in a number of ways using the group therapy format.

Group Model of Intervention

Ehrlich and Sipes (1985) present a model of group intervention designed to increase the pragmatic abilities of persons with head trauma. A communication group comprising therapists and clients with head injury provides the therapy setting. Therapists facilitate the generation of group communication goals. Clients receive feedback on the effectiveness of observed communication including positive social reinforcement to encourage appropriate communication as well as feedback regarding problem behaviors. A modular format is utilized within the group wherein each module includes the particular pragmatic behaviors to be addressed in treatment. The following four modules are addressed within this group format:

1. Nonverbal communication: vocal inflection, facial expression, eye gaze, body posture, and gestures
2. Communication in context: topic maintenance, initiation and response during conversation, and awareness of social context
3. Message repair: awareness of communication breakdown, consideration of listener need, and clarification strategies
4. Cohesiveness of narrative: sequencing of information and comprehension and production of temporal and spatial concepts

Therapists introduce each module by describing and demonstrating the target behaviors to be learned. Role play initially between the therapists and then between clients is utilized to illustrate appropriate and inappropriate examples. Role plays are videotaped and reviewed by the group. Clients are helped to look at specific behaviors that increase communication success and failure. Ways to modify communication behavior are also discussed. Ehrlich and Sipes (1985) suggest the following procedural outline:

1. Introduction of the module—the therapist defines target behaviors and provides videotaped role-play samples modeling appropriate and inappropriate behaviors.
2. Client role-play exercises—the clients perform role plays of assigned social situations that are videotaped. The group reviews the role play and discusses relevant aspects of communication, including ways to modify and improve observed communication behaviors.

Ehrlich and Sipes (1985) evaluated the success of the above intervention program by weekly assessments using the Communication Performance Scale. Comparison of pre- and posttreatment rating scales for six subjects indicated a significant overall improvement. As shown in Figure 5.1, the most change was evident in topic maintenance, initiation, syntax, cohesiveness, and repair. Less significant improvements were observed in intelligibility, listening, and lexical selection. Little or no changes were evident for body posture, interruptions, prosody, facial expression, and variety of language use. Ehrlich and Sipes concluded that the group format provided a successful therapy milieu to train pragmatic skills.

Individual Focus with Group Therapy

The authors' own clinical experience is consistent with the aforementioned findings. In their day-treatment postacute head injury rehabilitation setting, group therapy targeting pragmatic skills has been successfully completed with over 50 clients. In this setting, however, a more individualized approach has been adopted that allows for the targeting of particular pragmatic behaviors that are deficient in individual clients.

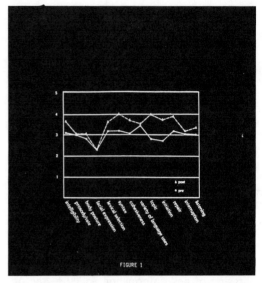

Figure 5.1. Clients' mean pre- and posttreatment scores for each scale item on the Communication Performance Scale. Endpoint descriptors of each scale are listed in Appendix B. (From Ehrlich, J., & Sipes, A. [1985]. Group treatment of communication skills for head trauma patients. *Cognitive Rehabilitation, 3,* 32–37; reprinted with permission.)

Initially, clients are videotaped in conversation with the therapist. The tapes are reviewed in group, and pragmatic goals and objectives are identified for each client. Two therapists independently rate each client on the Pragmatic Protocol (Prutting & Kirchner, 1983), which serves as a baseline measure of communication ability. Different clients have different goals and all are encouraged to assist each other in working on the specific communication objectives. Role-play activities are carried out during group therapy targeting relevant pragmatic skills.

It is felt that the key to success in working on restricted pragmatic abilities is to provide remediation across a broad range of naturalistic communication environments. Thus, it is important that clients receive feedback, not only during group therapy, but in individual therapy sessions and in settings outside the clinic as well. Other therapists working with the client, as well as those individuals within the home environment, receive descriptions of the communication goals and suggestions for how to provide appropriate feedback to the person with head injury.

Periodically, videotapes using the same therapist as a communication partner are recorded and again rated using the Pragmatic Protocol (Prutting & Kirchner, 1983). The group provides peer feedback regarding improvements and residual problems. Table 5.1 summarizes the steps of this approach to the remediation of pragmatic deficits.

Remarks

The treatment of pragmatic deficits requires structured feedback regarding communication performance across a wide variety of environments. Clients need intensive opportunities to practice appropriate behaviors and to modify existing problem areas, as well as to establish new, more effective modes of communication. Appropriate treatment goals are an extension of a thorough analysis of communication in naturalistic social situations. Peer input from a group therapy environment can provide a powerful clinical tool for assisting clients in understanding problem areas and for offering methods to improve their communication. Similarly, videotapes and role-play exercises offer a means to allow clients to recognize and practice target behaviors.

Table 5.1. Remediation of pragmatic deficits in a group format

1. Ten-minute conversation between client and therapist is videotaped.
2. Two therapists independently rate videotape samples using an appropriate pragmatic observational protocol. The most prominent areas of concern are identified.
3. Videotapes are reviewed in group, and individual goals and objectives are assigned.
4. Group members, adjunct therapists, and individuals in the home environment receive information on client communication goals and ways to give constructive feedback.
5. Role-play exercises targeting specific communication goals are conducted in regular group therapy sessions.
6. Periodic videotape samples are recorded, rated, and discussed in group. Progress is discussed.
7. Progress is monitored in settings outside the clinic by individual reports elicited from relevant persons.

Additional Group Activities

Our society has experienced a revolution and the ability to express oneself openly and clearly has become a valued skill. There are thus many resources and formats that address mechanisms for improving communication ability that can be adapted for communication group therapy. In addition to role-play exercises targeting individual pragmatic behaviors, there are a variety of communication activities to address specific components of communication. These include activities to increase: the awareness of the effects of different communication styles on the listener, the initiation of conversation in social settings, language specificity or the ability to communicate more concisely, the ability to read nonverbal cues, and so forth. Examples of group exercises follow.

The reader is encouraged to review the activities with any eye to determining which of the pragmatic behaviors in the Communication Performance Scale (Ehrlich & Sipes, 1985; see Appendix B) would be addressed in each of the exercises. Other activities can be designed or adapted from a variety of sources including "party game" descriptions and activities from seminars in how to improve communication.

Hat Communication Activity Group communication activity where people respond to each other in a specified style of communication.

Goals Increase awareness of the effects of different types of communication styles and behaviors.

Materials Communication hats. These are paper hats (the sort a fast-food service worker wears) with different directions written on the outside. Sample directions for five hats include: "Talk down to me," "Ignore me," "Interrupt me," "Compliment me," and "Ask me questions about myself."

Preparation Make the communication hats.

Procedure The therapist hands out the paper communication hats and instructs participants to put them on without looking at them. Time is given for everyone to review the others' hats. A topic is introduced, and the group members begin talking and responding to each other in the manner indicated on each individual's hat. After each topic, people try and guess what their hat said. The therapist directs discussion about how individuals felt when people responded to them in the specified manner. The group can trade hats and repeat the activity. The activity can be broken down and done in pairs. The rest of the group watches while one communication pair role plays a discussion and responds to each other according to the manner indicated on the hat. The group can make up a hat message for the group leader so that he or she can participate as well.

Party Activity Individuals assume hypothetical identities and role play a party situation trying to meet everyone in the room.

Goals Increase initiation of conversation in social settings; increase conversational skills.

Materials Identity cards listing hypothetical name, age, occupation, and family situation (e.g., marriage status/children) for each member in the group.

Preparation Make the identity cards.

Procedure Participants receive the identity cards. Everyone then role plays being at a party and introducing him or herself. Individuals may embellish on their life situation and provide additional information other than that on the card. At the end of the designated time, the group tries to recall everyone's identity. The group generates a discussion on social skills and initiating conversation, and might review what was hard or easy about the activity. A variation for a higher level group involves having participants write identities for each other (including the group leader).

Verbal Drawing Task Give/receive directions for drawing a multishaped form.

Goals Improve language specificity and comprehension of verbal commands by targeting the ability to follow and to give accurate directions.

Materials Three pieces of blank paper per person and two colored pens per person.

Preparation None.

Procedure Divide participants in pairs. Instruct one participant in each pair to make a drawing, involving three different kinds of shapes (e.g., rectangle, triangle, square) and two colors. Do not let the other person in the pair see the drawing. The participant who drew the picture gives instructions to the partner so that he or she can reproduce the drawing without seeing it. Participants then compare drawings and see if/where communication and/or direction following broke down. The pairs then switch roles. The person who received directions now gives directions to the other person. The therapist can then lead a discussion about accuracy of communication. He or she might ask participants which role they found more difficult and generate a discussion surrounding the answers. Tasks can be modified to increase or decrease the difficulty by changing the constraints on the drawing task or, if necessary, providing the models to be drawn.

Extemporaneous Speeches Participants present extemporaneous speeches to the group.

Goals Increase verbal expression skills, language specificity, and topic maintenance.

Materials None.

Preparation None.

Procedure The therapist helps participants generate a master list of speech topics on the board. Each person chooses a topic and has four (or more) minutes to prepare a minimum 2-minute speech. After each speech, the group offers information concerning strengths and weaknesses (e.g., "need better eye contact"). To make the task easier, the therapist can present a speech format that each participant should follow. For example, the therapist may write on the board: "1) Introduce topic. 2) Give information about topic. 3) Summarize your information and then give examples of short speeches following this structure."

Final Remarks The above communication exercises provide participants with opportunities to practice target communication skills. A few general group therapy principles serve to enhance their effectiveness. First of all, each exercise should be introduced by clearly outlining the goals of the activities. Closure of the activity should include repetition of the purpose of the activity. This helps to increase awareness of communication behaviors and styles and to reinforce the rationale for group participation. Second, mechanisms for generalization of gains in communication skills to settings outside the group therapy environment should be actively programmed. This might include extending communication training to more naturalistic settings such as community outings; the residence; and occupational, speech/language, and therapeutic recreation therapy sessions. Providing participants who are able with a structure for self-monitoring target communication behaviors (e.g., recording the number of times conversation is initiated with family members or recording the number of questions asked about other people's lives as a means of decreasing egocentricity in conversation) offers another generalization technique. Third, in settings where the same clients participate on a consistent basis, activities such as those described may be implemented several times to look at improvements. Difficulties with particular aspects of communication tasks can be documented and targeted on subsequent occasions.

Individual Communication Therapy

Therapeutic treatment of pragmatics can be carried out in individual sessions as well as in a group therapy format. The principles and videotape/role-play activities described earlier are applicable to this therapy format. An important tenet is that because most communication occurs in a dyadic interaction, deficits need to be treated in this context. In the case of individual therapy sessions, the therapist (usually a speech language pathologist) would play the role of a communication partner.

Pragmatic therapy involves three basic phases: 1) awareness training, 2) practice of target behaviors, and 3) training for generalization and maintenance. Initially, it is critical for the participant to be made aware of communication deficits. This is best accomplished via videotapes of conversational exchanges. Participants can be shown areas of difficulty by having them count frequency of target behaviors (positive or negative) while watching the videotape. For example, a common communication deficit in persons with head injury is egocentricity in speech. A client with this problem might be instructed to count the number of times he or she asks of a partner a question about his or her thoughts or interests.

Once a client has a good understanding of his or her deficits, exercises providing practice in skill areas can be implemented. For the most part, these should involve a dyadic exchange between therapist and participant. Protocols can be developed to document therapy progress. The collection of quantitative and qualitative data provides critical information to guide the continuation, modification, or cessation of therapy exercises. Examples of therapy protocols developed by Sprunk-Berlin and Metzelaar of Good Samaritan Hospital's Center for Cognitive Rehabilitation, Puyallup, Washington, that target different communication behaviors are presented in Figures 5.2 and 5.3.

The scoresheets shown in Figures 5.2 and 5.3 are utilized in conjunction with topic cards. Together, the participant and therapist choose a topic card. The therapist reminds the participant of his or her target communication goal. They engage in a dialogue on the chosen topic, and the therapist records relevant data during the conversation. Performance is reviewed with feedback from the therapist and a new topic is then chosen. The task protocols provide a means for documenting performance. In the protocol shown in Figures 5.3, where sample data have been recorded, the sequence of utterances is documented by numbering each consecutive statement that is produced. Thus, information on performance for both communication partners is recorded. This permits the examination of the sequence and contingent nature of conversational exchanges accounting for the dynamic nature of communication.

The importance of addressing generalization of target communication behaviors to environments beyond the therapeutic setting has already been emphasized in the context of group therapy. It is perhaps even more critical in individual therapy where there are fewer components common with more naturalistic settings. Again, providing therapy across a wide variety of settings and communication partners is important for encouraging generalization. Collection

Participant _____   Therapist _____

Date	Topic	Length of conversation (# of minutes)	Number of noncontingent statements (i.e., topic not maintained)	Number of interruptions	Number of questions/statements focusing on listener's thoughts or interests	Participant impressions	Therapist comments

Figure 5.2. Sample therapy protocol for collecting data on performance in a communication exercise emphasizing topic maintenance. Other communication parameters (e.g., duration of eye contact, appropriate facial expression) might be substituted depending on with which pragmatic behaviors an individual client required intervention. (Developed by H. Sprunk-Berlin & K. Metzelear, Good Samaritan Hospital's Center for Cognitive Rehabilitation, Puyallup, WA; reprinted with permission.)

Participant: JIM | Therapist: SUE

Date	Topic	Initiate new topic	Contingent remark to partner's comments	Contingent remark to self's comments	Question to partner	Initiate new topic	Contingent remark to partner's comments	Contingent remarks to self's comments	Question to partner	Therapist comments
11/1	Cars	5	2	3 6 8			7		1	Very egocentric, got off topic
11/3	School		3	4 5 6 7	1		2			egocentric, only asked the initial question
11/7	Politics		2	3 4 5	6		7		1	some improvement, asked an additional question
11/8	Jobs		4	5 6 7	1 8		2 9		3	much better. There was a good exchange between us.
11/10	Holiday		2 8	3	4 9		5 10	6	1 7	Continues to do well. Showing more interest in others.
11/14	Houses		3 6 9	10	1 6		2 7		8	Good exchange with comments. Not a need to always question.
11/16	Sports		2 7 10		3 8		4 9	5	1 6	Can see big changes! Good job!
11/18	Travel		3 7		1 4 8		2 6 9		6	Very smooth conversation!

Figure 5.3. Therapy protocol with sample data. This client exhibits particular difficulty with egocentric speech. Therapy is focusing on teaching him to acknowledge his communication partner's utterances and to ask questions of communication partner. Numbers refer to the order and classification of each utterance in the two-person exchange. (Developed by H. Sprunk-Berlin & K. Metzelear, Good Samaritan Hospital's Center for Cognitive Rehabilitation, Puyallup, WA; reprinted with permission.)

of quantitative and qualitative descriptions of performance in those settings is also essential for directing therapy efforts.

SUMMARY

Persons who have sustained head injuries may present with a variety of communication disorders. Although classic aphasias, apraxias, and dysarthrias are possible sequelae of head trauma, these do not represent the most prominent communication problems. When clients exhibit corresponding symptomatology of focal language or speech problems, intervention designed for these impairments should be implemented.

The greatest communication concern of persons with head injury relates to how language is used as a social tool. Pragmatics, a relatively new branch of speech/language pathology, provides a focus for intervention of communication deficits. Pragmatics refers to how meaning is communicated between people, and by definition depends upon the exchange between speaker and listener. Persons with head injury often have difficulty with pragmatic behaviors such as appropriate topic selection and maintenance and turn taking in conversation.

Assessment of pragmatic abilities may be completed by observing clients in conversation and rating communication performance on a variety of pragmatic behaviors. The essential components for evaluating pragmatic abilities include actually observing the clients in a communication exchange and having a method or checklist for rating a full range of pragmatic abilities.

Treatment of pragmatic deficits also needs to be conducted within the context of natural communication. Group therapy utilizing videotaped communication samples to establish communication objectives and specific role-play exercises to practice appropriate pragmatic skills offers a valuable clinical tool in this area. A variety of additional communication activities that emphasize selected components of communication can also be utilized. Therapy directed at improving pragmatic behaviors can also be conducted within an individual therapy context. Such therapy requires initial training to increase a client's awareness of deficits. This training phase would be followed by practice sessions using topic cards and data collection protocols. Regardless of whether therapy is conducted in a group or an individual therapy context, remediation of pragmatic deficits must extend beyond the clinical environment and include monitoring and feedback in a variety of natural communication settings.

REFERENCES

Austin, J. (1962). *How to do things with words.* Cambridge: Harvard University Press.

Bates, E. (1979). *The emergence of symbols.* New York: Academic Press.

Bloom, L., & Lahey, M. (1978). *Language development and language disorders.* New York: John Wiley & Sons.

Constantinovici, A., Arseni, C., Iliesciu, A., Debrota, L., & Gorgea, A. (1970). Considerations on post traumatic aphasia in peacetime. *Psychiatric Neurolo-Neurochir, 73*, 105–115.

Darley, F.L., Aronson, A.E., & Brown, J.R. (1975). *Motor speech disorders.* Philadelphia: W.B. Saunders.

Ehrlich, J., & Sipes, A. (1985). Group treatment of communication skills for head trauma patients. *Cognitive Rehabilitation, 3*, 32–37.

Groher, M. (1977). Language and memory disorders following closed head trauma. *Journal of Speech and Hearing Research, 20*, 212–223.

Groher, M. (1983). Communication disorders. In M. Rosenthal, E.R. Griffith, M.R. Bond, & J.D. Miller (Eds.), *Rehabilitation of the head injured adult.* Philadelphia: F.A. Davis.

Halpern, H., Darley, F., & Brown, J.R. (1973). Differential language and neurologic characteristics in cerebral involvement. *Journal of Speech and Hearing Disorders, 38*, 162–173.

Heilman, K., Safran, A., & Geschwind, N. (1971). Closed head trauma and aphasia. *Journal of Neurology, Neurosurgery, and Psychiatry, 34*, 265–269.

Levin, H., Grossman, R., & Kelly, P. (1976). Aphasia disorder in patients with closed head injury. *Journal of Neurology, Neurosurgery, and Psychiatry, 39*, 1062–1070.

Milton, S.B., Prutting, C.A., & Binder, G. (1984). Appraisal of communicative competence in head injured adults. In R.H. Brookshire (Ed.), *Proceedings from the Clinical Aphasiology Con-*

ference (pp. 114–123). Minneapolis: BRK Publishers.

Porch, B.E. (1967). *Porch Index of Communicative Ability.* Palo Alto, CA: Consulting Psychologists Press.

Prigatano, G. (1986). *Neuropsychological rehabilitation after brain injury.* Baltimore: Johns Hopkins University Press.

Prutting, C., & Kirchner, D. (1983). Applied pragmatics. In T. Gallagher & C. Prutting (Eds.), *Pragmatic assessment and intervention issues in language.* San Diego: College-Hill Press.

Sarno, M.T. (1980). The nature of verbal impairment after closed head injury. *Journal of Nervous and Mental Disease, 168,* 685–692.

Schuell, N.M. (1965). *Differential diagnosis of aphasia with the Minnesota Test.* Minneapolis: University of Minnesota Press.

Schwartz-Cowley, R., & Stephanik, M.J. (1989). Communication disorders and treatment in the acute trauma center setting. *Topics in Language Disorders, 9*(2), 1–14.

Searle, J. (1969). *Speech acts: An essay in the philosophy of language.* Baltimore: University Park Press.

Sohlberg, M.M., & Mateer, C.A. (1989). *Introduction to cognitive rehabilitation: Theory and practice.* New York: Guilford Publication.

Thompson, I.V. (1975). Evaluation and outcoming of aphasia in patients with severe closed head trauma. *Journal of Neurology, Neurosurgery, and Psychiatry, 38,* 713–718.

Tompkins, C., & Mateer, C. (1985). Right hemisphere appreciation of prosodic and linguistic indications or implicit attitude. *Brain & Language, 24,* 185–203.

Wapner, W., Hamby, S., & Garner, H. (1981). The role of the right hemisphere in the apprehension of complex linguistic materials. *Brain and Language, 14,* 15–33.

Wechsler, D. (1945). A standardized memory scale for clinical use. *Journal of Psychology, 19,* 87–95.

Weinstein, D., & Keller, W. (1963). Linguistic patterns of misnaming in brain injury. *Neuropsychologia, 1,* 79–90.

Pool of Pragmatic Behaviors

Taxonomy	Modality	Description and Coding
UTTERANCE ACT	Verbal/Paralinguistic	Trappings by which the act is accomplished.
1. Intelligibility		Extent to which the message is understood.
2. Vocal intensity		Loudness or softness of the message.
3. Voice quality		Resonance and/or laryngeal characteristics of the vocal tract.
4. Prosody		Intonation and stress patterns of the message; variations of loudness, pitch, and duration.
5. Fluency		Smoothness, consistency, and rate of the message.
6. Physical proximity	Nonverbal	Distance from which speaker and listener sit or stand from one another.
7. Physical contacts		Number of times and placement of contacts between speaker and listener.
8. Body posture		Forward lean is when the speaker or listener moves away from a 90-degree angle toward other person; recline is when one party slouches down from waist to head and moves away from the partner; side-to-side is when a person moves to the right or left.
9. Foot/leg movements		Any movement of foot/leg.
10. Hand/arm movements		Any movement with hand/arm (touching or moving an object or touching part of the body or clothing).
11. Gestures		Any movements that support, complement, or replace verbal behavior.
12. Facial expression		Positive expression is when the corners of the mouth are turned upward; negative is downward turn; neutral expression is when face is in a resting position.
13. Eye gaze		When one looks directly at the other's facial region; mutual gaze is when both members of the dyad look at each other.
PROPOSITIONAL ACT	Verbal	Linguistic dimensions of the meaning of the sentence.
1. Lexical selection/use A. Specificity/accuracy		Lexical items of best fit considering the context.
2. Specifying relationships between words A. Word order		Grammatical word order for conveying message.
B. Given and new information		Given information is that information already known to the listener; new in-

APPENDIX A (*continued*)

Taxonomy	Modality	Description and Coding
		formation is information not already known to the listener.
a. Pronominalization		Pronouns permit the listener to identify the referent and is one of the devices used to mark givenness.
b. Ellipses		Given information may be deleted.
c. Emphatic stress		New information may be marked by stressing various items.
d. Indefinite/ definite article		If new information is signaled, the indefinite article is used; if old information, then the definite article is used.
e. Initialization		Given information is stated prior to new information.
3. Stylistic variations A. Varying of communicative style	Verbal, paralinguistic, nonverbal	Adaptations used by the speaker under various dyadic conditions (e.g., polite forms, different syntax, vocal quality changes).
ILLOCUTIONARY AND PERLOCUTIONARY ACTS	Verbal	Illocutionary (intentions of the speaker) and perlocutionary (effects on the listener).
1. Speech act pair analysis		Ability to take both speaker and listener role appropriate to the context. Directive/compliance—personal need, imperatives, embedded imperatives, permissions, directives, questions directives, hints. Query/ response—requests for confirmation, neutral requests for repetition, requests for specific constituent repetition. Request/response—direct requests, indirect requests, inferred requests, request for clarification, acknowledgment of the request, perform the desired action. Comment/ acknowledgment—descriptions of ongoing activities in immediate subsequent activity, of state or condition of objects, persons; naming; acknowledgments that are positive, negative, expletive, indicative.
2. Variety of speech acts		Variety of speech acts or what one can do with language such as: comment, assert, request, promise, and so forth.
A. Topic a. Selection		Selection of a topic appropriate to the context.
b. Introduction		Introduction of a new topic in the discourse.

(*continued*)

APPENDIX A (*continued*)

Taxonomy	Modality	Description and Coding
c. Maintenance		Maintenance of a topic across the discourse.
B. Turn taking		Smooth interchanges between speaker and listener.
a. Initiation		Initiation of speech acts.
b. Response		Responding as a listener to speech acts.
c. Repair/ revision		Ability to repair a conversation when a breakdown occurs and the ability to ask for a repair when misunderstanding, ambiguity, and so forth have occurred.
d. Pause time		When pause time is excessive or too short between words or in response to a question or between sentences.
e. Interruption/ overlap		Interruptions between speaker and listener; overlap is when two people talk at the same time.
f. Feedback to speaker		Verbal behavior to give the speaker feedback such as "yeah," "really"; nonverbal behavior such as head nods up and down can be positive; side-to-side nods can express negative effect or disbelief.
g. Adjacency		Utterances that occur immediately after the partner's utterance.
h. Contingency		Utterances that share the same topic with the preceding utterance and that add information to the prior communicative act.
i. Quantity/ conciseness		Contribution should be as informative as required, but not too informative.

From Prutting, C., & Kirchner, D. (1983). Applied pragmatics. In T. Gallagher & L. Prutting (Eds.), *Pragmatic assessment and intervention issues in language* (pp. 32–41). San Diego: College-Hill Press; reprinted with permission.

Pragmatic Behaviors from the Communication Performance Scale

1. INTELLIGIBILITY		
Difficult to understand; requires repetition	1 2 3 4 5	Always understandable
2. PROSODY/RATE		
Choppy rhythm, uneven; too fast or slow	1 2 3 4 5	Appropriate stress patterns
3. BODY POSTURE		
Away from others; limited gestures	1 2 3 4 5	Body oriented toward others; appropriate gestures
4. FACIAL EXPRESSION		
Limited affect and eye gaze	1 2 3 4 5	Shows emotions and appropriate eye gaze
5. LEXICAL SELECTION		
Limited word selection; ambiguous words	1 2 3 4 5	Good variety of words; clear referents
6. SYNTAX		
Ungrammatical; uses only short phrases	1 2 3 4 5	Uses mature sentence patterns, phrases, clauses and conjunctions
7. COHESIVENESS		
Random, diffuse, and disjointed verbal style	1 2 3 4 5	Planned, sequential expression of ideas; concise
8. VARIETY OF LANGUAGE USES		
Limited use of language; stereotypical language	1 2 3 4 5	Uses language to express feelings, share information, social interaction
9. TOPIC		
Abrupt shift of topic; perseveration	1 2 3 4 5	Can appropriately introduce, maintain, and change topic
10. INITIATION OF CONVERSATION		
Limited initiation of talk; restricted response to conversation	1 2 3 4 5	Freely initiates and responds to conversational leads
11. REPAIR		
Inflexible; unable to change message when communication failure occurs	1 2 3 4 5	Able to revise message to facilitate listener comprehension; flexible
12. INTERRUPTION		
Frequently interrupts others	1 2 3 4 5	Appropriate interruption; good conversation flow
13. LISTENING		
Limited listening; listener shows restricted reaction to speaker	1 2 3 4 5	Attends well; listener provides verbal and nonverbal feedback to speaker

From Ehrlich, J., & Sipesk, A. (1985). Group treatment of communication skills for head trauma patients. *Cognitive Rehabilitation, 13,* 32–37; reprinted with permission.

CHAPTER 6

An Experimental Comparison of Neuropsychological Rehabilitation

Ronald M. Ruff and Christine A. Baser

NEED FOR RESEARCH IN REHABILITATION

In this chapter, the field of neuropsychology is used as an example for "why," "what," and "how" research is of value for rehabilitation. However, from a research perspective most issues addressed herein can be generalized to other disciplines. In the final analysis, the goal is to achieve an orchestration between all the disciplines involved in rehabilitation.

Why Do Research?

The most fundamental reason for conducting experimental research in the field of rehabilitation is to facilitate the outcome of the client. The therapeutic services rendered should be based as much as possible on scientifically proven methods. Therefore, it is not only the experience per se of a seasoned clinician that is valuable, but rather it is the juxtaposition of such experience with empirically proven techniques that yields the most promising outcome.

In an experimental framework, postulated treatment expectations are subjected to the qualifications in order to falsify or verify these expectations. On this basis, valuable modifications can be systematically achieved. In other words, if the treatments are not subjected to this process, then clinicians are forced to select treatments based on mere tradition or intuition. It is simply

no longer feasible to rely only on trial-and-error procedures, doing whatever one may think works, allowing generations of newcomers without experience to continue to make the same type of mistakes. It is, therefore, the role of the rehabilitation team to delineate what works and what does not work, with what type of client.

The rehabilitation field is predominantly staffed with clinicians who frequently are not involved in the collection of empirical data. There are many reasons for this, among them a lack of education, confidence, or most often a hectic schedule that allows for little or no time to integrate empirical science and clinical practice. In part, the health care administrators are at fault for not giving their staff an appropriate amount of time for research and the advancement of systematic study of clinical phenomena. Such a dichotomization of research and practice is surely short sighted and remains a challenging chasm to be bridged by the committed professional.

Every clinician documents the progress of his or her client. The more accurate and detailed this documentation is, the more reliably subtle changes can be quantified. For example, if an individual with head injury is participating in treatment and is exerting effort and energy toward reaching a certain goal, it is important to establish whether such a goal has been reached. Frequently such goals must be stated within small increments such as a 5%–10% gain over

This study was supported by a grant provided by the Robert Wood Johnson Foundation (09056) to Ronald M. Ruff, Ph.D. Portions of this material previously appeared in Neuropsychological rehabilitation: An experimental study with head injured patients by R.M. Ruff, C.A. Baser, J.W. Johnston, L.F. Marshall, S.K. Klauber, M.R. Klauber, and M. Minteer, 1989, *Journal of Head Trauma Rehabilitation*, *4*, pp. 20–36. Copyright 1989 by Aspen Publications. Reprinted by permission.

baseline. Therefore a quantifiable system needs to be developed to capture such changes in a reliable fashion. This allows for adequate goal setting, and provides an incentive to motivate the client. Furthermore, good client care and documentation of progress, if combined with discipline in a standardized fashion, can provide the starting point for a research protocol. In the long term, this in turn holds the potential for higher quality client care.

Experience in rehabilitation is a most valuable commodity and research can provide a framework to effectively communicate this experience. In this framework, the experienced clinician communicates in a standardized fashion the type of technologies, methods, and interaction styles that have proven to be most effective. Thus the experiences can be transferred to students in the field. Moreover, the process of publication frequently provides peer review, and the accessibility of journals readily provides a network with other professionals, which in turn establishes an assimilation and accommodation of information. Therefore, research should be regarded as one of the most efficient teaching tools in the clinical setting.

It is not sufficient just to collect standardized data points—instead, two-dimensional quantifications must be creatively woven into the three-dimensional life of the client. To achieve this, theories of rehabilitation need to be developed by relying on the field of neuroscience. If the brain is to be rehabilitated, then an understanding of the central nervous system as well as the consequences of neuropathology is paramount. Moreover, rehabilitation is based on changes, and if behavior is to be modified, then an acquaintance with the behavioral sciences is equally important (see Figure 6.1). Based on the integration of neuroscience and behavioral science, theories of rehabilitation need to be developed according to specific hypotheses that then can be falsified or verified according to data.

The scientific study of rehabilitation serves a very practical purpose, namely to secure the future and progress of rehabilitation. For clients with traumatic brain injury, there has been a mushrooming of rehabilitation centers in the 1980s throughout the United States. These centers must be encouraged to continue and new programs need to be developed, particularly for those individuals with limited financial re-

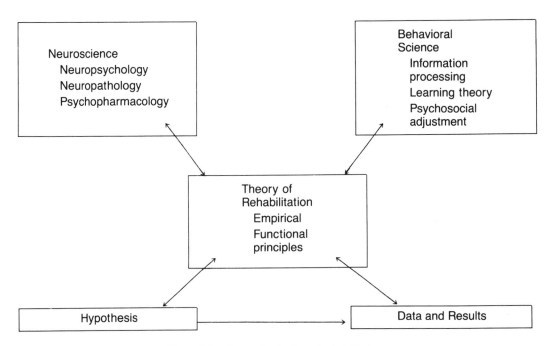

Figure 6.1.   Conceptualization of rehabilitation.

sources. However, for the insurance and medical communities to accept and support these programs, research will need to document their efficacy. It is only on this basis that government support can be obtained for all individuals with traumatic brain injury independent of their financial backing. The early 1990s will be a grace period, but the sooner research can rigorously document the scientific efficacy of rehabilitation, the better the needs of all who need rehabilitation will be met.

What Needs to be Researched?

In working with interns and doctoral students at the University of California Medical Center in San Diego, the following question is frequently posed: "What research project should I conduct?" Most often, a review of the literature does not provide the answer to that question. For example, if an author in the discussion section of an article recommends future projects, one is left to wonder whether these are already in progress. Moreover, the most original questions are typically kept secretive, as to not be "scooped" by a competing team of investigators.

The advice we give our students is to assure them that in the field of rehabilitation there is an abundance of relevant questions that need to be researched and that the problem should only be one of selection. The best possible source of generating and selecting important and relevant questions is found when working with a challenging client, who presents a problem for which there are no apparent answers. In other words, the best research questions most often stem from the challenge to find a more efficient and valuable treatment for a particular client. Once such a question has been formulated, then of course it is important to fine tune this question further, discuss it with colleagues, and review the appropriate literature.

ROLE OF NEUROPSYCHOLOGY
IN REHABILITATION

Neuropsychology is the scientific discipline that investigates the relationship between brain and behavior. The discipline has grown out of a tradition of psychometrically assessing behavior and,

on this basis, localizing cortical damage. In recent years a relatively small percentage of neuropsychologists have become increasingly interested in also entering the rehabilitation field. Most often the emphasis has been on providing comprehensive neuropsychological evaluations and not necessarily on providing treatment. No doubt this will change. The clinical utility of localizing specific cortical regions based on behavioral measures has dwindled in the clinical setting based on the introduction of modern neuroimaging techniques. Nonetheless, a combination of behavioral and neuroimaging techniques is the preferred mode, particularly when faced with determining the potential outcome of a specific client (e.g., Langfitt et al., 1986; Levin et al., 1985; Ruff, Cullum, & Luerssen, 1989).

Neuropsychological assessments have evolved into function-specific descriptions of cognitive domains (see Table 6.1). For the most apparent deficiencies, namely language and motor disturbances, therapies have been available for decades. Therefore, every major medical center throughout the United States utilizes speech/language, occupational, and physical therapists. However, the empirical data to support the efficacy of such therapies, particularly for the language-related ones, are relatively sparse (e.g., Basso, Capitani, & Vignolo, 1979;

Table 6.1. Specific cognitive domains in neuropsychology

Sensory perceptual	Processing sensory input
Motor abilities	Processing motor output
Attention	Processing of information according to alertness, selective focusing, capacity, and speed
Memory and learning	Storing and retrieval of information
Language	Communicating by receiving and expressing verbal information
Spatial and constructional abilities	Processing and manipulating spatial information
Executive functioning	Modulating other cognitive processes to achieve goal-directed activities

Hagen, 1973). More research is definitely needed in this area.

In addition to the motor and language difficulties, it has been known for years that neurological disorders cause attentional disturbance, amnesia, and difficulties in spatial integration and executive functioning (Levin, Benton, & Grossman, 1982; Rosenthal, Griffith, Bond, & Miller, 1983). Therefore neuropsychologists need to systematically develop treatments in the area of attention, memory, and executive functioning. Occupational therapy has been effective with spatial integration and extending training to functional (everyday life) activities. However, more research is needed to establish efficacious treatments in the area of spatial integration.

Before addressing a pilot study that sought to evaluate the efficacy of such neuropsychological treatments, three different models of neurobehavioral recovery underlying rehabilitation are briefly discussed.

THEORIES OF NEUROBEHAVIORAL RECOVERY

Three major theories have been proposed to explain the basis for neurobehavioral recovery: substitution, compensation, and relearning. All three recognize that once the central nervous system (CNS) has been compromised, a permanent and irreversible component of the damage will remain. In persons with traumatic brain injury,

anatomic and structural damage permanently affecting the CNS is caused, for example, by brain lacerations or lesions secondary to subdural or intracerebral hematomas. Moreover, more diffuse and microscopic lesions are caused by the shearing of neurons, which in turn can lead to disconnection of neural pathways (Gennarelli et al., 1982). In addition to the anatomical damage, traumatic brain injury can result in neurophysiological and neurochemical damage causing seizure disorders, hypersensitivity to stimulation, lower tolerance to drugs and alcohol, a variety of disinhibition syndromes, and so forth. None of the proposed theories is capable of dealing with this complexity, and the focus has been primarily limited to considering anatomical models for rehabilitation.

Substitution

The theory of substitution proposes that an intact or less damaged region can take over for a permanently damaged area of the brain. Gazzaniga (1978) suggests that it is possible to "shunt" around a brain lesion by setting up environmental contingencies, which thereby require a different part of the brain to be used in the solution of the problem. Figure 6.2 depicts an information-processing model where input is encoded hierarchically before the decoding of output is possible. Substitution will allow the information to be processed via a different routing, circumventing the damaged region.

The substitution theory implicitly assumes

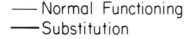

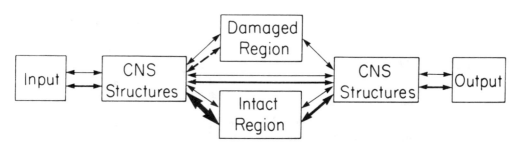

Figure 6.2. Processing according to substitution model.

a flexible communication system between the brain structures. No doubt the cortical systems are richly interconnected, but the shunting does assume that alternate or redundant pathways allow for this rerouting. A second assumption implies that the CNS in its normal state is underutilized, and that a reserve exists that allows for the substitution. The third assumption is that of a certain flexibility across functions within the CNS, analogous to Lashley's notion (1937) of equipotentiality for the associative cortex. None of these assumptions has been empirically proven. Moreover, the model of substitution has not been empirically validated in the field of rehabilitation.

Compensation

The theory of compensation proposes that lower levels within the CNS carry out, to some extent, higher level functioning (see Figure 6.3). This theory assumes an explicit hierarchy of functions that correspond with anatomical structures. The second assumption is based on the notion that damaged higher levels release lower level stations (i.e., top-down inhibition is implied). The third assumption associated with the compensation hypothesis is the notion that the damage to the CNS leads to a regression of skills. For example, if an individual is injured at the age of 25, there will be a setback to an earlier stage of development, leaving the client to be, in some areas of functioning, at the level of a 10-year-old. Therefore, the regression is thought to correspond with the ontogenesis of functioning. None of these assumptions has been empirically proven.

Relearning

The concept of relearning implies that through exposure of activities, which are combined with feedback, behavior can be modified (see Figure 6.4). The assumptions underlying this theory are by far the least controversial (Luria, 1966). The first primary notion is that relearning is possible despite serious brain damage such as an amnesia, agnosia, and aphasia. Second, new strategies can assist in compensating for impaired functions. At the present time, this notion appears to be the most parsimonious and, in the context of clinical work, the most relevant.

If relearning is the principal theory behind rehabilitation therapy, then it is important that the treatment be placed in the following framework. In step one, it is imperative to assess the client's current level of functioning in the area where relearning is to take place. In step two, the overall objectives need to be identified and specific goals must be set. These goals must be different from but close to the present level of functioning (knowledge) of the client. Finally, in step three the treatment must allow the client to test, evaluate, and modify his or her current knowledge with the new objectives so that ongoing adaptation is achieved. Depending on the individual client's functioning levels, different relearning techniques should be applied; the in-

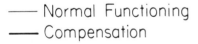

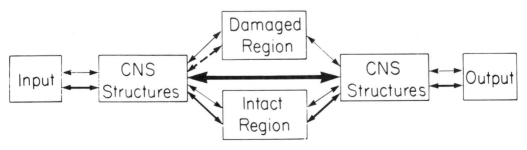

Figure 6.3. Processing according to compensation model.

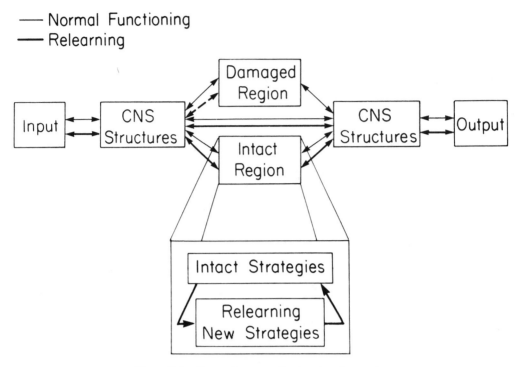

Figure 6.4.   Processing according to relearning model.

terested reader is referred to an informative description by Gross and Schutz (1986) of applying different strategies dependent on both client variables and aim of treatment.

In summary, if rehabilitation relies on relearning, then appropriate goals must be set that need to be associated with appropriate feedback. The generic feedback in the form of praise or encouragement most often used in the therapeutic context is of limited value. Instead clients need to be challenged in small, incremental steps and success as well as failure in relation to therapeutic objectives needs to be communicated in a supportive environment.

PILOT STUDY OF ALTERNATE TREATMENTS: HOW EFFICACIOUS IS NEUROPSYCHOLOGICAL REMEDIATION?

Rationale

The main interest and question motivating the authors' study was very fundamental: Taking a "first things first" approach, the thrust was to determine if a treatment modeled after neuropsychological processes would be the most efficacious in producing improved cognitive outcome. An alternative treatment needed to be selected. It was felt that a comparison using a "day treatment" program as an alternate was both reasonable and useful. Day treatment programs—where the patients spend most of the day involved in various activities that emphasize different aspects of everyday functioning—have been popular in recent years. While the ultimate goal for treatment outcome research on neuropsychological interventions would be to specify those treatment components and client/therapist interactions and attributes that lead to successful outcome (Kazdin, 1986), it was first necessary to challenge the notion that neuropsychologically based models were efficacious.

Design Overview

The pilot study called for a comparison between two alternate treatments, and thus 20 persons with head injury were assigned to each treatment condition. Because of space, equipment, and staff constraints, the groups were subdivided and the four subgroups were treated in an ABBA sequence, beginning and ending with the day treatment condition.

As seen in Table 6.2, the protocol lasted for 22 weeks for each participant, involving two baseline assessments separated by an 8-week waiting period, 8 weeks of treatment (totaling 160 hours of intervention), and one posttreatment assessment. The waiting period before treatment served as a control for the possible confounding effect of spontaneous recovery occurring during a comparable 8-week period. Despite the additional exposure to test measures, and consequently the possible practice effects, it was important to control for changes due simply to the passage of time and natural healing.

Selecting the Client Sample

Subject selection is particularly challenging in such a new field as neuropsychological rehabilitation, to anticipate who will best be served by treatment when most reports of clinical efficacy have not been rigorously tested. Sampling bias in psychotherapy research has long been identified as a threat to external validity (Meltzoff & Kornreich, 1970). Krupnick, Shea, and Elkin (1986) address the particular hazards of using solicited subjects in outcome research, but provide a qualified "thumbs up" for this method of securing subjects and suggest several good cautionary measures to reduce Type I and Type II errors.

For the purpose of this study it was neces-sary to rely upon several sources of referrals that ultimately generated a sample with differing motivations and expectations for treatment. Generally people came to know about the study in one of three ways: solicitation announcements through the local head injury organization, doctor (neurosurgeon, physiatrist, psychiatrist, or psychologist) referral, or solicitation through the community college program for brain-impaired adults. Thus while all candidates knew the study involved treatment of the cognitive sequelae from their head injury, some wished to participate in hopes of changing their behavior and others professed more altruistic reasons such as "to help other head-injured victims" or "so professionals will know more about head injury" and did not explicitly indicate expectations for a personally favorable outcome.

To counteract the differing motivations and expectations of the subjects several steps were taken. First, screening of potential candidates included an interview to assess the person's cooperation or resistance to the idea of treatment. Once a candidate had passed the screening and was offered an opportunity to participate in the study, a verbal commitment was secured from each individual that he or she would complete the entire program. Bearing in mind the ethical principles applicable for research with human subjects regarding the use of undue influence, this verbal commitment was intended to promote an alliance between the investigators and the participants whereby each understood the other's

Table 6.2.   Design of treatment timetable

Group	Baseline testing 1	8 weeks	Baseline testing 2	8 weeks	Posttreatment testing
Group A_1	Test forms A	Waiting period	Test forms B	Day treatment condition	Test forms A
Group B_1	Test forms B	Waiting period	Test forms A	Neuropsychological treatment condition	Test forms B
Group B_2	Test forms A	Waiting period	Test forms B	Neuropsychological treatment condition	Test forms A
Group A_2	Test forms B	Waiting period	Test forms A	Day treatment condition	Test forms B

Total N = 40 for each treatment condition. However, the treatment program was run with 10 subjects at one time, necessitating the formation of four successive groups, two for each treatment condition.

Two alternative versions of memory and learning measures, forms A and B, were used over repeated administrations. In addition, the groups were counterbalanced for order of forms administered.

dedication and seriousness of intent. Also, throughout the program participants outlined their individual goals and were encouraged to discuss their experience of progress or obstacles to treatment. It was the consensus of the staff that all participants could potentially benefit from treatment and that despite some use of denial and rationalization as to why they chose to participate, all subjects ultimately did identify their own personal expectations and goals.

An attempt was made to address motivation and expectancy as an ongoing part of the treatment. Since the participants were blind to the main hypotheses of the study (i.e., a comparison of alternate treatments), there was not a differential influence for motivation in the two treatment conditions.

Screening for Neuropsychological Impairments

Potential candidates who inquired about the study were sent a questionnaire regarding demographic and medical information to provide an initial screening. Based upon clinical rationale it was determined that all subjects must meet the following criteria: 1) age between 17 and 65; 2) at least one functional hand; 3) at least 50% field of vision; 4) ability to communicate verbally, regardless of whether dysarthria, mild aphasia, or anomia were present; 5) a head injury of at least moderate severity as defined by Glasgow Coma Score when available, or retrospective estimation of length of unconsciousness and posttraumatic amnesia; 6) at least 1 year postinjury; 7) the capacity to withstand 5 hours of treatment daily; and 8) the absence of major psychiatric diagnoses or premorbid history of other neurological or neuropsychiatric disorders.

Those individuals who met these criteria were then scheduled for a psychometric screening to: 1) identify and eliminate those persons who did not evidence significant cognitive sequelae, and 2) provide quantification of potential confounding variables to be used in random assignment to treatment conditions. Measures for the screening battery (see Table 6.3) were intended to provide an estimation of level of cognitive functioning.

Group assignment was achieved by con-

Table 6.3. Measures used to screen potential candidates from sample pool

Test measure	Description
Galveston Orientation and Amnesia Test (Levin, O'Donnell, & Grossman, 1979)	Assesses orientation to person, place and time; establishes periods of retrograde and anterograde amnesia based on client's report of events
Mattis Dementia Rating Scale (Mattis, 1976)	Assesses attention, initiation/perseveration, construction, memory, and conceptualization
Sensory Perceptual Examination	Included testing visual fields, unilateral and bilateral stimulation of visual, auditory, and tactile modalities
Ruff Language Screening Examination (Ruff, 1986)	Assesses repetition, comprehension, visual naming, spelling, calculations, and expression
Brief Clinical Interview	Addressed motivation for participation, past treatment efforts and outcome, cooperation, interpersonal comfort, social skills, and emotional functioning

sulting a statistician who was not acquainted with any of the potential clients. The selection process was quasi-random, attempting to balance gender, age, sex, and particular neurobehavioral measures selected from the screening. Two or three alternate participants were also specified in case of early attrition or nonavailability of a candidate.

Subjects

A total of 40 subjects were admitted to the study, with an attrition rate of only 1 person. The demographic and neurological characteristics are summarized in Table 6.4 for the neuropsychological treatment group and for the day treatment group.

Staff

The majority of the staff hired for this project remained throughout its 2-year length, thus min-

Table 6.4.   Demographic and neurological data on treatment groups

	Patient number[a]	Age at time of program completion	Gender	Years of formal education	Occupation at time of injury	Months from injury to first testing	Days in coma[b]	Neurosurgery	Clinical diagnosis
Neuropsychological treatment group	1	60	M	15	Title officer	63	<1	No	MCC
	2	30	F	15	Flight attendant	40	35	No	SCC and BSC
	3	41	M	12	Boiler maker	61	<1	Yes	MCC
	4	31	M	14	Construction worker	70	25	Yes	Penetrating injury
	5	22	F	12	Junior college student	41	30	No	SCC and BSC
	6	23	M	12	High school student	85	42	Yes	SCC and BSC
	7	26	M	13	Landscaper	41	42	No	SCC
	8	48	M	15	General contractor	40	28	Yes	SCC
	9	34	M	15	Salesperson	18	9	No	SCC
	10	28	F	13	Waitress	85	14	Yes	SCC
	11	33	M	14	Supervisor	17	<1	No	MCC
	12	29	M	16	Freelance writer	20	42	No	SCC
	13	20	M	14	Junior college student	18	28	No	SCC and BSC
	14	18	M	13	High school student	45	47	No	SCC
	15	26	M	12	Unemployed	19	<1	Yes	Penetrating injury
	16	19	M	12	Part-time cook	12	28	Yes	BSC
	17	25	F	13	Receptionist	25	21	No	SCC
	18	26	M	14	Auto detailer	23	35	No	SCC and BSC
	19	28	F	12	Housewife	33	28	Yes	SCC and BSC
	20	30	F	13	Dental assistant	43	28	No	SCC
Day treatment group	1	39	M	16	Accountant	64	21	No	SCC and BSC
	2	20	F	11	High school student	46	70	Yes	SCC and BSC
	3	42	M	12	Truck driver	44	31	No	SCC and BSC
	4	28	F	14	Horse groomer	80	59	No	SCC
	5	45	F	12	Waitress	59	115	No	SCC
	6	36	M	14	Deep sea diver	90	105	No	SCC
	7	18	M	11	High school student	33	122	No	SCC and BSC
	8	23	M	10	High school student	85	61	Yes	SCC
	9	24	M	12	Juggler/entertainer	27	35	Yes	SCC
	10	37	M	18	Accountant	80	59	No	SCC and BSC
	11	26	M	12	Welder	54	65	Yes	SCC and BSC
	12	41	M	14	Sous chef	38	26	No	SCC
	13	32	F	12	Secretary	38	62	No	BSC
	14	46	F	14	Housewife	59	64	Yes	SCC and BSC
	15	24	M	14	Carpenter	23	60	Yes	SCC and BSC
	16	23	M	12	Truck driver	52	120	Yes	SCC and BSC
	17	23	F	12	File clerk	62	5	No	SCC
	18	40	M	14	Truck driver	25	5	No	SCC
	19	24	F	12	Beautician	60	65	Yes	SCC
	20	24	M	11	Construction worker	92	3	Yes	SCC

[a]N = 20 for each treatment group.
[b]Days in coma determined by relative's account or medical records.
MCC = moderate cerebral contusion.
SCC = severe cerebral contusion.
BSC = brain-stem contusion.

imizing the impact of staff turnover. The staff comprised the following team of people:

Principal investigator—neuropsychologist; oversaw all aspects of the project and provided training to staff

Two postdoctoral neuropsychology fellows; organized scheduling and data collection, administered test batteries, provided some training, and delivered treatments

Two predoctoral psychology interns; assisted with data collection and treatment delivery

Two mental health volunteers; assisted with treatment delivery

The staff were trained to provide the treatments, particularly those involving new computer-assisted techniques. Daily staff meetings facilitated processing of therapeutic issues and resolution of problem areas. Formal supervision was done once a week to review cases more thoroughly. Daily progress notes were kept on each client to assist in communication among the staff and provide a written record of therapeutic efforts.

Setting

The treatments were administered in an outpatient clinic in close proximity to the University of California, San Diego Medical Center. The facilities were most conducive to small group sessions, and differing areas were devoted to specific treatment functions (computer room, group therapy room, etc.). A full-time administrative assistant provided the necessary support functions. Because this facility was devoted exclusively to providing cognitive remediation and no other professional disciplines shared the space, a strong identity formed whereby many clients viewed the facility as similar to a school or work setting rather than a medical center. Lunch time was typically a group affair with staff and clients eating together, which further contributed to a "fraternity" atmosphere.

Aspects of Treatment

The neuropsychological treatment condition was divided into four 2-week segments, progressing from attention training to visuospatial training, memory training, and logical thinking training.

Table 6.5 delineates the most prominent aspects of treatment for each of the four modules.

The day treatment condition was structured to provide a stimulating environment that encouraged reflection, action, and interaction. Choosing which components to include in this treatment condition was based upon introducing a broad range of interesting activities, but not attempting to retrain specific cognitive abilities. Thus many aspects focused upon daily living skills and creative exercises. Table 6.6 outlines the specific content areas chosen for inclusion in this treatment condition.

Daily Schedules

In both treatment conditions the days were divided into 50-minute sessions, with the clients rotating through each "class" so that each person participated in every type of intervention offered for that day. The structure was much like that of a school setting, where students attend each academic subject every day. With this structure every client worked with each staff member at least once during the day. Schedules for the day were given to each client and posted in each room to facilitate transitioning among classes.

Techniques Used

Owing to the growing popularity of computer applications in rehabilitation and the practical advantages of computer-assisted training, computerized interventions were used for both treatment groups, holding constant the time spent per day on the computer. For the neuropsychological treatment condition new computer programs were developed specifically for this project and when consistent with the treatment approach, commercially available software was used. One of the major advantages to using computer-assisted techniques was the precision of the feedback that could be given to the user and the ability to select among varying conditions, such as level of difficulty, speed, exposure time, amount of stimuli, and so forth, as part of the software's features.

While the neuropsychological treatment condition included computer-assisted techniques that trained cognitive functions, the day treatment condition included computer and video

Table 6.5. Primary aspects of the neuropsychological treatment condition

Module 1—Attention

Reaction times	Improving speed of information processing through simple detection and response tasks
Vigilance	Sustaining attention over time
Selective attention	Focusing on relevant stimulus dimensions; control of automatic response tendencies
Alternating attention	Shifting from one cognitive set to another based upon rapidly alternating cues

Module 2—Spatial integration

Localization	Orienting to a single source of visual or auditory stimuli based upon intrapersonal space
Mapping	Integration of two or more points in space using extrapersonal reference, involving progressively longer sequences of stimuli forming "pathways"
Transfigured mapping	Extends the use of mapping by adding a component of symbolic representation of space that promotes development of planned or anticipated image representation
Visuospatial analysis	Various tasks that emphasized perceptual accuracy, figure-ground determination, and size estimation

Module 3—Memory

Encoding strategies	Implementation of various mnemonic aids to promote the initial learning and registration of information; specific techniques such as imagery, method of vanishing cues, chunking, chaining, and so on were taught and practiced using differing levels of complexity and amounts of information
Retrieval strategies	Implementation of cuing methods to facilitate recall; both external aids and self-cuing were used to maximize the retrieval of previously learned information

Module 4—Logical thinking

Categorization	Generation, maintenance, and shifting of cognitive sets
Problem solving	Using a five-step procedure, which was mnemonically learned, clients systematically worked through problems and analyzed outcomes
Convergent thinking	Reasoning using a deductive process to formulate specific conclusions
Divergent thinking	Reasoning using an inductive process to brainstorm alternatives and assist generalization from specific to broad contexts

games as an alternate intervention. The computer and video games, such as "Ping Pong," "Barnstormers," and "Blackjack," emphasized psychomotor speed and attention, but in addition, a large element of luck was included in most games so that skill alone did not determine the outcome. Nonetheless, the video and computer games did provide feedback to the user by way of scores, although somewhat less precise than the performance feedback given to the neuropsychological treatment group.

Another factor was held constant between the alternate treatment groups. Both conditions included daily group psychotherapy to address the psychosocial issues and personal adjustments inherent during head injury rehabilitation. From the clinical experience of the investigators it was determined that an outlet for discussing stress, coping skills, emotional reactions to disability, interpersonal relationships, and other psychological issues was essential during any intensive remedial treatment. Rather than disregard the psychosocial component and attempt to provide intensive treatment without an opportunity for ventilation and group support, it was decided that addressing the psychosocial issues

Table 6.6.   Primary aspects of the day treatment condition

Computer and video games	Adventure and "action" games were available that emphasized visuo-motor speed but not reasoning, problem solving, or memory.
Health and coping	Topics concerning physical and emotional well-being were addressed in open discussion.
Current events and topical discussion	Participants reported to the group on news stories gathered from various media sources.
Independent living	Workbook exercises concerning reading labels, following directions, using transportation, banking, budgeting, preparing résumés, and other skills dependent upon reading, writing, and math were used.
Art and recreation therapy	Art projects and parlor games were introduced for individual or group participation.

would be a natural part of most treatment approaches and warranted inclusion in both treatment conditions.

A description of all the various tasks and their modifications is beyond the scope of this chapter. Some tasks were taken from previously published rehabilitation materials (Craine & Gudeman, 1981; Ruff, Evans, & Green, 1986; Wilson & Moffatt, 1984), but many were devised specifically for this project using materials available at educational supply stores, which were then modified. One of the most challenging aspects of this project was to organize enough therapeutic tasks (over 100 hours of treatment sessions), with varying levels of difficulty, and training the staff to be competent in the delivery of the interventions. It was an enormous undertaking given the fact that few resources were readily available to guide the development of comprehensive programs, few established programs served as prototypes, and the materials are generally expensive. For the most part, however, few of the materials required much training beyond familiarization to use them effectively. The exceptions were the computer software programs, which required a good deal of hands-on experience to become knowledgeable about all the options and subroutines that were available.

Although the content and structure of the neuropsychological and day treatment groups were very different, an attempt was made to ensure a therapeutic environment for both conditions. Staff, although not blind to the treatment condition, provided support, encouragement, feedback, and assistance to all subjects in an effort to develop strong alliances. Staff meetings were utilized as a forum to discuss therapeutic approaches and to monitor and maintain the integrity of the treatment conditions. Thus, nonspecific treatment factors were held constant between both groups, although it remains uncertain how much, if any, bias was introduced through differential conduct of staff.

Fundamental principles were incorporated into every treatment intervention in the neuropsychological treatment condition and thus provided a foundation for systematically approaching the remediation (see Table 6.7). Going beyond an understanding of task content, the staff was trained to administer interventions using basic premises consistent with behavioral and neurotraining theories. An excellent source for the description and application of these principles is Craine and Gudeman's text (1981), and the reader is referred to that book for more information.

Results

The first question to be considered was whether a treatment effect emerged for either group. In a comparison between the average pretreatment and posttreatment scores, both groups improved significantly: multivariate analysis of variance, $p < 0.001$ (Ruff et al., 1989). Thus regardless of treatment approach used, subjects improved when provided with intensive therapy aimed at affecting cognitive functioning.

To determine whether a treatment based upon neuropsychological principles was more effective than a treatment that provided general stimulation and activity, first a p-plot was generated to identify nonchance findings when con-

Table 6.7. Principles of neurotraining

1. Recovery from brain damage is possible due to the plasticity of function and compensatory processes that are characteristic of the central nervous system.

2. The cerebral cortex is an open system with a dynamic process of organization that responds to external influences of deprivation, thereby slowing or halting learning, or stimulation, which heightens learning and adaptation.

3. The process of learning is achieved through repetitive and structured activity that becomes organized into functional behaviors and mastery of complex routines.

4. Neurotraining activities should follow the hierarchical developmental stages of whatever skill or behavior is being relearned. Basic skills are overlearned to lay the foundation for more complex skills dependent upon earlier mastery.

5. When possible, multisensory presentation and cortical integration of modalities should be utilized to facilitate the more complex aspects of cortical functioning.

6. The emphasis of neurotraining should promote the fundamental processes of learning and information utilization rather than specific task contents.

7. Identification of individual cognitive strengths and weaknesses, through comprehensive and systematic assessment, should precede neurotraining and be used to specify and structure a retraining program.

8. Consistent, immediate, comprehensible feedback should be given to clients throughout training to assist their adaptations in performance.

Adapted from Craine, J.F., & Gudeman, H.E. (1981). *The rehabilitation of brain functions: Principles, procedures, and techniques of neurotraining.* Springfield, IL: Charles C Thomas.

sidering numerous dependent measures (Schweder & Spjotvoll, 1982). Those values determined to be above chance are found in Table 6.8 and confirm that the changes in the neuropsychological treatment condition were significantly greater than in the day treatment group along several dimensions.

Perhaps most encouraging were the findings of significantly improved memory and attention in the neuropsychological treatment condition based upon the scores of a measure of selective attention (Ruff 2 & 7 Test; Ruff, Evans, & Light, 1986) and verbal learning (Selective Reminding Test; Buschke, 1973). Given marked improvements in both of these areas, it can be inferred that subjects exposed to neuropsychological remediation may demonstrate greater accuracy in attention and more efficient encoding of information. Significant improvement on other measures, placement errors on the Rey Complex Figure and the comprehension subtest of the WAIS-R, may reflect greater planning and conceptual organization that could be attributed to the neuropsychological treatment emphasis on implementation of methodical strategies and monitoring the appropriateness of one's responses. Continued study is needed to account for these specific changes and to integrate these findings with other reports of successful outcome.

While the results did provide preliminary support for the hypothesis that a neuropsychologically based treatment targeting specific cognitive functions may effect greater improvements than an alternate treatment emphasizing general stimulation, caution must be exercised not to magnify these findings beyond the scope of the current data. While careful statistical analysis provided controls for spurious chance findings, it is still notable that improvements in the posttreatment measures were not more consistent in those areas of cognitive functioning targeted by the neuropsychological treatment. Thus, while a treatment effect was seen on some measures of attention, memory, and logical thinking, there were other dependent measures where this effect was not realized as would be anticipated if the functional improvements were fairly global. This inconsistency in measurement of treatment outcome remains to be explained by additional studies and improved methods for operationalizing outcome.

Consideration of Treatment Integrity and Generalization

As with any empirical study, the alternate hypothesis is accepted and the null hypothesis is rejected only when analysis of the results indicates a very small probability of obtaining findings by chance. However, even when the prem-

Table 6.8.   Measures reflecting greater improvement in the neuropsychological treatment condition than the day treatment condition, using pre-post difference scores

Test measure	Day treatment			Neuropsychological			p value[b]
	Avg Pre	Post	Dif[a]	Avg Pre	Post	Dif[a]	
Ruff 2 & 7 Selective Attention Letters: Errors							
Mean	8.8	9.1	0.3	10.5	7.8	−2.7	0.06
Standard dev.	(6.14)	(8.69)	(5.21)	(12.1)	(8.60)	(5.90)	
Rey Complex Figure 3-Minute Recall— Placement Score							
Mean	1.8	2.7	0.9	1.6	1.4	−0.2	0.03
Standard dev.	(1.35)	(1.91)	(1.76)	(0.80)	(0.94	(1.18)	
Rey Complex Figure 60-Minute Recall— Placement Score							
Mean	2.0	2.7	0.7	1.6	1.5	−0.1	0.01
Standard dev.	(1.20)	(1.80)	(1.81)	(0.98)	(1.01)	(1.43)	
Selective Reminding Test Long-Term Storage							
Mean	83.7	79.9	−3.8	82.9	92.5	9.6	0.001
Standard dev.	(27.1)	(28.1)	(8.46)	(20.4)	(19.3)	(10.18)	
Selective Reminding Test Sum of Consistent Long-Term Retrieval							
Mean	38.8	42.1	3.3	32.1	43.6	11.5	0.03
Standard dev.	(36.0)	(38.1)	(13.48)	(27.9)	(33.3)	(14.92)	
Digit Symbol Scaled Score							
Mean	5.0	5.1	0.1	4.6	5.7	1.1	0.09
Standard dev.	(2.35)	(2.89)	(0.91)	(1.61)	(2.20)	(0.82)	
Verbal IQ Score							
Mean	92.4	92.6	0.2	92.6	96.2	3.6	0.02
Standard dev.	(11.1)	(11.5)	(4.03)	(12.0)	(4.41)		
Comprehension Scaled Score							
Mean	89.9	8.7	−0.2	8.7	9.8	1.1	0.04
Standard dev.	(1.97)	(2.66)	(1.33)	(2.14)	(2.70)	(1.49)	
Full Scale IQ Score							
Mean	86.8	89.8	3.0	87.8	92.9	5.1	0.07
Standard dev.	(9.55)	(11.5)	(3.37)	(12.2)	(13.3)	(4.00)	
Figural Fluency Test Number of Unique Designs							
Mean	11.9	13.1	1.2	10.3	13.4	3.1	0.10
Standard dev.	(4.55)	(5.59)	(2.54)	(2.86)	(4.16)	(2.81)	

[a]Difference score (Dif) was calculated by subtracting the average of the two pretreatment scores (Avg Pre) from the posttreatment performance (Post); level of $p = 0.065$ was selected (according to the p-plot procedure) for the significance level for comparisons of the difference scores between the control and the experimental group.

[b]Only those values of $p \leq 0.10$ are shown. On other dependent measures the changes in scores in the group means were not sufficient to obtain significant differences between treatment groups. All significant findings were in the same direction of the neuropsychological treatment condition achieving improved performance.

ises of a controlled experiment are accepted as true findings there is the issue of generalizability of these results to other subjects and settings, and ultimately the replicability of the findings over time. In this pilot study there emerged several issues to consider in evaluating these results and planning for further investigations.

First is the issue of treatment integrity, that is, whether the experimental conditions were delivered as intended and whether they were representative of procedures used in clinical practice (Kazdin, 1986; Yeaton & Sechrest, 1981). Based upon other studies and reports of neuropsychological remedial techniques, the present program was developed and executed. Thus existing precedent was used to organize both treatment conditions, but in a single-blind study it may have been prudent to determine at the onset that biases were not inadvertently introduced into the treatment conditions. It may be clearly warranted in future studies to determine that the proposed methods are in fact consistent with state-of-the-art neuropsychological remediation. As Kazdin (1986) recommends, this may be accomplished through consultation with colleagues and ratings of treatment techniques by experts who provide the same clinical services. Unfortunately, neuropsychological remediation is such a new field and so few techniques have been empirically studied that defining the purity and representation of treatments may be biased and imprecise even when done by experts.

Decisions regarding the length and intensity of the treatment program were also made based upon clinical "common sense" and logistical considerations. While it was not totally unreasonable to propose treatments of 8-weeks duration, 20 hours per week, it is unlikely that this schedule would be practical in a clinical setting. For the most part, 20 hours a week solely of cognitive remedial treatments exceeds what most settings could provide and would surely be challenged on a cost-effectiveness basis. Likewise, an 8-week period may not be long enough to ensure substantial changes in the majority of individuals with head injury, whose learning and adaptation of behavior is slowed. Thus, creating realistic and optimal conditions of treatment delivery is an important and frequently overlooked aspect of successful outcome.

While the debate concerning the relative influence of client and therapist characteristics in psychotherapy treatment outcome has a long history (Bandura, 1977; Frank, 1979, 1981; Telch, 1981), these issues are equally germane to neuropsychological interventions. Subject variables such as rate of learning, flexibility, perceptual accuracy, anosognosia, emotional well-being, and self-monitoring capacity will need to be sorted through carefully, particularly in regard to whether these characteristics should be targets of treatment or primarily considered influencing variables. Decisions regarding which subject variables should be held constant to reduce extraneous variance and which variables should be more thoroughly studied as interacting with remedial interventions will be paramount in producing effective and utilitarian research.

Therapist variables affecting remedial treatment outcome may be somewhat different from those found to have an impact on the psychotherapeutic process. Certainly there are similarities among therapeutic processes, such as expectancy for change, therapeutic alliance, empathy, and so forth, yet at this time it is pure speculation as to which therapist characteristics and aspects of the treatment process are most important to remedial work. The authors' experience in this pilot study was that a minimum knowledge of head injury and its behavioral affects was essential for all therapists. Beyond this, however, flexibility in the therapists to make adaptations in their approach, and patience to endure the necessary repetitions and overlearning were important attributes that facilitated client interaction. Of course there were many other essential traits observed to contribute to good client-therapist relations, but which of these actually influenced outcome cannot be assumed solely from observation. As Telch (1981) points out, it may be more efficacious to focus upon the therapist's proficiency in implementing the interventions than upon client or therapist attributes. Ensuring adequate training of the treatment providers is often given cursory consideration at best in many studies, and not addressed at all in others. In a treatment as comprehensive and intensive as the present one, ensuring equal, if not similar, proficiency and skill among all therapists in all aspects of the treatment was an overwhelming task. Certainly if the treatments were to be considered representative and implemented most carefully, the issue of therapist training and competence bears greater examination.

As a pilot study this investigation seemed to raise more questions than it answered, and as such has paved the way for future refinements in second-and third-generation research. Problems inherent in administering a treatment "package" that was true to the proposed condition under study, yet was sensitive to individual needs provided a major challenge. While the clinician recognizes the need for flexibility and individually tailored treatment interventions to achieve successful outcome, the researcher is also bound to maintain the integrity of the independent variable and not compromise or obfuscate the conditions under study. Balancing both of these needs was paramount and ongoing. A priori decisions regarding treatment length, the sequencing of administration of treatment modules, frequency of sessions, client and therapist variables, sampling bias, and how best to measure change remain important methodological issues to consider and incorporate in future research.

FUTURE DIRECTION OF RESEARCH

Based on the present pilot study, the first conclusion is that training in the areas of attention and memory appear to be the most promising to pursue. Consequently, the authors are presently investigating a set of more refined remediation techniques in the areas of attention and memory. Two groups of individuals with head injury are being remediated with either attention or memory training. The aim is to study the specific gains possible with either alternate treatment module.

A second decision was to fine tune and modify the dependent measures. Assessments before and after treatments appear not to be sufficiently sensitive to capture the treatment effects. One of the reasons is due to the fact that most neuropsychological test procedures have been poorly normed without standard error of measures available, and there is a limitation to the availability of alternate versions. Therefore the

authors decided to add a third control group that was tested across the same three time intervals as the subjects in the pilot study. Comparisons across all three groups will provide further refinement of separating treatment effects from changes due to practice effects from repeated testing with relatively close time intervals. In addition, dependent measures often fail to capture subtle performance changes and do not reflect the dynamic processes involved in retraining. Rather than using measures that are more static and based upon the achievement of certain scores, traditionally an approach of absence/ presence of deficits, outcome measures may need to be revised to capture the process of learning and adaptation that the client has acquired. Ultimately it may be more vital to place a greater emphasis on assessing metacognitive abilities and their relation to outcome and specific cognitive functions.

A third hurdle for neuropsychological remediation in the future will be to determine which gains are clinically meaningful. Should one expect statistically significant gains following treatment? Should these gains be measured according to group means or on an individual basis? If a patient is more severely impaired should one expect greater gains? Since individuals with head injury as a population are heterogeneous, it is more therapeutically meaningful to set specific goals on an individual basis (i.e., evaluate undesirable states prior to treatment and determine the desired outcome on an individual basis). The outcome would therefore focus on whether the desired goals have been reached for the individual. This, however, creates a challenge on how to empirically evaluate an innovative therapy program.

A fourth challenge is the selection of an appropriate research paradigm. In treatment research the experimental design should not dictate the treatment approach, but rather the emphasis must be on the most clinically relevant treatment. Experimental designs must be selected and created to evaluate gains for groups of clients while at the same time being sensitive to change for the individual across treatment phases. Thus in ongoing studies the authors have introduced a single case design juxtaposed with pretreatment and posttreatment testing. This yields information with respect to the gains that individual clients make. Such information is vital if one is to determine which type of treatment is most valid for a specific deficit. While large-group comparisons provide information on overall efficacy of a treatment approach, knowledge of whether that approach was successful with certain individuals is lost. Therefore research efforts need to be focused at several levels to gain a perspective on broad as well as specific implementation of treatments. Macroscopic (large-group comparisons) and microscopic (individual case studies) investigations can offer differing, but complementary insights regarding treatment efficacy.

A fifth challenge, which will be the most difficult, is to document scientifically how neuropsychological remediation changes everyday functioning. Some clinicians have proposed that training modules in memory or attention should be avoided altogether, and instead the focus should be on practical skills. However, simply training individuals on everyday tasks is clearly not the answer to this immense challenge. Teaching is based not only on providing an individual with skills, but also on enabling the student to understand the principles and rules behind the skills. This will promote generalization so that the skills can be adapted to the varying environmental demands. For example, a treatment goal cannot be limited to having an individual navigate only one set of stairs because

it is likely that this individual will have to climb different types of stairs. Thus, generalization must be built into treatment goals. Accordingly, cognitive training must ultimately serve the purpose of generalization of skills that demonstrate meaningful gains in everyday functioning. Therefore a modular approach that trains attention and memory, for example, must be part of the future in neuropsychological rehabilitation. Both of these particular cognitive functions are building blocks for other treatments and extensive research is needed to delineate what level of impairment can best be treated with what types of learning strategy.

The field of rehabilitation must be transdisciplinary if it is to be successful. Models need to be developed that actively integrate the disciplines (i.e., case management systems). Moreover, it is critically important that some treatments be tailored to the individual and made relevant to their long-term living plan. Individual motivators, and family and social circumstances must be integrated if any treatment approach is to be effective. Therefore, researchers are faced with the immense challenge of not only evaluating the outcome of rehabilitation, but validating the long-term outcome according to behavioral observations in the individual's environment. This challenge should, however, not sabotage individual therapists from exploring and scientifically validating specific treatment modules that can stock the shelves of therapists dedicated to rehabilitation.

REFERENCES

Bandura, A. (1977). Toward a unifying theory of behavior change. *Psychological Review, 84,* 191–215.

Basso, A., Capitani, E., & Vignolo, L.A. (1979). Influence of rehabilitation on language skills in aphasic patients. *Archives of Neurology, 36,* 190–196.

Buschke, H. (1973). Selective reminding for analysis of memory and learning. *Journal of Verbal Learning and Verbal Behavior, 12,* 543–550.

Craine, J.F., & Gudeman, H.E. (1981). *The rehabilitation of brain functions: Principles, procedures, and techniques of neurotraining.* Springfield, IL: Charles C Thomas.

Frank, J. D. (1979). The present status of outcome studies. *Journal of Consulting and Clinical Psychology, 47,* 310–316.

Frank, J.D. (1981). Reply to Telch. *Journal of Consulting and Clinical Psychology, 49,* 476–477.

Gazzaniga, M.S. (1978). Is seeing believing: Notes on clinical recovery. In S. Finger (Ed.), *Recovery from brain damage* (p. 409). New York: Plenum.

Gennarelli, T.A., Thibault, L.E., Adams, J.H., Graham, D.I., Thompson, C.J., & Marcincin, R.P. (1982). Diffuse axonal injury and traumatic coma in the primate. *Annals of Neurology, 12,* 564–574.

Gross, Y., & Schutz, L.E. (1986). Intervention models in neuropsychology. In B. Uzzell & Y. Gross

(Eds.), *Clinical neuropsychology of intervention* (pp. 179–204). Boston: Martinus Nijhoff Publishing.

Hagen, C. (1973). Communicative abilities in hemiplegia: Effect of speech therapy. *Archives of Physical and Medical Rehabilitation, 54,* 454–464.

Kazdin, A.E. (1986). Comparative outcome studies of psychotherapy: Methodological issues and strategies. *Journal of Consulting and Clinical Psychology, 54,* 95–105.

Krupnick, J., Shea, T., & Elkin, I. (1986). Generalizability of treatment studies utilizing solicited patients. *Journal of Consulting and Clinical Psychology, 54,* 68–78.

Langfitt, T.W., Obrist, W.D., Alavi, A., Grossman, R.I., Zimmerman, R., Jaggi, J., Uzzell, B., Reivich, M., & Patton, D.R. (1986). Computerized tomography, magnetic resonance imaging, and positron emission tomography in the study of brain trauma. *Journal of Neurosurgery, 64,* 760–767.

Lashley, K.S. (1937). Functional determinant of cerebral localization. *Archives of Neurology and Psychiatry, 38,* 371.

Levin, H.S., Benton, A.L., & Grossman, R.G. (1982). *Neurobehavioral consequences of closed head injury.* New York: Oxford University Press.

Levin, H.S., Kalisky, Z., Handel, S.F., Goldman, A.M., Eisenberg, H.M., Morrison, D., & Von Laufen, A. (1985). Magnetic resonance imaging in relation to the sequelae and rehabilitation of diffuse closed head injury: Preliminary findings. *Seminars in Neurology, 5,* 221–231.

Levin, H.S., O'Donnell, V.M., & Grossman, R.G. (1979). The Galveston Orientation and Amnesia Test: A practical scale to assess cognition after head injury. *Journal of Nervous and Mental Disorders, 167,* 675–684.

Luria, A.R. (1966). *Higher cortical functions in man.* New York: Basic Books.

Mattis, S. (1976). Mental status examination for organic mental syndrome in the elderly patient. In L. Bellak & T.B. Karasu (Eds.), *Geriatric psychiatry,* (pp. 77–121). New York: Grune & Stratton.

Meltzoff, J., & Kornreich, M. (1970). *Research in psychotherapy.* Chicago: Aldine.

Rosenthal, M., Griffith, E.R., Bond, M.R., & Miller, J.D. (Eds.). (1983). *Rehabilitation of head injured adults.* Philadelphia: F.A. Davis.

Ruff, R.M. (1986). *San Diego Neuropsycological Battery.* Unpublished test manual, University of California, San Diego.

Ruff, R.M., Baser, C.A., Johnston, J.W., Marshall, L.F., Klauber, S.K., Klauber, M.R., & Minteer, M. (1989). Neuropsychological rehabilitation: An experimental study with head injured patients. *Journal of Head Trauma Rehabilitation, 4,* 20–36.

Ruff, R.M., Cullum, C.M., & Luerssen, T.G. (1989). Brain imaging and neuropsychological outcome in traumatic head injury. In E.D. Bigler, R.A. Yeo, & E. Turkheimer (Eds.), *Neuropsychological function and brain imaging* (pp. 276–280). New York: Plenum.

Ruff, R. M., Evans, R., & Green, R. (1986). Long term remediation of head injured patients. In J.A. Blumenthal & D.C. McKee (Eds.), *Applications in behavioral medicine and health psychology: A clinician's source book* (pp. 271–298). Sarasota, FL: Professional Resource Exchange.

Ruff, R. M., Evans, R.W., & Light, R.H. (1986). Automatic detection vs. controlled search: A paper and pencil approach. *Perceptual and Motor Skills, 62,* 407-416.

Schweder, T., & Spjotvoll, E. (1982). Plots of *p*-values to evaluate many tests simultaneously. *Biometrika, 69,* 493–502.

Telch, M.J. (1981). The present status of outcome studies: A reply to Frank. *Journal of Consulting and Clinical Psychology, 49,* 472–475.

Wilson, B., & Moffatt, N. (1984). *Clinical management of memory problems.* Rockville, MD: Aspen Publications.

Yeaton, W.H., & Sechrest, L. (1981). Critical dimensions in the choice and maintenance of successful treatments: Strength, integrity, and effectiveness. *Journal of Consulting and Clinical Psychology, 49,* 156–167.

SECTION III

Aspects of Rehabilitation in the Community

CHAPTER 7

Daily Living Skills
The Foundation of Community Living

Robin McNeny

The performance of activities of daily living requires a complex balance of physical, cognitive, and perceptual skills. Head injury typically disrupts many of these skill areas and results in a loss of functional ability (Panikoff, 1983). The process of retraining the specific skills and regaining the fine balance required for independence can take a considerable period of time. Essential to this process is the intervention of trained professionals who guide and direct recovery. Helpful to the process is a network of supportive family and friends eager to be trained.

The best foundation is laid for community reintegration when the adult with head injury has achieved independence in basic self-care and in some advanced living skills. Those for whom independence is not possible are best prepared when a compensatory system that allows for needs to be met and tasks completed has been firmly established. These compensatory systems can take many and varied formats and are the product of collaborative efforts between client, family, and clinician.

Addressing the needs of the adult with head injury seeking community reintegration is quite complex. Much time, talent, and energy from many sources must be devoted to the recovery of daily living skills. Because the intervention is so multifaceted, the best assessment and intervention is provided by a specialized team of clinicians sensitive to the unique needs of those with head injury.

ASSESSMENT

The assessment of activities of daily living is a continual process. When a person with head injury is first seen in the acute care setting, the occupational therapist is most concerned with the individual's ability to feed him or herself, the individual's ability to attend to basic grooming, and the many physical problems associated with acute head injury. During the rehabilitation phase, therapy is directed toward maximizing independence in basic self-care. As improvements in function occur, rehabilitation may be focused on retraining advanced living skills. The retraining continues in the outpatient or day rehabilitation setting and may still be addressed in the transitional living program.

Many functional assessments have been developed to allow measurement of daily living skill performance. Among these are the Functional Capacity Evaluation (Jette, 1980), the Klein-Bell Scale (Klein & Bell, 1982), the PECS (Harvey & Jellinek, 1983), and the Comprehensive Evaluation of Basic Living Skills (Casanova & Ferber, 1976). There is at present no widely used assessment, standardized or nonstandardized, designed strictly for persons with head injury though research is headed in that direction. Until such an instrument is available, it is important that the head injury treatment team determine the type of functional assessment best suited to its needs and utilize it consistently.

When assessing the daily living skills of a person with head injury, the clinician should carefully observe task performance, analyzing it to determine the cause of breakdown in independence. It is critical to successful retraining that the therapist know where the individual is experiencing difficulty so therapy can be focused on that specific skill area. For example, if the individual has difficulty opening boxes and packages during meal preparation due to decreased fine motor skills, a portion of therapy can be directed toward improving fine motor skills.

BASIC SELF-CARE SKILLS

The essentials of day-to-day function are the basic self-care skills of feeding, dressing, hygiene, and transfers. Clearly, maximal independence in these skills is important for successful community reintegration.

Feeding

Feeding involves three components: oral-motor ability, physical ability, and cognitive/behavioral skills. Deficits in any of these areas will impair independent function in feeding.

Oral-motor deficits such as dysphagia, poor control of secretions, or weakened musculature are addressed by the treatment team early in rehabilitation (Logemann, 1983). For most persons with head injury, improvements do occur in oral-motor skills and the diet is normalized in time to ordinary food. There are those, however, who must remain on pureed diets or who continue with specific oral-motor problems. These individuals find a return to social dining more difficult. The treatment team therefore should provide such an individual and his or her family with instructions on meal preparation and ideas for managing public dining with a minimum of inconvenience and embarrassment.

Coordination deficits, hemiplegia, spasticity, and decreased strength are physical deficits that limit utensil use during feeding. In addition, impaired balance, sensory deficits, facial fractures, and visual disorders may interfere as well. Intensive intervention by the treatment team typically yields improvements in these areas. At times, adaptive aids may be employed to facilitate independence when physical problems interfere. The treatment team should attempt to make these aids and devices as innocuous as possible to increase their acceptability to the client. Likewise, it is important to successful community reintegration that the individual be comfortable using these aids in all feeding situations.

Deficits in behavior, cognitive function, and perceptual function typically have the greatest impact on reintegration into social dining. Specialized environments may be necessary to enhance successful feeding. Therapy should be directed toward retraining acceptable table behavior, reducing agitation, and reducing impulsivity if these are problematic. Certainly this is best done when peer pressure from other head-injured and perhaps noninjured individuals of similar age are present in a group for meals. Inappropriate behaviors such as burping, messiness, and open-mouth chewing are discouraged. Self-monitoring of table behavior is encouraged.

Among the last feeding subskill to return following head injury is the ability to sustain social conversation during meals. When less attention is required by the individual to accomplish the mechanics of self-feeding, the therapist is wise to institute social dining components into meals. Families should do likewise. Mastering this skill is very important to community reintegration, as much social and even business interaction occurs around the table (McNeny, 1990).

Dressing

The perceptual, cognitive, and physical sequelae of head injury may well limit independence in dressing. The occupational therapist typically evaluates dressing skills during the inpatient rehabilitation phase. While physical deficits such as hemiplegia, impaired balance, and incoordination may slow performance, they usually do not prevent independence in dressing (Baum, 1981). While many perceptual deficits seen early do improve, such as impaired body scheme and right/left disorientation, there are others that linger and if severe, may prohibit full independence. These might include an apraxia, a neglect, or a figure-ground misperception. Impaired memory, sequencing, and organization; impulsivity; and decreased initiation and problem solving will all limit dressing skills. To facilitate independence, the therapist should focus on techniques to overcome the cognitive deficits found to limit function. The ideal goal of this retraining is to enable the individual to dress independently, in a functional amount of time, without the assist of another. However, achievement of this goal is not always possible.

Regardless of the amount of training, some adults with head injury fail to become fully independent with dressing and undressing. While for some individuals the primary problem limiting dressing is physical, it is usually cognitive impairment that limits them. A failure to monitor quality during dressing may result in a sloppy appearance. Also, because planning skills are impaired, the individual may fail to purchase the proper clothes for a social or business event.

Involved clinicians need to be alert to the specific needs of the adult with head injury and provide specialized intervention to meet these needs. As the individual progresses from one facility to the next toward community reintegration, clinicians should establish contact and discuss these specialized treatment programs to facilitate carry-over. Naturally, families should be instructed in these programs to ensure carry-over in the home.

Hygiene

One's physical appearance plays an important role in the social and business world. For this reason, it is advisable that intervention focused on hygiene needs begin early in rehabilitation and be refined as recovery proceeds.

Adaptive aids will usually address any physical impairment impeding performance. However, lack of initiative, disinterest, impaired organization and sequencing, impulsivity, and poor quality control are much more difficult to remediate. It is important for hygiene to become a part of the daily routine, whether in the hospital, at home, or in a transitional facility. Establishing a routine is particularly important if time management is a problem. A cue card or checklist in the bathroom is helpful for some persons. Others benefit from keeping all tools and products needed for hygiene in a central location.

Family and staff are of most benefit when they reinforce the importance of the hygiene schedule. Also, the family can and should provide feedback to the individual on his or her appearance, particularly when he or she looks well groomed. Likewise, the individual should receive feedback when shoddy efforts have resulted in an less-than-optimal appearance.

Transfers

Impaired mobility following head injury need not exclude independent living. Many mobility-impaired adults with head injury can learn independent and safe transfers to and from the bed, wheelchair, tub, toilet, and car/bus. If equipment is necessary for bathroom transfers, it should be available both in the living environment and at work or school. Environmental barriers in the workplace should be addressed by the occupational therapist in conjunction with the employer. In addition, attention should be given to transfers to a car or public transportation, whichever is pertinent.

Clearly, the ability to cross streets or at least obtain help in crossing intersections is a major aspect of community integration. Rusch and Mithaug (1980) present an instructional program sequence of skills necessary for street crossing in Figure 7.1.

Throughout transfer training, independence and safety should be stressed. Equipment should be convenient and unobtrusive. Also, those with whom the individual will be working, socializing, and living should be comfortable with the transfers with which they may be involved.

ADVANCED LIVING SKILLS

Advanced living skills are those activities that enable one to function within the home and community. Independence in these skills contribute to successful community reintegration (Neistadt & Marques, 1984). Adults with head injury who suffer from moderate to severe cognitive, perceptual, and/or physical deficits will have the most difficult time regaining independence in these skills. Predictions regarding the individual's ultimate level of independence are impossible to make as there are many variables that affect the final outcome. In addition, the recovery process can be quite lengthy and progress slow.

Domestic and home-living skills constitute a significant part of independent living. The cat-

Date: _____ Phase: _____ Session: _____

Trainer: _____ Trainee: _____

INSTRUCTIONAL ASSISTANCE

Code	Level of assistance	Specific physical assistance	Verbal cue
5	None	None	None
4	Verbal cue	None	"Listen"
3	Verbal cue and model	Point prompt	"Watch me"
2	Verbal cue and prompt	Nudges	"You do it"
1	Verbal cue and physical assistance	Total	"Do it with me"

	Tasks/trials	1	2	3	4	5	6	7	8	Total	Average
Approach	1. Walk to curb										
	2. Stop at curb										
Look	3. Look behind										
	4. Look in front										
	5. Look left										
	6. Look right										
Step	7. Wait for cars										
	8. Step off curb										
Walk	9. Walk quickly across street										
	10. Step on curb										

Figure 7.1. Crossing uncontrolled intersection recording form. From *Vocational training for mentally retarded adults: A behavior analytic approach* (p. 136) by F.R. Rusch and D.E. Mithaug, 1980, Champaign, IL: Research Press. Copyright © 1980 by the authors. Reprinted by permission.

egorization of these skills found in Table 7.1 may be helpful to the practitioner who is helping the head-injured client assess his or her needs.

As part of the planning process, the therapist, the person with head injury, and the family should meet to fully assess the life-style of the individual and to establish relevant goals. Those activities vital to the individual should be highlighted. Without this step, much time, money, and effort may be wasted pursuing irrelevant goals.

Communication Skills

Communication skills involve writing, phone use, and typing. Writing difficulties may arise from incoordination of the upper extremities, loss of dominance, impulsivity, and perseveration. Perceptual dysfunctions (i.e., inattention, field cuts, and constructional apraxia) also may impair writing performance. These areas are typically addressed during rehabilitation but they can persist over the long term and thus contribute to trouble at school or work.

When illegibility or slow performance are problems in writing, then alternatives to writing as a mode of expression or record keeping should be explored. A hand-held memo-writing device may be of assistance if illegibility is the problem. Using a tape recorder rather than taking notes or writing messages may be an alternative at work, school, or home.

Managing difficulties with the telephone is also relatively easy. The local phone company can be of assistance if physical deficits are interfering. Therapists should work with head-injured persons to ensure consistently accurate dialing/button pushing and the use of appropriate phone features (e.g., putting callers on hold, transferring calls). Phone etiquette including taking messages, soliciting information, and

Table 7.1. Domestic/home-living activities and skills

Safety skills[a]

1. Simple first aid
2. Use of phone for emergencies (e.g., fire, police, doctor)
3. Avoiding hazardous substances and activities
4. Requesting assistance when necessary

General housekeeping/maintenance skills[a]

1. Dusting
2. Vacuuming
3. Mopping
4. Sweeping
5. Emptying trash in appropriate receptacle
6. Cleaning windows
7. Changing light bulbs and fuses
8. Caring for/maintaining equipment

Clothing, care and use

1. Sorting, washing, and drying clothes
2. Ironing
3. Folding
4. Putting clothes in appropriate storage
5. Mending
6. Selecting weather-appropriate clothes
7. Selecting color/pattern-coordinated clothes
8. Selecting activity-appropriate clothes
9. Selecting age-appropriate clothes
10. Dressing

Bathroom activities

Personal care
1. Washing face and hands
2. Bathing and drying
3. Washing hair
4. Brushing hair
5. Brushing teeth
6. Shaving
7. Using deodorant
8. Menstrual care
9. Using the toilet

Cleaning
1. Washing tub/shower and sink
2. Scouring toilet
3. Cleaning mirror
4. Mopping
5. Storing supplies

Bedroom activities/skills

1. Making bed
2. Changing bed linens regularly
3. Engaging in solitary leisure activities
4. Dressing for bed
5. Sleeping
6. Cleaning room

(continued)

Table 7.1 (*continued*)

Kitchen skills

Food preparation
1. Selecting appropriate foods
2. Following a recipe
3. Measuring
4. Using utensils (e.g., spatula, mixing spoon)
5. Using appliances
6. Using stove
7. Setting the table

Kitchen organization
1. Identifying needed kitchen supplies for purchase
2. Categorizing food groups for storage (e.g., freezer foods, canned goods, refrigerator foods)
3. Storing dishes, pans, utensils, and supplies

Meal planning
1. Identifying food groups
2. Planning menus of nutritious combinations of food
3. Selecting appropriate recipes

Clean-up
1. Clearing table
2. Disposing of trash
3. Storing leftovers
4. Washing and drying dishes
5. Returning dishes to appropriate storage places
6. Scouring sink and cleaning counters
7. Sweeping
8. Mopping floor

Eating
1. Using utensils (e.g., spoon, fork, knife, cup)
2. Using napkin
3. Passing food dishes
4. Serving appropriate protions
5. Using table manners
6. Communicating food needs/preferences

Living room/family room activities/skills

1. Socializing with others
2. Engaging in leisure activities such as operating and watching television, operating record player, and operating radio
3. Cleaning (listed under General housekeeping/maintenance skills[a])

Yard care skills

1. Grass mowing
2. Pruning
3. Shoveling snow
4. Planting
5. Weeding
6. Watering

making emergency calls should be assessed and trained. If memory is a problem, a strategy notebook used for troubleshooting can be devised and kept handy. Use of a phone directory is also important but if cognitive deficits interfere with proficiency with the directory, alternative systems may be established. A small personal phone directory or a list of commonly called numbers kept by the phone can be helpful. An electronic phone dialer also can aid clients with cognitive impairments by eliminating the need to recall phone numbers.

If typing is a required skill for school or office functions, retraining may be needed. Competency in machine operations and the importance of accuracy and proofreading should be emphasized. Ever-advancing technology has made available typewriters suitable for nearly all physically disabled persons. In addition, features such as spelling checks, memories, and display screens can aid with some cognitive deficits.

Money Management

Many cognitive skills are required for independent money management. The physical deficits that make picking up coins, writing checks, and using a calculator difficult are fairly easily managed through specific therapy and adaptive aids. However, when impaired attention, impulsivity, decreased organizational skills, illogical reasoning, and impaired decision making are problems, retraining is much more difficult (Kreutzer, Coulter, Lent, & McNeny, 1986).

A logical progression of retraining from simple to complex skills should be employed. Once competency is attained using bills and coins in a clinic setting, then shopping trips can be incorporated into the program. It is important to observe how well the individual shops. Does the person examine merchandise for quality? Is the budgeting of available resources satisfactory? Do the heightened noise and distractions of the typical retail environment interfere with performance? Is a written shopping list required? Is topographical orientation adequate? Does the person stay on task and avoid distractions? Repeated excursions should serve to enhance performance in all of these areas.

Managing checking and savings accounts should be reviewed as appropriate. Accuracy in check writing, register maintenance, and handling banking transactions and reconciliation should be stressed. The individual's family should be involved throughout the process so they can encourage the proper amount of independence with banking.

Even with the best training, however, complete independence in financial management may be an unattainable goal for some persons with head injury. When it appears supervision and/or assistance will be needed from another person, the clinician should guide the family. Through education, the family can learn to offer the proper amount of assistance while allowing the individual maximal control of his or her finances.

Time Management

Vital to independent living is the ability to schedule one's day incorporating work, self-maintenance, home maintenance, and social/leisure pursuits. Following head injury, it is often difficult for individuals to perform this task without assistance. Intervention should begin as the clinician guides the individual to establish and maintain a daily schedule. The entire day should be scheduled, from waking to bedtime. Writing down the schedule aids with memory deficits and provides a concrete, consistent source of information for the individual.

The individual should be given increasing responsibility for establishing the schedule and selecting appropriate activities. It is important for persons with head injury to relearn how to make decisions about the use of their time. It is also important to teach them how to balance activities to allow sufficient time for completion of all necessary activities (e.g., too much time spent with friends playing cards may result in too little time devoted to doing laundry or grocery shopping).

Homemaking

When the issue of independent living arises after head injury those involved begin to question who will fix the meals, take care of the laundry, and perform cleaning chores. For some persons with head injury the best solution is to arrange for help with these tasks. However there are many head-injured persons who can relearn these skills and perform them quite ably.

Physical and/or cognitive deficits may limit performance in homemaking. Adaptive aids or compensatory techniques may solve the physical problems. Unfortunately, addressing the cognitive problems is not always so simple.

Cooking requires that the individual be oriented, able to follow at least simple directions, and able to perform the task safely. Each person will have his or her own set of deficits related to cooking. Therefore, the best clinical management and intervention is done on an individual basis. When instruction is tailor-made to meet the particular need of an individual, then specific suggestions can be employed to enhance success.

If supervision is needed for meal planning and grocery shopping, the therapist might suggest this be done weekly at a specific time. To minimize effort and time spent preparing meals, the therapist might propose the use of boxed mixes and frozen foods. Having a hot lunch in the employee cafeteria and a sandwich at home for supper might be a solution for another individual.

Time should also be set aside on the weekly schedule for doing laundry. As needed, vacuuming, dusting, mopping floors, and other home maintenance tasks should be taught. Throughout the training period, safety, quality control, initiative, problem solving, and time management should be addressed.

Driving and Transportation

Driving is a complex, multidimensional activity requiring finely tuned motor, cognitive, and perceptual abilities. The decision regarding a head-injured person's readiness to drive should be made by a knowledgeable treatment team after careful consideration of the individual's assets and liabilities. Though our society depends heavily on the private car for mobility, the health care professional should not feel pressured to permit driving too early in recovery.

Once driving is permitted, a comprehensive driving evaluation must be performed by a driving evaluator. This evaluation should include assessment of physical skills, visual skills, perceptual function, speed of motor responses, and judgment. Deficits in any of these areas may well prohibit driving (Jones, Giddens, & Croft, 1983).

There are other aspects of driving that should be considered. The individual should be able to judge traveling time to allow for punctual arrivals. He or she should be able to follow travel directions, whether in written or verbal form. Some skill reading a map should be developed. In addition, routine automobile maintenance (e.g., dispensing gasoline and changing tires) and the management of automotive crises (e.g., sudden breakdown or an accident) should be reviewed. Even recalling where one's car keys have been placed or where the car is parked can be problematic. Clients with head injury may be taught to place keys in the same spot upon entering the house, or always to park in a specific spot at work or at the mall. Written reminders might be necessary to facilitate use of these strategies.

For some persons with head injury, driving is not a viable option whether due to post-traumatic epilepsy, severe motor deficits, or visual disturbance. These persons may well benefit from training in the use of public transportation. The mechanics of using a bus or cab should be taught and may be sufficient for many individuals. Others will require specific remediation strategies to aid them in managing a particular problem area. It might be suggested that the individual keep the bus or cab company's phone number by the phone or in his or her wallet. It might also be necessary for the individual to write down the fees for the bus or cab services to keep them handy. Always boarding and disembarking at the same stops for specific trips (e.g., shopping, work, or a visit home) might aid someone who is easily confused. It might be helpful to keep this information written down and stored in a wallet as a backup. Routinely keeping fare money in a specific pocket might also improve organization at the moment of boarding. The clinician should assist the individual in establishing, adapting, and learning his or her own unique transportation routine.

Social Skills

A head injury often changes very dramatically the personality and social nature of a person. Inappropriate and socially insensitive behavior may become the rule rather than the exception. Childlike behavior may replace the mature demeanor of a middle-age adult; consequently, role reversals within the family unit often occur. Self-confidence may be replaced with fear, anxieties, and self-doubt. The treatment team needs to address these issues, and aid the individual and the family and employer as well in coping with them. This is a continual process that may continue for years as new problems arise.

Family education should begin early and continue throughout the recovery process. Family concerns should be welcomed by the clinician and addressed promptly. Further, family members should be taught to keep their relationships with the head-injured person as normal and age appropriate as possible (Lezak, 1978). Treatment staff should model appropriate interactions with head-injured persons. Families and employers can be taught how to cope with head-injured individuals' unreasonable and demanding behavior, agitation, confusion, childishness, fearfulness, and/or frustration. Community-based support groups are also helpful for some families.

In addition, care should be given to teaching social skills strategies to the individual with head injury. A group training approach is often useful for such training. The training should include programing designed to heighten the individual's social perceptiveness and attention to social situations. Practice in specific situations involving vocational, avocational, and social scenario may serve to improve the individual's competency. Videotaping social encounters can provide useful, concrete feedback on performance. Allowing others in the social skills group a chance to critique one another's performance provides additional feedback for each participant while providing an opportunity for each person to practice giving feedback.

Throughout the social skills training process, the treatment staff should offer immediate cues and/or assistance when social problems arise. As community reintegration occurs, responsibility for providing the head-injured persons with feedback should shift to the family, colleagues, and/or friends.

CONCLUSION

The process of retraining competency in daily living skills is complex and stretches over a considerable period of time. Before the retraining process is completed, a host of professional clinicians, as well as the head-injured person's family, friends, employer, and co-workers may find themselves involved in the process to some degree.

Not every person with head injury reaches full independence in all aspects of daily living skills, but a high level of function is possible for many. Adaptive aids or techniques, specific cognitive remediation strategies, and/or some creative use of alternate approaches to function may be necessary. It is hoped that the head-injured person and his or her support system can learn to live with these alternative plans. However, if they are found to be awkward, uncomfortable, or embarrassing, new solutions should be sought.

Rehabilitation professionals, the person with head injury and his or her family must work cooperatively to meet the challenges posed by head injury. Deficits in daily living skills are not quickly or easily remediated and require the vigilance, responsiveness, and creativity of all involved. Although many obstacles to progress may arise, many head-injured persons will experience accomplishments leading them on the road to successful reintegration.

REFERENCES

Baum, B. (1981). Relationship between constructional praxis and dressing in the head injured adult. *American Journal of Occupational Therapy, 35,* 438.

Casanova, J.S., & Ferber, J. (1976). Comprehensive Evaluation of Basic Living Skills. *American Journal of Occupational Therapy, 76,* 101.

Harvey, R., & Jellinek, H. (1983). Patient profiles: Utilization in functional performance assessment. *Archives of Physical Medicine and Rehabilitation, 64*, 268–271.

Jett, A.M. (1980). Functional Capacity Evaluation: An empirical approach. *Archives of Physical Medicine and Rehabilitation, 61*, 85.

Jones, R., Giddens, H., & Croft, D. (1983). Assessment and training of brain-damaged drivers. *American Journal of Occupational Therapy, 37*, 754.

Klein, R.M., & Bell, B.J. (1982). Self care skills: Behavioral measurement with the Klein-Bell Scale. *Archives of Physical Medicine and Rehabilitation, 63*, 335.

Kreutzner, J., Coulter, S., Lent, B., & McNeny, R. (1986). A glossary of cognitive rehabilitation terminology. *Cognitive Rehabilitation, 4*, 10.

Lezak, M.D. (1978). Living with the charac-

teriological altered brain injured patient. *Journal of Clinical Psychiatry, 39*, 592.

Logemann, J. (1983). *Evaluation and treatment of swallowing disorders.* San Diego: College-Hill Press.

McNeny, R. (1990). Activities of daily living. In M. Rosenthal, E.R. Griffith, M.R. Bond, & J.D. Miller (Eds.), *Rehabilitation of the adult and child with traumatic brain injury* (2nd ed.) (pp. 193–205). Philadelphia: F.A. Davis.

Neistadt, M.E., & Marques, K. (1984). An independent living skills training program. *American Journal of Occupational Therapy, 38*, 671.

Panikoff, L. (1983). Recovery trends of functional skills in the head injured adult. *American Journal of Occupational Therapy, 37*, 735.

Rusch, F., & Mithaug, D. (1980). *Vocational training for mentally retarded adults: A behavior analytic approach.* Champaign, IL: Research Press.

CHAPTER 8

Transitional Living Centers in Head Injury Rehabilitation

Corwin Boake

The need for postacute rehabilitation for survivors of head injury is dictated by the nature of recovery after severe head injury. The average 45-day length of stay in acute head injury rehabilitation (Carey, Seibert, & Posavac, 1988) is sufficient to advance most severely injured patients beyond the need for hospital care, but too short to gain the maximal benefit from rehabilitation. Although most individuals can live at home after discharge from acute rehabilitation and attend therapies on an outpatient basis, it is generally difficult to provide or coordinate the appropriate services within a multidisciplinary clinic serving many disability groups. There is a large gap between the skills taught in most outpatient clinics and the skills needed to live and work in the community.

Postacute head injury rehabilitation programs provide day or residential services that are designed to bridge this gap between institutions and the community. The rationale for postacute residential treatment programs (better known as "transitional living centers") is that they are the most appropriate or feasible method of postacute rehabilitation for some clients. In particular, clients who require intensive training may be most effectively treated in a 24-hour residential program. Many other clients do not require such intensive treatment, but rather are appropriate for residential programs because they cannot live at home or do not have access to postacute day treatment programs in their communities.

Recognition of the need for postacute rehabilitation has involved changes in the accepted goals and time span of head injury rehabilitation. First, the scope of postacute rehabilitation includes training of functional skills such as daily living activities and work performance, and is broader than the basic abilities typically addressed in acute rehabilitation. Functional skills training seeks to improve clients' competence in community settings, rather than to reverse the severity of their underlying impairments. Second, the time span for postacute rehabilitation is much longer than for acute rehabilitation. This view was not supported by earlier studies of recovery from head injury, which showed that clients' level of functioning usually reached a plateau by 6 months or at most 1 year postinjury (Bond & Brooks, 1976). However, these studies did not directly measure change in performance of functional, goal-oriented activities needed to maintain a residence or job. It is now known that improvement in performance of functional skills may occur over a much longer time span. For example, in Thomsen's (1984) study of severe head injury survivors in Denmark, considerable improvement was seen over a long interval between an initial follow-up at 2½ years postinjury and a later follow-up 10–15 years postinjury, although most of the clients did not receive formal rehabilitation during this time. The percent of individuals living independently increased from 8% at the first follow-up to 48% at the

The author would like to thank Nancy Seward for sharing her survey results, and Dr. Randall Evans and Patti Thomas for their helpful comments.

second. Thus the time span for recovery of functional skills may be much longer than for basic neurological and neuropsychological capacities.

Since 1978 there has been a rapid increase in the number of transitional living centers for survivors of head injury. The rate at which new centers have opened is difficult to estimate because there have been few formal surveys. However, some indication of the growth rate can be obtained by comparing two recent surveys. Seward (1985) listed a total of 34 transitional living centers located in the United States. These centers had been in operation an average of 2 years at the time of the survey. By comparison, the two most recent editions of the *National Directory of Head Injury Rehabilitation Services* (National Head Injury Foundation [NHIF], 1988, 1989) listed respectively, 103 and 137 transitional living centers in this country. The fact that the Center for Comprehensive Services, the oldest existing transitional living center for adults with head injury, opened in 1977 illustrates the brief history of this form of rehabilitation. Transitional-type programs were used in the rehabilitation of head-injured veterans of World War II (e.g., Rowbotham, 1945) but these programs were closed soon after the war and have had little impact on contemporary transitional centers.

The goal of this chapter is to outline the basic principles of transitional living centers for clients with head injury and to discuss important issues such as admission criteria, goal setting, and strategies of retraining living skills. The final section in this chapter discusses the need for program evaluation and the impact of newer postacute rehabilitation programs on the future of transitional centers. (Further discussion and alternative viewpoints about transitional living centers can be found in Fralish, 1988, and Moore & Plovnick, 1988.)

DEFINITION AND GOALS OF TRANSITIONAL LIVING CENTERS

The NHIF (1988) *National Directory of Head Injury Rehabilitation Services* defines the goals of a transitional living program as follows:

> . . . primary emphasis is to provide training for a living situation of greater independence. There is a

greater focus on compensating for skills that cannot be restored in an emphasis on functional skills to live in the community as a transitional step into the community. The typical length of stay is 4 to 18 months. (p. 347)

This length of stay is in agreement with the average of 12 months noted in Seward's (1985) survey of transitional living centers. Some of the questions left open by the NHIF definition are better specified in a definition provided by Sachs (1986):

> A transitional living program for head injured adults provides a short-term set of treatments that promote evaluation and development of the clients' practical independence and psychological independence within a supervised residence that challenges the clients with daily living activities and adult responsibilities, and leads to reentry into the community or to a long-term supervised program. (p. 6)

Both definitions agree that the goal of the transitional living center is to train clients to live in more independent, community-based living situations. The transition may be from a rehabilitation hospital to the family home, or from the family home to a supervised apartment. The transition may even be within the home, to a lesser degree of dependence on assistance or supervision by family members. In Seward's (1985) survey, most of the clients in transitional centers were discharged to their family homes or to independent community residences.

The concept of transition distinguishes the transitional center from other types of postacute rehabilitation programs that are primarily oriented toward behavioral change, employment, or long-term residential placement. In behavioral programs, the primary goal is to change the behavioral problems that prevent clients from progressing in other rehabilitation programs. In vocational programs, the primary goal is to improve clients' employability and not to change clients' living situations. The goal of long-term residential programs is to provide living settings that are not time limited and do not necessarily lead to living settings that are more independent.

Location of Transitional Centers

A point that is not fully specified by either of the previous definitions is the type of physical facility and area where transitional centers should be located. Sachs (1986) specified that programs should be housed in supervised residences (i.e., dormitories, group homes, and apartments with availability of staff supervision or assistance for daily living activities), so that clients could be given more responsibility for performing daily living skills. Seward (1985) reported that transitional centers maintained an average of 18 beds, in both private and double rooms, but did not report the types of facilities in which these were located. A widespread view is that transitional centers should be housed in family homes or apartment buildings because most clients must generalize skills to similar settings after discharge (Giles & Shore, 1988; Sachs, 1986). This view is also consistent with the normalization philosophy (Condeluci & Gretz-Lasky, 1987), which seeks to avoid institutionalized settings and other cues that stigmatize persons with disabilities.

A related and controversial issue is the type of area where transitional centers should be located. Obviously clients will have more opportunities to practice skills independently if the center is linked to community resources by public transportation routes. Giles and Shore (1988) recommended that transitional centers should be located within walking distance of banks, shopping, and other essential community resources to be used in retraining. However, many transitional centers are located in rural areas or in areas not reached by public transportation, so that in these centers it is probably more difficult to practice some of the community-related skills needed after discharge. The corresponding view is that it is difficult to meet the staffing and travel requirements for supervised clients, and that it is more cost-efficient to simulate community resources within the transitional center for training purposes (Leland, Lewis, Hinman, & Carrillo, 1988). Centers that contain vocational workshops or "affirmative industries" are consistent with this approach. One issue that has not been considered in this debate is that urban centers are more accessible for clients to receive follow-up services after discharge.

Admission Criteria

Seward (1985) found that most clients were admitted to transitional centers from either re-

habilitation hospitals or their family homes. However, a transitional center will not be appropriate for all individuals upon discharge from acute rehabilitation or even at later times. Transitional centers can use admission criteria to identify clients who are ready to begin the transition into the community. First of all, clients must consent to treatment and must be free of medical problems that would prevent a successful transition. The center may exclude clients who have certain medical problems (e.g., uncontrolled seizures), are not bowel or bladder continent, or need physical assistance for self-care. An age cutoff may automatically apply if state laws require that clients younger than 18 years old attend school. Many centers are not accessible to clients who use wheelchairs, but more centers may wish to accommodate clients who have both head and spinal cord injuries. Most centers accept clients with brain disorders other than head injury (e.g., anoxia, cerebrovascular accident) if the disorders are not progressive.

Additional criteria can be used to set a minimal potential for progress and a maximal risk for problems that could prevent successful transition. The criteria for progress often include sufficient physical endurance to participate in the therapy schedule (e.g., 6 hours per day), functional two-way communication, and sufficient learning ability to show carry-over from training. Some centers have attempted to specify learning potential by requiring that clients' IQs must be above 70 or 80, or that clients must be functioning above Level V on the Rancho Los Amigos Scale (Malkmus, Booth, & Kodimer, 1980). Such IQ-based criteria can be criticized because there is so little evidence about the validity of IQ as a predictor of postacute rehabilitation outcome in persons with head injury.

The usual risk criteria exclude clients who are dangerous to themselves or others; have behavioral problems that might disrupt the operation of the program; or have significant, persisting substance abuse problems. Centers may also exclude clients with histories of major psychiatric disorders. Many clients have unsuccessful transitions because of noncompliance related to poor motivation or unawareness of impairments, but it is unclear how to specify criteria to limit the number of such clients. One controversial solution is to delay admission until 6 months or 1 year postinjury, in the hope that longer postinjury experience will improve clients' awareness and particularly their willingness to accept changes in social or work status. There is evidence for the view that unawareness leads to poorer outcome after acute rehabilitation (e.g., Najenson, Groswasser, Mendelson, & Hackett, 1980), but it might still be the case that some clients would make faster progress if transfer from acute rehabilitation to transitional centers occurred early rather than after a delay.

PROCESS OF TRANSITIONAL REHABILITATION

Clients in rehabilitation transitional centers must have an explicit, consensual goal for their level of independence after discharge. The transitional center can then provide the necessary program of services to enable the client to make the transition to the new living situation.

Outcome Goals

Clear outcome goals are necessary to plan the training programs, secure clients' and families' participation, track clients' progress, anticipate the time of discharge, and arrange supports and services needed after discharge. Outcome goals may also be important for contracting with payers and for maintaining accountability among parties involved (i.e., transitional center, family, and payer). For example, a client's outcome goals might be to live alone in an apartment near his or her family, receive weekly supervision, and return to his or her former workplace in a modified position. If clear goals cannot be determined or agreed upon soon after admission, then optional goals should be identified and a choice made among these when possible. Without goals for the eventual transition, there is a danger the training program will be conducted in an undirected, open-ended fashion until time or funding is exhausted.

Goals that are feasible for clients to reach in transitional rehabilitation depend not only on clients' residual abilities, but also on their available time and funding, motivation, and support systems. For example, if a client requires 2 years of

retraining in order to live independently, but can remain at the transitional center for only 1 year, the goal should be reconsidered. Time limitations can result from motivation and support systems as well as from funding. Often clients are unwilling to commit for long periods of time, and lengthy separations may weaken marital or family relationships. The goal of improving quality of life should not be sacrificed to achieve the highest level of independence possible. Motivation and support systems must also be considered in setting outcome goals. Motivation will affect the rate of progress, and discharge plans should not require the client's support system to provide unrealistic amounts of assistance or supervision.

Transitional Strategies

The goal of transitional centers is to train clients to live in more independent settings than before admission. Different living settings can be ranked according to level of independence, as in Table 8.1. Similar lists are provided by Baker, Seltzer, and Seltzer (1977) and by Sohlberg and Mateer (1989). Each level of independence corresponds with a living setting in the community and requires the client to perform certain living skills, with a given degree of assistance or supervision. Each client's level of functioning upon admission corresponds with one of the living settings, and the client's projected living setting after discharge corresponds to a higher level of functioning. As clients reach higher levels of functioning through rehabilitation, they should become capable of residing in living settings that are more independent. The particular skills required for each living setting can serve as short-term goals or intermediate objectives during transitional rehabilitation. Progress in transitional rehabilitation can be measured by the client's successful performance in more independent residential settings. To complete the client's transition, the center must provide a final residential setting similar to the client's projected postdischarge living setting.

However, transitional centers generally can provide residential settings corresponding to some, but not most, levels of independence. For example, a center might include a dormitory, a

Table 8.1. Levels of independence in living settings

Level	Example of living setting
Independent	Live in own home or family home without monitoring
Monitoring	Live in own home; daily to weekly monitoring visits by family members or aide
Part-time supervision	Live in family home without daytime supervision (caregivers may work outside home), or live in supervised apartment with supervision or assistance as needed; independent in community mobility
Group home	Live in group home with full-time staff; partly independent in community mobility
Full-time supervision	Live in family home with full-time supervision or assistance by family member, or live in own home with full-time attendant
Institution	Requires nursing care, or restricted from community due to behavior

group home, and a few supervised apartments. Another center might include a group home, supervised apartments, and one or two unsupervised transitional apartments. The fewer the number of residential settings a center can provide, the more the center will be forced to place clients at different levels of functioning into the same residential settings. The extreme case occurs in centers that can provide only one residential setting (e.g., dormitory, group home) for all clients. When clients living in the same setting are at significantly different levels of functioning, the center may use an incentive system in which higher functioning clients are rewarded with privileges to exercise greater independence and choice of activities. Blackerby (1988) described an incentive system used in a transitional living center in which clients gained higher levels of privileges by earning points for appropriate social behaviors.

For programs that can provide more residential settings, there are at least three paths for clients to make the transition to their projected living settings. First, clients can enter the program at the least independent residential setting and move to more independent settings as their level of functioning improves. For example, if a center includes a dormitory, a group home, and supervised apartments, all clients are first admitted to the dormitory. The major advantage of this strategy is that clients can be closely evaluated during the first weeks following admission, especially when there are risks from behavioral problems. In addition, many clients might be rewarded by frequent promotions to more independent living situations. The major potential disadvantage is that clients can become demoralized if they must sacrifice independence compared with their preadmission living setting. For example, a client who lives in his or her family home, requires no daytime supervision, and is independent in neighborhood mobility might be admitted to a dormitory with 24-hour supervision and less independence and responsibility than at home. A second disadvantage is that clients' time may be used unproductively before they are challenged to reach higher levels of functioning. Centers using this strategy may compromise by having an initial evaluation period, during which clients' may have limited independence, and then placing clients in the appropriate residential setting once the evaluation is complete.

A second transition path is to admit clients to the living settings corresponding to their current levels of functioning. For example, the client in the previous example could be admitted to the group home or supervised apartment, if available, rather than to the more restrictive dormitory. The advantages of this strategy are that time is spent productively and that the procedure appears logical and fair. The major disadvantages are that opportunities for close evaluation may be missed and that the initial living situation may be assigned incorrectly, because of faulty information about clients' levels of functioning. However, these difficulties might be avoided if clients go through an initial evaluation period.

A third transition path is to place clients into

apartments directly upon admission, while providing needed assistance and supervision for them to reside there successfully. Living skills training takes place in the apartment setting throughout the length of stay at the center. As clients gain in skills, less staff assistance is offered, in the same way that job coaching is faded in supported employment. This approach requires that clients have a viable outcome goal of living independently or in a supervised apartment. The advantages are that clients might be motivated by living in their own apartments and might take more initiative in completing their own daily routines than in following a group schedule. The major disadvantage is that the approach is labor-intensive for staff and therefore not cost-effective for some centers and clients. There is an important need to determine which transition path is most effective, and for which type of client.

Strategies for Training Living Skills

The largest component of therapeutic programming in transitional centers consists of living skills training to prepare clients to live in more independent settings. Perhaps the most obvious difference between transitional centers is whether living skills training is accomplished through formal therapy sessions or through functional activities. Therapy sessions include speech therapy, cognitive retraining, physical therapy, occupational therapy, recreational therapy, social skills training, and other treatments. Functional activities are the goal-oriented work duties, chores, errands, and leisure activities that constitute most of one's daily routine. In some transitional centers, clients follow a schedule of chores and work duties (e.g., Seaton, 1985), and may attend no therapy sessions other than group discussions. The staff in such centers may consist largely of paraprofessionals who receive consultation from a smaller number of licensed therapists. In other centers, clients receive much of their training through formal therapy sessions scheduled by the hour. The content of therapy sessions changes over the course of training to address more integrative skills. The staff of such centers must include a sufficient number of licensed therapists to conduct the therapy ses-

sions. Therapy sessions are generally deemphasized during later stages of training, when the priority is to provide clients with community experiences similar to those they encounter after discharge. Most centers fall between these two extreme cases and provide training programs based on a mixture of functional activities and therapy sessions (e.g., Belanger, Berrol, Cole, Fryer, & Lock, 1985; Sohlberg & Mateer, 1989).

Rather than reject therapy sessions categorically, it should be considered whether there are any instances in which this form of training might be helpful. For example, impairments such as dysarthria and hemiparesis can profoundly affect clients' level of independence, yet can often be ameliorated through appropriate therapy. Discharge from acute rehabilitation does not necessarily mark the endpoint of benefit from formal therapy, and one should be cautious not to reject any form of treatment that might raise the level of independence to a significant degree.

However, therapy sessions can be counterproductive if overutilized or if used in place of community practice (Falvey, 1986). Mayer, Keating, and Rapp (1986) discussed how common impairments in head-injured clients, particularly those involving memory and executive functions, can prevent generalization of skills from clinical settings to the community. They recommended that many functional skills be learned as fixed routines, through practice in settings similar to those where the same skills will be used after discharge. To learn food preparation, for example, it is probably more valuable for clients to fix meals in a kitchen than do measurements or sequencing exercises in a classroom. The same reasoning may apply to mobility training through practicing pedestrian and public transportation skills directly in the community (Milton, 1985; Signorat, 1984), as compared to classroom map-reading and time-management exercises. Behavioral issues such as appropriateness, judgment, and work habits might be more difficult to address within the framework of hourly therapy sessions. In training certain skills, however, classroom exercises may be an important step toward community practice. For example, preparation in basic money-management skills (e.g., calculator, checkbook, budgeting form) may help many clients to manage larger sums of money.

Living skills training is a complex subject that involves many issues that cannot be discussed within the scope of this chapter (e.g., access, equipment needs, safety). Detailed discussions of living skills training in postacute rehabilitation are available in Giles and Clark-Wilson (1988) and McNeny (Chapter 7, this volume). Falvey (1986) provided an excellent overview of functional skills training in the education of developmentally disabled students.

Vocational Training

Transition to a more independent living setting is a necessary but not sufficient condition for achieving an adequate quality of life. It is widely accepted that some form of productive activity is also a necessary condition for life satisfaction. For this reason, transitional centers should provide training for clients to engage in vocational or avocational (i.e., unpaid) activity after discharge. Another reason is that clients who do not become employed after discharge from transitional centers generally remain financially dependent and thus cannot afford to live independently. (Vocational training issues are discussed in Chapters 11, 12, and 13 in this volume.)

Vocational training can be conducted in the same transitional approach as living skills training; that is, clients should have vocational outcome goals and should be trained toward transitioning to these work settings. One transitional strategy is for clients to work in community-based "occupational trials" positions (Ben-Yishay, Silver, Piasetsky, & Rattok, 1987) similar to those they will hold after discharge, in the hope of maximizing transferable work experiences. Unfortunately it is difficult to arrange for clients to be paid for working in these temporary placements, which may also involve considerable job coaching by co-workers. In comparison, affirmative industries or workshops may provide more realistic work experiences, in terms of compensation and responsibility, but cannot generally train clients in work skills applicable after discharge. Because many clients will not be eligible for gainful employment after

discharge, the transitional center must prepare such clients for avocational pursuits such as volunteer work. A discussion of issues related to avocational pursuits was provided by Gobble, Dunson, Szekeres, and Cornwall (1987). The most important issue in vocational outcome, however, is obtaining and maintaining clients' job placements in their home communities after discharge, and this may be difficult to accomplish for clients without access to vocational follow-up services.

Socialization and Leisure

Long-term follow-up surveys of survivors of head injury have revealed that social isolation is among their most common problems (Oddy, Coughlan, Tyerman, & Jenkins, 1985). These findings suggest that for clients to achieve an adequate quality of life, transitional centers must provide retraining in social/leisure activities as well as living and work skills. Following a transitional strategy for retraining socialization skills, similar to vocational and living skills, transitional centers should try to engage clients in socialization and leisure activities they can maintain after discharge in their home communities. Responsibility for retraining these skills is usually handled by therapeutic recreation specialists (Fazio & Fralish, 1988), although leisure activities also involve mobility, money-management, and social skills. There is a great need for interventions that can reintegrate clients into the social network of their nondisabled peers and provide alternative leisure and socialization opportunities.

Behavior Management

Clients who are appropriate for transitional centers do not usually have major neurobehavioral syndromes such as explosive rage and hypersexuality. However, milder syndromes of disinhibition, lack of initiative, and denial or unawareness of impairment are common. Because these neurobehavioral problems are often major obstacles to progress and eventually to successful transitions, many transitional centers have adopted elements of the "therapeutic community" model (Ben-Yishay et al., 1985). Recently there has been increased interest in behavior modification as an intervention approach in postacute rehabilitation (e.g., Burke, Wesolowski, & Guth, 1988). Implementation of behavioral programs in transitional centers requires many changes from similar programs in restrictive settings, as discussed by Hogan (1988) and Muir et al. (1983). For example, the desired client behaviors may be rewarded by greater opportunity for independence rather than consumable rewards. External incentives may need to be used carefully to avoid "overcompensating" desired behaviors and distorting natural consequences.

Related Issues

The scope of transitional rehabilitation includes many important issues not discussed in this chapter, among them accreditation (Arakaki, 1988), case management (Dixon, Goll, & Stanton, 1988), family training (Diehl, 1983), substance abuse, and training of paraprofessional staff. Family issues are especially important in transitional centers because family members are usually the clients' long-term advocates and caregivers (Jacobs, 1988), and transitional centers may provide the last opportunity for many family members to be trained for these roles. The fact that paraprofessional staff are responsible for implementing skills training and behavioral interventions in most transitional centers requires centers to make special, ongoing efforts to prepare them for these responsibilities (Moore & Plovnick, 1988).

CONCLUSIONS

The role of transitional living centers in head injury rehabilitation is to provide intensive living skills training to enable clients to live in more independent community settings. Although there is consensus about the goal of transitional rehabilitation, the field has developed rapidly and many fundamental issues remain unresolved. The evidence to resolve these issues is lacking because, as Cope (1985) noted, postacute rehabilitation programs evolved without outcome data to guide program development or demonstrate effectiveness. In the absence of firm evidence, referral and funding of clients in tran-

sitional centers may depend mainly on anecdotal evidence and on the wish to exhaust all therapeutic modalities (Kreutzer & Boake, 1987).

However, there are several program evaluation methods that could easily be implemented in transitional centers to measure their effectiveness. The simplest method is to build a data base that measures clients' levels of independence at the time of admission, discharge, and after some follow-up interval. For example, a center could report the number of clients residing in different types of living settings at discharge and follow-up. A common pitfall, as Goldstein (1942) noted many years ago, is that rehabilitation centers tend to be compared by the proportions of clients living independently or holding competitive employment, without regard to their severity of injury or level of functioning at admission. An alternative approach to program evaluation is to demonstrate cost savings due to postacute rehabilitation compared to no treatment (Sohlberg & Brock, 1985). In any case, pre-post comparison studies of clients' independence (e.g., Fryer & Haffey, 1987) may remain the main source of evaluation data on transitional centers, given the difficulties of recruiting a control group (Aronow, 1987).

Ultimately the role of transitional living centers in head injury rehabilitation will depend not only on evaluation research, but on the availability and cost-effectiveness of alternative postacute rehabilitation programs. Newly developed independent living (Condeluci, Cooperman, & Seif, 1987) and supported employment programs (Wehman, Kreutzer, Wood, Morton, & Sherron, 1988) have the advantage of providing long-term services to clients in their home communities. It would be a major advance in head injury rehabilitation if these long-term, community-based programs could solve the placement and follow-up problems that are so difficult to address in time-limited transitional centers located away from the communities to which clients are discharged. If these new programs are successful, future transitional centers would be encouraged to become community-based resource centers providing long-term placement and follow-up, in addition to their traditional role as centers for retraining living skills.

REFERENCES

Arakaki, A.H. (1988). Traumatic brain injury (TBI): The new delivery system. *Journal of Insurance Medicine, 20*(3), 5–9.

Aronow, H.U. (1987). Rehabilitation effectiveness with severe brain injury: Translating research into policy. *Journal of Head Trauma Rehabilitation, 2* (3), 24–36.

Baker, B.L., Seltzer, G.B., & Seltzer, M.M. (1977). *As close as possible: Community residences for retarded adults.* Boston: Little, Brown.

Belanger, S., Berrol, S., Cole, J., Fryer, J., & Lock, M. (1985). Bay Area Head Injury Recovery Center: A therapeutic community. *Cognitive Rehabilitation, 3*(4), 4–7.

Ben-Yishay, Y., Rattok, J., Lakin, P., Piasetsky, E.B., Ross, B., Silver, S., Zide, E., & Ezrachi, O. (1985). Neuropsychologic rehabilitation: Quest for a holistic approach. *Seminars in Neurology, 5,* 252–264.

Ben-Yishay, Y., Silver, S., Piasetsky, E.B., & Rattok, J. (1987).Relationship between employability and vocational outcome after intensive holistic cognitive rehabilitation. *Journal of Head Trauma Rehabilitation, 2*(1), 35–48.

Blackerby, W.F. (1988). Practical token economies. *Journal of Head Trauma Rehabilitation, 3*(3), 33–45.

Bond, M.R., & Brooks, D.N. (1976). Understanding the process of recovery as a basis for the investigation of rehabilitation for the brain injured. *Scandinavian Journal of Rehabilitation Medicine, 8,* 127–133.

Burke, W.H., Wesolowski, M.D., & Guth, M.L. (1988). Comprehensive head injury rehabilitation: An outcome evaluation. *Brain Injury, 2,* 313–322.

Carey, R.G., Seibert, J.H., & Posavac, E.J. (1988). Who makes the most progress in inpatient rehabilitation? An analysis of functional gain. *Archives of Physical Medicine and Rehabilitation, 69,* 337–343.

Condeluci, A., Cooperman, S., & Seif, B.A. (1987). Independent living: Settings and supports. In M. Ylvisaker & E.M.R. Gobble (Eds.), *Community re-entry for head injured adults* (pp. 301–347). Boston: College-Hill Press.

Condeluci, A., & Gretz-Lasky, S. (1987). Social role valorization: A model for community reentry. *Journal of Head Trauma Rehabilitation, 2*(1), 49–56.

Cope, D.N. (1985). Traumatic closed head injury: Status of rehabilitation treatment. *Seminars in Neurology, 5,* 212–220.

Diehl, L.N. (1983). Patient-family education. In M. Rosenthal, E.R. Griffith, M.R. Bond, & J.D. Miller (Eds.), *Rehabilitation of the head injured adult* (pp. 395–401). Philadelphia: F.A. Davis.

Dixon, T.P., Goll, S., & Stanton, K.M. (1988). Case management issues and practices in head injury re-habilitation. *Rehabilitation Counseling Bulletin, 31,* 325–343.

Falvey, M.A. (1986). *Community-based curriculum: Instructional strategies for students with severe handicaps.* Baltimore: Paul H. Brookes Publishing Co.

Fazio, S.M., & Fralish, K.B. (1988). A survey of leisure and recreation programs offered by agencies serving traumatic head injured adults. *Therapeutic Recreation Journal, 22*(1), 46–54.

Fralish, K. (1988). Transitional living programs. In P.M. Deutsch & K.B. Fralish (Eds.), *Innovations in head injury rehabilitation* (Ch. 14). New York: Matthew Bender.

Fryer, L.J., & Haffey, W. J. (1987). Cognitive rehabilitation and community readaptation: Outcomes from two program models. *Journal of Head Trauma Rehabilitation, 2*(3), 51–63.

Giles, G.M., & Clark-Wilson, J. (1988). Functional skills training in severe brain injury. In I. Fussey & G.M. Giles (Eds.), *Rehabilitation of the severely brain-injured adult: A practical approach* (pp. 69–101). London: Croom Helm.

Giles, G., & Shore, M. (1988). The role of the transitional living center in rehabilitation after brain injury. *Cognitive Rehabilitation, 6*(1), 26–31.

Gobble, E.M.R., Dunson, L., Szekeres, S.F., & Cornwall, J. (1987). Avocational programming for the severely impaired head injured individual. In M. Ylvisaker & E.M.R. Gobble (Eds.), *Community re-entry for head injured adults* (pp. 349–380). Boston: College-Hill Press.

Goldstein, K. (1942). *After-effects of brain injuries in war.* New York: Grune & Stratton.

Hogan, R.T. (1988). Behavior management for community reintegration. *Journal of Head Trauma Rehabilitation, 3*(3), 62–71.

Jacobs, H.E. (1988). The Los Angeles Head Injury Survey: Procedures and initial findings. *Archives of Physical Medicine and Rehabilitation, 69,* 425–431.

Kreutzer, J.S., & Boake, C. (1987). Addressing disciplinary issues in cognitive rehabilitation: Definition, training, and organization. *Brain Injury, 1,* 199–202.

Leland, M., Lewis, F.D., Hinman, S., & Carrillo, R. (1988). Functional retraining of traumatically brain injured adults in a transdisciplinary environment. *Rehabilitation Counseling Bulletin, 31,* 289–297.

Malkmus, D., Booth, B.J., & Kodimer, L. (1980). *Rehabilitation of the head injured adult: Comprehensive cognitive management.* Downey, CA: Professional Staff Association of Rancho Los Amigos Hospital.

Mayer, N.H., Keating, D.J., & Rapp, D. (1986). Skills, routines, and activity patterns of daily living: A functional nested approach. In B.P. Uzzell & Y. Gross (Eds.), *Clinical neuropsychology of intervention* (pp. 205–222). Boston: Martinus Nijhoff.

Milton, S.B. (1985). Compensatory memory strategy

training: A practical approach for managing persisting memory problems. *Cognitive Rehabilitation, 3* (6), 8–16.

Moore, M.K., & Plovnick, N. (1988). Post-acute programs. In P.M. Deutsch & K.B. Fralish (Eds.), *Innovations in head injury rehabilitation* (Ch. 5). New York: Matthew Bender.

Muir, C., Haffey, W.J., Ott, K.J., Karaica, D., Muir, J.H., & Sutko, M. (1983). Treatment of behavioral deficits. In M. Rosenthal, E.R. Griffith, M.R. Bond, & J.D. Miller (Eds.), *Rehabilitation of the head injured adult* (pp. 381–393). Philadelphia: F.A. Davis.

Najenson, T., Groswasser, Z., Mendelson, L., & Hackett, P. (1980). Rehabilitation outcome of brain damaged patients after severe head injury. *International Rehabilitation Medicine, 2,* 17–22.

National Head Injury Foundation. (1988). *National directory of head injury rehabilitation services, 1988 edition.* Southborough, MA: Author.

National Head Injury Foundation. (1989). *National directory of head injury rehabilitation services, 1989 edition.* Southborough, MA: Author.

Oddy, M., Coughlan, T., Tyerman, A.W., & Jenkins, D. (1985). Social adjustment after closed head injury: A further follow-up seven years after injury. *Journal of Neurology, Neurosurgery, and Psychiatry, 48,* 564–568.

Rowbotham, G.F. (1945). *Acute injuries of the head: Their diagnosis, treatment, complications and sequels* (2nd ed.). Baltimore: Williams & Wilkins.

Sachs, P.R. (1986). A family guide to evaluating transitional living programs for head injured adults. *Cognitive Rehabilitation, 4*(6), 6–9.

Seaton, D. (1985). Community reentry for the head injured adult. *Cognitive Rehabilitation, 3*(5), 4–8.

Seward, N.T. (1985). *Residential treatment program survey.* Unpublished manuscript, Mount Vernon Hospital, Alexandria, VA.

Signorat, M. (1984). Orientation and mobility training for the head injured patient. *Cognitive Rehabilitation, 2*(2), 4–7.

Sohlberg, M.M., & Brock, M.S. (1985). Taking the final step: The importance of post-medical cognitive rehabilitation. *Cognitive Rehabilitation, 3* (5), 10–13.

Sohlberg, M.M., & Mateer, C.A. (1989). *Introduction to cognitive rehabilitation: Theory and practice.* New York: Guilford Publications.

Thomsen, I.V. (1984). Late outcome of very severe blunt head trauma: A 10–15 year second follow-up. *Journal of Neurology, Neurosurgery, and Psychiatry, 47,* 260–268.

Wehman, P., Kreutzer, J., Wood, W., Morton, M.V., & Sherron, P. (1988). Supported work model for persons with traumatic brain injury: Toward job placement and retention. *Rehabilitation Counseling Bulletin, 31,* 298–312.

CHAPTER 9

Day Rehabilitation Programming

A Theoretical Model

Randall W. Evans and Brian K. Preston

There is no theoretical "model" for day rehabilitation programming for persons with neurobehavioral sequelae from traumatic brain injury and that is unfortunate. It is unfortunate because, without a sound theoretical perspective for service provision, it is very difficult, if not impossible, to assess program effectiveness or to develop innovative treatment systems.

For the most part, the current situation that prevails in existing day rehabilitation programs is one that emphasizes the provision of traditional therapies (e.g., physical, occupational, speech, psychological, and prevocational) within a "disciplinary" framework. This framework is, no doubt, consequent to an extension of the acute care, medical model mentality. It is the authors' contention that this is a wholly inadequate approach for day treatment, one that will not provide many brain-injured individuals with the necessary skills and training challenges to make a meaningful, generalized impact upon their overall community reentry outcome. Therefore, it the intent of this chapter to present an alternative approach or model with respect to day programming for individuals with brain injury.

With respect to the presentation of an alternative model to day programming, the authors recognize that in this proposal they present components, or ideas, of day *and* residential programs that are familiar to the reader. This is particularly evident when treatment techniques are discussed. However, the model presented is also one that places a genuine emphasis on *management* of the provision of service itself, in addition to the customary *provision* of treatment options. The chapter describes this emphasis on management and, when appropriate, gives examples of program execution within the model.

BACKGROUND INFORMATION

A day *program* for an individual suffering from neurobehavioral sequelae of traumatic brain injury is therapeutically distinct from *outpatient* services. According to the National Head Injury Foundation (NHIF) and the Commission on Accreditation of Rehabilitation Facilities (CARF) a day program "allows the individual to return home to his or her family while continuing to receive intensive rehabilitation" (NHIF, 1985, p. viii). The primary distinction then between day programs and outpatient services for individuals with traumatic brain injury lies within coordination, comprehensiveness, flexibility, and accountability for the management of all these components. Outpatient services per se do not provide for such coordination or management and therefore outpatient services, unless they are clearly integrated, do not constitute a managed program.

For example, in traditional outpatient programs discipline-specific services are provided (e.g., occupational, speech, and physical therapies) with little emphasis on the *interaction* of these services with respect to the long-term vocational, interpersonal, and psychosocial needs of the individual. It is a situation of "splintered" efforts with little or no coordination among the various therapists. This treatment approach may be adequate for rehabilitation circumstances where few services are needed or in circumstances where the clients' cognitive abilities permit them to be their own "manager." However, this is rarely the case in traumatic head injury rehabilitation.

Additionally, in most outpatient programs, therapy rarely exceeds 10 hours per week and there is usually little or no consistent communication between the various therapists involved in the treatment effort. Furthermore, traditional outpatient services are performed in "contrived" settings (i.e., in an office or gym) with little or no conducting or extension of treatment in the community itself. Again this may not be an issue if a person's cognitive abilities permit him or her to generalize the acquired skill, but such is usually not the case in individuals with traumatic head injury.

In summary, it is speculated that outpatient services, if not performed in a coordinated, intensive, and ecologically valid environment offer little prospect for long-term behavior change in persons with traumatic head injury.

A comprehensive day program (the key word may be *program*) ideally would offer therapeutic services that are specifically designed to meet the wide variety of needs of the population it serves, as would any program for that matter. The targeted needs would ideally extend far beyond the traditional repertoire of the rehabilitation disciplines and may include: access to financial planning, advocacy, legal counsel, family services, substance abuse counseling, job coaching, and other nontraditional services. The approach may then be called *client centered,* though not necessarily discipline centered.

Again, there is no model in the theoretical sense for day programming. Discipline-centered treatment is not really based on theory, but rather it represents a comprehensive approach to a group of individuals who are *likely* to need the services of a well-rounded team. It is the authors' contention that a theoretical day program would first assess the likely needs of the population and then try to assemble a "team" of individuals who possess the skills necessary to address those needs—the proverbial cart before the horse issue.

In an attempt to construct a day program that is theoretically (e.g., client centered) driven, a number of assumptions must first be addressed about the population to be served. These assumptions require elaboration and justification. As studied herein, these assumptions form the basis of the authors' theoretical model for day programming for persons with traumatic brain injury.

UNDERLYING ASSUMPTIONS

Healing

It is common knowledge that the brain experiences a natural, physical *healing* process following traumatic injury. In generic terms, this healing process is often called "spontaneous recovery," which implies that, with proper life support and some therapeutic involvement, (beyond basic life support), the brain will undergo at least partial restoration of lost functions (Levin, Grossman, & Eisenberg, 1987). It has been speculated that this natural healing or recovery process can last anywhere from 3 months to 2 years, depending upon the severity of the injury.

It is also recognized that, while certain brain regions may experience spontaneous recovery, other regions may not recover at similar rates and in some instances neurological or behavioral regression is possible, as in the case of delayed post-traumatic epilepsy, psychosis, hydrocephalus, dementia, and so forth. It is important to recognize both the healing and regression phenomena when executing a day program (or any other traumatic brain injury program for that matter). For example, some neurological events may accelerate or alternatively may override treatment interventions. The potential for these influences must be understood when developing the treatment plan. In summary, appreciation for the healing, or course of recovery, process is critical when predicting or proving program effectiveness or outcome.

Learning

Much has been written about the memory and *learning* abilities of persons with traumatic brain injury (for review see Brooks, 1984). When viewed collectively, the literature is rather nihilistic in that memory and learning deficits are discussed in close association with permanent, irreversible brain damage. This inherently implies, and usually assumes, that individuals with memory deficits from traumatic brain injury are incapable learners. While it is technically true that individuals with traumatic brain injury are often less efficient learners than their noninjured counterparts, the authors posit that the overwhelming majority of all persons with traumatic brain injury, mild to severe, maintain objective, verifiable learning abilities. There are even reports of persons learning without the awareness of learning (J. Ewert, personal communication, August, 1987).

Furthermore, an assumption is made that previously reported learning abilities (or lack thereof), in persons with traumatic brain injury, as reported in the literature, are only modestly correlated with the acquisition of essential instrumental "ecologically valid" living skills (e.g., space management, personal hygiene, fitness) and basic prevocational and vocational skills. In other words, a notable gap exists between neurometric "scores" on memory measures and memory skills exhibited in normal community living.

The authors consider an individual's learning abilities as an important factor when designing day rehabilitation program. There are little meaningful data available from the rehabilitation or the neuropsychological literature of predictor variables relating psychometric memory and learning functions to matters of daily living. Therefore, it is prudent to expand one's definition of learning to other areas, including, but not limited to, the individual's ability to learn or relearn skills such as ambulation, balance, communication, problem solving, activities of daily living, and the like. In other words, learning and memory assessment and treatment should not be considered the domain left solely to the neuropsychologist.

Compensation

The brain injury itself may reduce, or in severe cases, place an absolute ceiling upon an indi-

vidual's ability to reacquire a certain skill. In these instances, the individual must then learn a *compensatory* means to achieve a task or function. Compensating techniques are best utilized in circumstances where a skill (e.g., smooth, coordinated movement of an extremity) is permanently lost or altered, or in circumstances where the reacquisition of the skill would require such an extensive effort that such effort would distract from the reacquisition of other important skills. It is noted that the acquisition of compensatory strategies and the reacquisition of other "lost" skills often occur simultaneously. That is, learning ability per se should not be thought of in absolute terms; rather, it is accurate to affirm that persons with traumatic brain injury are likely to have altered learning curves relative to the content of the stimulus or task to be learned and to the degree of inflicted brain damage. Compensatory strategies are *learned* strategies.

Summary

To review, there are necessary assumptions to understand that underlie the authors' model with respect to day programming, and with respect to brain injury rehabilitation in general. First, the therapist/program must have a thorough understanding and appreciation for the natural, spontaneous recovery phenomena as well as for the regression phenomena that can occur following traumatic brain injury (i.e., actual physical or healing properties of the brain). Second, at the core of all therapies, there must be an appreciation of and an emphasis upon careful analysis of the individual's ability to remember and to learn. The author's definition of memory and learning is broad based, and considers learning and memory abilities in various environments, in various treatment modalities, and even at various times. No longer is it sufficient to rely upon psychometric test data to define a person's memory and learning ability across all domains. (Learning capacity is addressed further in the following section.) Third, the acquisition (through learning) of compensatory skills is often helpful in assisting the individual toward functional improvement. By definition, compensation is a substitute-oriented strategy; that is, individuals may learn to add a new skill to their repertoire in substitution for a lost skill.

CRITERIA FOR CANDIDATE SELECTION

The variables/issues that determine whether an individual is a proper candidate for day programming are rather straightforward. They should take into account the issues raised in the previous section and, therefore, the initial diagnosis should not automatically qualify or disqualify day program interventions. Rather, an evaluation process is needed to determine the clinical fit for day treatment. A preadmission evaluation (PAE) should be performed that focuses, at a minimum, upon the following three variables that will likely have a dramatic impact upon the candidate's overall potential for success in the program: capacities for insight, motivation, and learning (Bond, 1984; Levin et al., 1987; Lishman, 1973; Prigatano, 1987). These three characteristics are not often linked together, or considered predictor variables of rehabilitation outcome in the traditional sense. It is even more difficult to measure objectively the presence or absence of same. Nonetheless, since individually each has been linked to treatment success (see Brooks, 1984), it is hypothesized that when considered together, these three variables can provide the program staff with valuable information concerning the likelihood for success in the day program. Therefore, they require careful assessment and review prior to program enrollment. A note of caution is also given here—it is quite likely that the individual with severe brain injury may have some temporary compromise in one or all of these areas. This situation does not necessarily eliminate an individual from program eligibility, but rather may be the immediate target for treatment. However, preliminary short-term and long-term goals must reflect the candidate's functioning within these variables. Further elaboration of the importance of these variables follows.

Insight

The candidate's capacity for accurate self-assessment, (i.e., insight) into his or her abilities

and deficit areas, can be the single most important factor for the client's ultimate success in a day program. Insight, or lack thereof, is usually considered to be determined by psychological factors (e.g., repression or denial of information) and/or determined by neurological factors (e.g., agnosia, which is basically defined as a neurological inability to self-assess accurately). Ben-Yishay and Diller (1983) and others (e.g., Bond, 1984) emphasize the importance of the client's insight as to the ultimate success of the rehabilitation effort. For example, it is the authors' experience that individuals with head injury and their families consider rehabilitation as most effective when it is clearly associated with goals that are easy to observe and assess (i.e., allowing for greater insight). These goals may be reality based—return to work, return to independent or semi-independent living, or return to school. Treatment effectiveness is usually enhanced when the relationship between treatment effort and outcome is clearly delineated, which usually allows for increased likelihood for insight. Unless some "real-world" activity is part of the therapeutic effort, head-injured clients have considerable difficulty understanding how therapy in an office setting has bearing upon their ability to succeed in the real world.

Motivation

It is assumed that all individuals, with brain injury or not, possess factors in their life that can be considered as "motivators." Briefly defined, motivators are known goals or conditions, usually easily measurable, toward which an individual strives. It is hypothesized that individuals with traumatic injury who have identified motivators or goals and who have limitations placed upon them secondary to an injury can nonetheless be provided with a strategy to achieve objectives/goals through the prudent use of those motivators. On the contrary, an individual without identified motivators or goals is at considerable risk for inertia or to drift in therapy. Therefore, a critical aspect of the preadmission evaluation is to attempt to define potential client motivators and goal states. Precious therapy time is likely to be wasted if this is not done.

Learning

As mentioned earlier in this chapter, the importance of the client's core memory and learning abilities must be assessed prior to day program enrollment. Assessment of these abilities should, at a minimum, include: 1) objective formalized assessment, as is often performed in neuropsychological evaluation procedures; and 2) analysis of the candidate's past responses to attempts at learning. This assessment may include review of the client's previous progress at other rehabilitation efforts and careful review of the circumstances in which the client learned most effectively.

OUTCOME ORIENTATION AND FUNCTIONAL EQUIVALENCIES

In discussing the outcome of any treatment intervention, some clarification regarding the precise definition of the term "outcome" is in order (Fuhrer, 1987). In scientific papers, outcome is often synonymous with "results." That is, the outcome of a study may be reported in statistical terms with reference to levels of significance, to the statistical power of a given intervention, to the validity and reliability of the findings, and the like. In these circumstances, comparisons of differently treated groups determine the outcome of a given intervention. It is important to have such an appreciation of outcome when evaluating overall program effectiveness or when comparing the treatment strategies between programs. When used appropriately these outcome studies can redirect and redefine treatment approaches, substitute the need for continued treatment, and/or validate the program's treatment philosophy. The problem with this definition of outcome is obvious—it is likely to be insensitive to the *individual's* response to treatment. It is the authors' contention that each and every individual engaged in a day treatment program must have an individualized, well-defined, and objectifiable treatment plan, a plan loaded with outcome-oriented statements. Furthermore, these statements, and the treatment process necessary to accomplish them, must have direct and verifiable relevance to what is considered real-world

functioning. When stated properly, outcome-oriented treatment goals can be understood by professionals and lay persons alike. In other words, treatment outcome statements should be defined in terms of *functional equivalencies;* this is also known as being ecologically valid. This outcome orientation is well supported in the literature (for review see Fuhrer, 1987).

For example, consider the following rehabilitation goals: 1) "The client will ambulate with moderate assistance" or 2) "The client will increase memory functioning by 50%." Such goal statements are not uncommon in the medical and treatment charts of persons with traumatic brain injury. Unfortunately, these, and similarly worded goal statements have little or no meaning to the nonprofessional and they in no way communicate how the client will actually perform in his or her community setting. While this may appear to be a simplistic example of confusing rehabilitation goal statements, it is the unfortunate truth that such statements are often present in standard charts and treatment plans.

Alternatively, outcome-oriented goal statements with a functional equivalency (i.e., ecologically meaningful statements) may read: 1) "The client will rely only upon the use of a rolling walker for ambulation" or 2) "The client will utilize a daily planner to attend scheduled daily activities." Such minor modifications in outcome statements will clarify exactly when goals have been reached, will more than likely motivate the client toward success, and will educate other concerned parties about overall program progress and effectiveness.

It is thus clear that all day programming interventions should have clearly stated goals that are outcome oriented. There is, however, a larger, system-wide issue relevant to outcome achievement. This issue concerns the relationship of effort (which may be defined in terms of hours in treatment, money spent, etc.) to the individual's overall outcome in a day program. Economists refer to this relationship as the "law of diminishing returns." The relationship is as follows and is illustrated in Figure 9.1.

Point A. In catastrophic cases (i.e., traumatic brain injury) a small amount of effort usu-

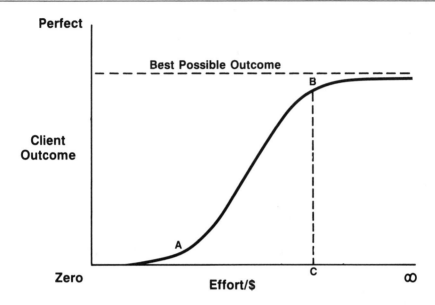

A = Critical amount of effort ($) to show increase in outcome
B = Best possible outcome per effort ($ spent)
C = Ideal level of effort ($) necessary to maximize outcome

Figure 9.1.   Graphic representation of the relationship of effort to outcome. (See text for further discussion.)

ally only "buys" a small amount of outcome. For example, 1 hour of day programming per day may have only a negligible
effect in a severe traumatic injury case.

Points A–B. There exits a point in a person's
rehabilitation where the treatment effort is
clearly producing a desired, measurable
outcome. In such circumstances, increasing the effort usually results in a more desirable outcome.

Point B. The individual has either achieved, or
is close to achieving, the desired outcome
state. At this point additional effort may
have little or no overall impact on outcome;
that is, more is not necessarily better.

Point C. This should be the focus of all therapeutic interventions—to identify the point
of maximally efficient use of a person's resources and simultaneously the attainment
of the best possible outcome.

This theoretical model can actually be applied in any treatment setting. In the situation of
a day treatment setting, the client usually has a

limited amount of time to attend therapies each
day and the overall time in the program is obviously restricted by such factors as funding
availability, program resources, prioritized problems, community opportunities, and so forth.
There is, therefore, a need to prioritize treatment
goals and objectives. This is accomplished
through the development and execution of a
treatment plan or "problem list," which is discussed next.

TREATMENT PLANS/PROBLEM LISTS

Treatment plans in rehabilitation settings can be
constructed in several ways. An obvious choice
in many settings is to expose the client to disciplinary assessments (occupational therapy,
physical therapy, speech/language, psychology,
etc.) and for the results of these assessments to
be coalesced into the treatment plan. This approach has characterized rehabilitation efforts
for many years and is considered comprehensive
in nature. Day treatment programs, if staffed appropriately, are fully capable of providing these

services within these contingencies. Therefore, when developing and staffing such programs it is prudent to assume that those "necessary" disciplines are represented in the treatment team. It is further assumed that the provision of a multidisciplinary team will allow the client adequate access to clinical services and personnel that will increase the likelihood for a positive outcome. As mentioned earlier, though, this is probably an inadequate approach.

An alternative approach to the development of the treatment plan, however, may exist. That is, instead of staffing a day treatment program by disciplinary means, the authors recommend that programs first consider a formal assessment of the likely needs of its clientele, in functional terms, and then provide treatment staff that can accurately address those needs. This distinction is conceptually and, it is hoped, genuinely more client centered. The authors assert that this approach must be made in earnest in order for the day program to be maximally effective. A brief discussion of this approach to treatment follows.

Recent studies have consistently suggested that those factors that often form the ultimate barriers to successful community reintegration for persons with traumatic brain injury center around the individuals' psychosocial and family functioning (Prigatano et al., 1986; Ylvisaker & Gobble, 1987). This being the case, it would seem wise for day rehabilitation programs to provide ready access to psychological and family therapies for their clients. The fact of the matter remains that psychological and family treatment, until very recently, have been viewed as ancillary forms of therapy in the rehabilitation setting. In this circumstance, the real needs of individuals may have been held in abeyance and in deference to a traditional view of rehabilitation as discipline centered (versus client centered). Recreation therapy, academic counseling and tutoring, and life planning tend to be similarly neglected by traditional rehabilitation disciplines. There is little doubt, however, that these are needed services in day rehabilitation.

So then, the authors suggest that day treatment programs be staffed and managed with a direct appreciation for and an investigation of the true functional needs of the clientele they are to

serve. If, for example, a day program expects to serve mostly persons with chronic needs then the needs of that population should first be addressed prior to program establishment. If it is likely to serve persons with more acute needs, then it should be staffed according to those needs, and so on.

That is, this becomes a comprehensive problem-solving model, staffed by individuals familiar with the probable clinical needs of the population. In that regard, a treatment plan is really a descriptive *problem list*—the "problems" being those surmountable barriers that the client must overcome in order to make a meaningful advancement toward independence or whatever goals are established. Granted, the treating individuals will likely have training specific to a given discipline. Nonetheless, the therapist's decision of whether to treat should not be solely bound by administration of treatment that is "proper" for that discipline. Rather, the therapist should self-critique his or her own repertoire of skills and determine if his or her skills and teaching ability coincide with the individual client's needs. For example, a neuropsychologist working with a memory-impaired client in a supermarket (e.g., choosing a weekly menu) characterizes this approach. Until recently this may have been quite an unlikely event. Fortunately, postacute rehabilitation appears to be moving in the problem-solving direction, although several philosophical barriers, with regard to which discipline performs which therapeutic activity, remain.

In summary, treatment plans should not necessarily be structured according to various, traditional disciplines. Rather, a day program must first assess the likely needs of its clientele (vocational training services, advocacy or legal counseling, etc.) and personnel should be secured who can meet these needs. This may seem a simplistic notion—it is. Unfortunately, it is the authors' experience that staffing patterns between various types of brain injury programs (inpatient versus outpatient) vary little. This lack of variation does not appear to be sensitive to the changing needs of the individuals served.

One final comment upon establishing the problem list or treatment plan is that the law of diminishing returns phenomenon and proper resource management clearly prevail when a prioritized list (or plan) is established. Those problems that have the most significant impact upon the individual's eventual ability to function independently must demand sufficient attention and effort. The client's access to the day program is finite and his or her time in the program must be used in accordance with the barriers or problems that have the greatest negative impact. For example, a client may have deficits in independent living skills, but because vocational reentry is considered attainable within a narrow time frame, the living skills training may be deferred. At some level this practice of prioritization is always implicitly performed; however, it is the authors' belief that this prioritization should be actively attended to and managed in the day program. Prioritization leads to effective clinical case management, which is vital to an individual's success. This is discussed next.

CLINICAL CASE MANAGEMENT

A poorly designed treatment intervention can lead a brain-injured individual down a path of clinical failure, as may be the case when subtle cognitive deficits are neglected for an individual who is attempting to return to a complex vocational challenge. Similar failure can occur when the same individual's care is not properly managed; for example, when a decision is made in a vocational program to focus upon a more observable deficit (e.g., an orthopedic injury) at the expense of giving a cognitive problem a low treatment priority.

In cases of catastrophic insult (e.g., brain injury), the occasion is set for the possibility of several rehabilitation professionals to assume accountability for solving many injury-related problems. The questions become: Who's in charge of the treatment plan? Who determines the prioritization of problems to be addressed? Who assists the client in the treatment decisions and the effect (i.e., use of limited resources)? In the sections to follow, that individual is referred to as a clinical case manager. Hembree (1985) succinctly defined the clinical case manager's role:

". . . the combination of activities designed to insure appropriate use of medical care facilities, improve quality of care, control or reduce costs, insure proper referrals, provide primary care, and manage patients' episodes of care, disability, and rehabilitation." (p. 11)

In a day treatment setting, where a dozen or more rehabilitation specialists are likely to be involved in the treatment effort of each individual, a single point of accountability must exist regarding the overall direction and ultimate outcome of a client's program. Although the concept of case management is not new in rehabilitation, psychiatry, and other disciplines where chronic disability is common, the postacute head injury field is becoming increasingly reliant upon individuals to fulfill the roles of the above definition.

Dixon, Goll, and Stanton (1988) describe the various environments in which case managers are likely to practice. In the context of this chapter, case management services are facility based; that is, case management functions, in the day rehabilitation program, as the service accountable for outcome. It is particularly prudent to have a case manager assigned to each client in a day program setting as the possibility exists that "nonprogram" personnel (e.g., private physicians, family members) may exert significant influence upon the overall rehabilitation process and inadvertently function as the case manager.

In summary, case management services must be made available for individuals in day programming. Case management significantly reduces the risk for errors of omission in treatment planning; furthermore, the literature is quite convincing that expert case management significantly reduces cost overruns, and greatly improves the likelihood for appropriate use of and access to resources (for review see Dixon et al., 1988).

TREATMENT MODALITIES

Allowing persons with physical, cognitive, behavioral, and/or psychological problems following traumatic brain injury to live in an environment of their choosing, and in a life-style to which anyone would aspire, is the heart of rehabilitation treatment, day treatment or otherwise. What treatment modalities then should exist in a day treatment program? Ideally, persons in a day treatment program would be afforded access to rehabilitationists expert in problem solving for the population in question, whether those experts hold "staff" positions at the program or whether they are utilized as contract staff on an as-needed basis to address specific, albeit lower frequency problems.

As discussed earlier in this chapter, the preadmission evaluation sets the occasion for the appropriateness of the client admission to the day program and for the initial treatment plan. In most circumstances, clients enrolled in a day treatment program will either live within the structure/support of the family or extended family environment or, in "advanced" cases, live independently while seeking services to increase other areas of independent function (e.g., seeking specialized vocational training and placement). Generally, clients are referred to day treatment who: 1) are medically stable; 2) demonstrate significant capacity for insight, motivation, and/or learning potential (i.e., have a clinical "fit"); 3) have the funding support adequate to complete a program that results in significant, measurable clinical gains; 4) live within a relatively short (e.g., less than 30-mile) distance of the program, so that treatment can occur within his or her community; and 5) demonstrate the physical, cognitive, and behavioral skills to live in a home-like environment. (Note: If this last point is in question, the client may be an appropriate candidate, at least for an evaluation, for residential-based rehabilitation.)

Once these five criteria have been established, and given the situation that the program has adequately investigated the anticipated needs of the population it is to serve, the following services (at a minimum) should be included as a part of the day treatment program:

1. Basic *life support services,* including completely accessible environments, meals (lunch), recreational outlets, and rapid access to general health and medical care.

2. *Transportation* (private or public) access necessary to achieve treatment objectives.

3. *Assessment and treatment planning,* including, but not limited to, cognitive deficits, problematic learned behavior, sensory deficits, psychomotor deficits, mental health problems, and other functional problems relating to the conduct of everyday life. Additionally, baseline optometric, dental, general medical, and neuropsychiatric assessments are usually indicated.

4. *Individualized treatment programming* conducted by expert, accredited, and/or licensed staff. Appropriate equipment and materials necessary to conduct treatment should be included as part of the comprehensive plan.

5. *Recreational and community activities* are essential and ideally would be conducted within or close to the client's own community. Social interaction is critical secondary to the considerable problems with social isolation encountered in persons with traumatic brain injury.

6. *Clinical case management and quality control* services necessary to ensure accountability and optimal outcome attainment. Ideally, independent case record clinical auditors would provide feedback/instruction to assure that the client is "on track" and that his or her resources (see Figure 9.1) are properly utilized and managed.

7. *Client status reporting* to the financial provider, family, legal authorities, and other concerned parties. Usually, monthly reports that are clearly outcome oriented (i.e., a prioritized problem list) are sufficient to communicate client progress and achievements. A special report, in terms of the client's long-term living needs/arrangements, is usually needed to assist the client and others as an effort to anticipate and plan for future needs. This long-term plan, with reference to specific needs (i.e., income potential, living arrangements, anticipated daily activities) often serves as a guide for outcome planning while a client is enrolled in the day program.

8. *Family counseling/training and respite ser-*

vices are frequently indicated, to ensure a smooth, reliable transition for the client into family activities. Neglect of family needs, whether the program is residentially based or day based, significantly increases risk for regression.

9. *Prevocational and vocational training,* including immediate access to appropriate vocational treatment options including work-hardening skill development, job coaching, employer training, job placement and follow-through training, "troubleshooting" once the placement has been made, and follow-up services. For example, the Carolina Community Re-Entry Program has developed a "phase" vocational program that takes into account the client's insight, motivation, and learning abilities and employs the individual in appropriate vocational context in relation to those skills (see Figure 9.2).

It is quite likely that a significant portion of candidates appropriate for day treatment will have vocational training and placement as a key factor of their programming; consequently, comprehensive, expert access to a wide variety of vocational services is indicated. Again, the issue of ecological validity is paramount; therefore, actual training in the community setting is ideal prior to program completion.

The reader may note that in this description of necessary services for a day treatment program, the recommended program is not only *functional* in its description, but also *comprehensive*. The fact that an individual may reside in a setting elsewhere from where "therapies" occur usually does not significantly reduce the individual's need to have ready access to a team of professionals capable of providing intensive problem-solving options. Additionally, the management needs remains significant for overall program accountability.

Furthermore, because the services needed remain comprehensive in nature, there is also the issue of basic funding (i.e., Where does the money come from?) and the funding options

(e.g., fee-for-service, per diem, blended funding) available. This is discussed next.

FUNDING THEORY AND OPTIONS

Payment for day rehabilitation services can potentially be derived from public and/or private sources. For example, individuals with brain injury have obtained treatment as "outpatients" for decades from each of these sources. However, the postacute options for comprehensive brain injury rehabilitation have expanded; this expansion has created considerable confusion in the payer community. A primary source of confusion resides in the new terminology used to describe innovative treatment programming, as this new nomenclature does not match existing terminology in modern-day payer policies. For example, "community reentry," "cognitive remediation," and "job coaching" are terms essentially foreign to the insurance industry; understandably, the industry's response is to decline payment for such services. Therefore, the need to marry current technology and its nomenclature to payer nomenclature and expectations is in order.

Consider the insurance industry, for example. Insurance companies are financial institutions, plain and simple. They collect monies, usually in the forms of premiums; they invest these monies in various ventures; and they pay out settlements, in the form of coverage for various illnesses and injuries. Additionally, each insurance office offers different "product lines" (Keane, 1985); some are more or less favorable toward the product line of rehabilitation. Since many insurance policys were written without knowledge or appreciation for postacute (i.e., "nonmedical") rehabilitation, this aspect of rehabilitation is often not included in the product line—essentially is not "covered." How then can clinically indicated services rendered by the rehabilitation community be paid for? Two critical variables to gain access to these funds are education (about the services to be provided) and assurances for cost management should the "product" be purchased. At present, it is relatively easy to educate about the need for services; cost management, which is analogous to

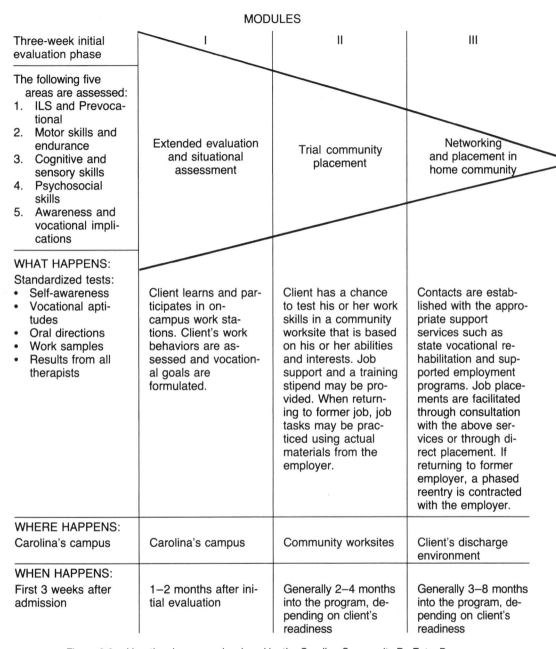

	MODULES		
Three-week initial evaluation phase	**I**	**II**	**III**
The following five areas are assessed: 1. ILS and Prevocational 2. Motor skills and endurance 3. Cognitive and sensory skills 4. Psychosocial skills 5. Awareness and vocational implications	Extended evaluation and situational assessment	Trial community placement	Networking and placement in home community
WHAT HAPPENS: Standardized tests: • Self-awareness • Vocational aptitudes • Oral directions • Work samples • Results from all therapists	Client learns and participates in on-campus work stations. Client's work behaviors are assessed and vocational goals are formulated.	Client has a chance to test his or her work skills in a community worksite that is based on his or her abilities and interests. Job support and a training stipend may be provided. When returning to former job, job tasks may be practiced using actual materials from the employer.	Contacts are established with the appropriate support services such as state vocational rehabilitation and supported employment programs. Job placements are facilitated through consultation with the above services or through direct placement. If returning to former employer, a phased reentry is contracted with the employer.
WHERE HAPPENS: Carolina's campus	Carolina's campus	Community worksites	Client's discharge environment
WHEN HAPPENS: First 3 weeks after admission	1–2 months after initial evaluation	Generally 2–4 months into the program, depending on client's readiness	Generally 3–8 months into the program, depending on client's readiness

Figure 9.2.   Vocational program developed by the Carolina Community Re-Entry Program.

the resource allocation phenomenon alluded to in Figure 9.1, is much more difficult to measure and, therefore, to market. Nonetheless, it remains a critical challenge for all postacute rehabilitation programs to prove clinical efficiency in a cost-management context.

Day rehabilitation programming appears to have an even greater challenge. In the author's proposal for the ideal day program, inclusive of comprehensive services, the program is asking for funding commitments for many services that are often not covered within the strict language of the policy. For example, family therapy, educational counseling, and community living training are rarely found within the language of acceptable (reimbursable) services. Should then a day program provide only reimbursable therapies, as is often the case under fee-for-service restrictions? For clinical reasons, the answer should be clearly "no"; otherwise, the program is not really a program, but rather an environment where splintered services are provided.

The problem of lack of understanding of the rewards of day programming for individuals with brain injury is not limited to the insurance industry. Publicly funded services, in their reimbursement policies, also presently show a lack of funding commitment to these nonmedical programs. Again, these reimbursement schedules were typically written many years ago, without any anticipation of rehabilitation extending beyond the acute medical stage of "recovery." A possible exception to this rule is the case of publicly funded vocational rehabilitation efforts. However, even in this situation, the need for intensive, comprehensive services for the individual with traumatic brain injury was not fully realized.

The resulting situation then is one of a lack of understanding and some confusion on both sides—provider and payer. Without a responsible exchange of information this is a disappointing situation in which both sides are potential losers. Education by both parties with regard to each other's resources and goals for the collaboration is clearly in order. On the provider side, the day program must prudently inform the potential payer about the type and outcome of services to be rendered. Furthermore, the provider should perform its own market-based program plan to reduce the potentially large gap between what the program wants to provide and what dollars may be available. On the payer side, attempts should be made to inform providers about potential limitations for reimbursement while keeping options available for going "out of contract" to provide payment. The obvious incentive for expanding the language of the policy or going out of contract would be to reduce long-term costs and to practice prudent cost management. The current climate of postacute rehabilitation mandates that creativity and flexi-

bility in reference to cost management must be practiced to secure funding for day programming.

Following are three potential funding options for day programming. In presenting these options, the authors are not necessarily addressing the funding source (e.g., workers' compensation, accident and health policy, self-pay), but rather are emphasizing funding strategy.

Per Diem Funding

Per diem reimbursement is typically a comprehensive fee schedule, a schedule in which "typical" or "expected" clinically needed services are covered under one predictable charge, based on a daily rate. There are clear advantages to this strategy, the most obvious of which is that a client receives whatever services he or she needs without restrictions imposed as to what is "covered." Most would agree that this is a "client-centered" reimbursement practice. Additionally, costs are predictable over time (for review see Evans, 1988).

A possible disadvantage to a per diem schedule is that this strategy is counter-intuitive to most insurance policies where fee-for-service practices abound. Payers may also be leary of paying daily rates for traditionally noncovered events such as meals, transportation, recreation, and the like. In essence, the per diem strategy violates the *process-driven* mentality of many insurance policies.

Fee-For-Service Funding

Fee-for-service is a reimbursement strategy familiar to most insurance companies. By definition, reimbursement is given for traditionally covered services—in the case of rehabilitation this may include reimbursement for physical, occupational, speech, and psychological treatments. This is a procedural-driven approach and one that allows payers to monitor closely the actual activity of the treatment effort.

Major potential disadvantages exist for day programming efforts under fee-for-service schedules, an obvious one being that the narrow confinements of many fee-for-service policies do not allow reimbursement for many nontraditional but needed treatments. Additionally, costs are less predictable, and the entire strategy is not really outcome oriented. Finally, many fee-for-service policies are written within a medical model framework and may not allow treatment to be held outside of a medical or office-based setting.

Blended Funding

Blended funding arrangements occur when two or more payers combine financial resources to pay for a given program. Each may provide co-payments for a per diem rate or each may combine on a fee-for-service schedule. The context in which blended funding often occurs is when each payer abides by its policy, yet each policy complements the other. This is a potentially creative solution to day programming reimbursement. For example, if the injury was consequent to a motor vehicle accident, the injured party's accident and health policy may pay for specific fee-for-service therapies, and the local vocational rehabilitation agency may pay for remaining vocationally related treatments. Thus, each payer reimburses for services within the language of the particular policy.

The strength behind the blended funding arrangement is for payers, who may have policy-driven limitations, to combine to share the financial burden. Blended funding arrangements are inherently logical in today's climate where lack of understanding and confusion about comprehensive coverage remains.

SUMMARY

In this chapter, a theoretical model for designing and managing a day rehabilitation program for persons suffering neurobehavioral consequences of traumatic brain injury was described. The model contains these basic features:

1. A clear understanding of the problems and deficits likely to be encountered by persons with traumatic brain injury must be in place. Clinical experience and attention to research literature will guide this understanding.
2. Appreciation for neurological development factors including recovery and regression curves will influence eventual outcome.
3. The preadmission evaluation must take into account the client's motivation, insight, and learning status.
4. Treatment methods must comprise ecologically valid components, necessitating the utilization of the community itself as an integral part of the program.
5. The program should be oriented toward problem solving, with an emphasis upon prioritization and resource allocation.
6. A single point of accountability for program direction and outcome achievement must be in place. A likely accountable individual is the clinical case manager.
7. Treatment modalities must avoid the temptation to become strictly discipline oriented. Rather, an appreciation for the "problems" that the individual is likely to have should guide the composition of the treatment team.
8. Finally, providers and payers need to understand the policies of each other's practices and to be flexible to each other's market demands, without violating the essential needs of the individuals they serve.

In summary, day treatment offers individuals access to a comprehensive shelf of services to help them solve complex problems and to overcome neurologically driven barriers on the road toward community reintegration. As we move into the next century, rehabilitation will surely have broken away from the confining practices of past decades. The ultimate treatment model for individuals with brain injury will provide unrestricted access to the options for successful living that noninjured persons enjoy.

REFERENCES

Ben-Yishay, Y., & Diller, L. (1983). Cognitive remediation. In M. Rosenthal, E.R. Griffith, M.R. Bond, & J.D. Miller (Eds.). *Rehabilitation of the head injured adult*. Philadelphia: F.A. Davis.

Bond, M. (1984). The psychiatry of closed head injury. In N. Brooks (Ed.), *Closed head injury: Psychological, social, and family consequences.* Oxford: Oxford University Press.

Brooks, N. (Ed.). (1984). *Closed head injury: Psychological, social and family consequences.* Oxford: Oxford University Press.

Dixon, T.P., Goll, S., & Stanton, K.M. (1988). Case management issues and practices in head injury rehabilitation. *Rehabilitation Counseling Bulletin, 31,* 325–343.

Evans, R. (1988, January 9). Brain-injured patients need broader insurance coverage. *Healthweek.*

Fuhrer, M.J. (Ed.). (1987). *Rehabilitation outcomes: Analysis and measurement.* Baltimore: Paul H. Brookes Publishing Co.

Hembree, W.E. (1985, July/August). Getting involved: Employees as case managers. *Business and Health Week,* pp. 11–14.

Keane, R.M. (1985). Providing rehabilitation services to the insurance industry. In L.J. Taylor et al. (Eds.), *Handbook of private sector rehabilitation.* New York: Springer.

Levin, H.S., Grossman, J., & Eisenberg, H.M. (Eds.). (1987). *Neurobehavioral recovery from head injury.* New York: Oxford University Press.

Lishman, W.A. (1973). The psychiatric sequelae of head injury: A review. *Psychological Medicine, 3,* 304.

National Head Injury Foundation (NHIF). (1985). *National directory of head injury rehabilitation services.* Framingham, MA: Author.

Prigatano, G. (1987). Neuropsychological deficits, personality variables, and outcome. In M. Ylvisaker, & E.M.R. Gobble (Eds.), *Community re-entry for head injured adults.* Boston: College-Hill Press.

Prigatano, G.P., Fordyce, D.J., Zeiner, H.K., Roveche, J.R., Pepping, M., & Wood, B.C. (1986). *Neuropsychological rehabilitation after brain injury.* Baltimore: Johns Hopkins University Press.

Ylvisaker, M., & Gobble, E.M.R. (1987). *Community re-entry for head injured adults.* Boston: College-Hill Press.

CHAPTER 10

Psychotherapeutic Treatment of the Client with Traumatic Brain Injury
A Conceptual Model

Robert J. Sbordone

It has been estimated that approximately 8.8 million Americans sustain head injuries each year. Approximately one fourth of these injuries include skull fracture and intracranial injury, which frequently result in long-lasting and often permanent alterations in cognitive, emotional, and behavioral functioning (Cooper, 1982). Until recently, the cognitive problems in persons with traumatic brain injury dominated both clinical and research studies (e.g., Mandelberg & Brooks, 1975). Since 1980, there has been a growing realization that emotional and social problems typically accompany cognitive difficulties in persons with traumatic brain injury. Lezak (1987, p. 57) has reviewed this literature and concluded that "the data of these studies suggest that traumatically brain injured patients are much more seriously handicapped by emotional and personality disturbances than by their residual cognitive or physical disabilities."

The methodology for assessing personality and associated behavioral changes following traumatic brain injury has been hindered by lack of a single acceptable theory of personality and measurement techniques relevant to the problems of clients with traumatic brain injury. As a consequence, researchers in this field have been left with descriptive and often idiosyncratic descriptions of behavior (Bond, 1986). Nonetheless, investigators such as Bond (1984, 1986) and Lezak (1978, 1987) have formulated five categories that define the emotional and behavioral problems of the client with traumatic brain injury: 1) emotional change (characterized by apathy, silliness, lability of mood, irritability, or changes in libido), 2) impaired social perceptiveness (characterized by selfishness, in which the feeling for others, self-criticism, and the ability to reflect are greatly diminished or absent), 3) impaired self-control (characterized by impulsivity, random restlessness, and impatience), 4) increased dependency (characterized by lack of initiative despite talk of action, and by impaired judgment and planning ability), and 5) behavioral rigidity (characterized by an inability to learn from experience even when the ability to learn new information is retained).

RELATIONSHIP BETWEEN LOCATION OF BRAIN INJURY AND EMOTIONAL PROBLEMS

Lishman (1968) has reviewed studies that examine the relationship between the location of the brain injury and resulting psychiatric and emotional problems. He found that left hemispheric injuries are more likely to produce psychiatric disability than right hemispheric injuries, although persons with right frontal lobe injuries were more likely to have psychiatric problems than those with left frontal lobe injuries. More recently, Sbordone (1985) has described an "atypical bipolar depression" that often follows right hemisphere diencephalic injuries consisting of manic and depressive swings lasting 1 or 2 days each. He also reported that this disorder typically did not occur until at least 6 months postinjury, and was frequently accompanied by the neurobehavioral manifestations of temporal lobe epilepsy. Lishman has also pointed out that temporal lobe injuries are more likely to produce psychiatric disability than frontal, parietal, or occipital lobe injuries. This association was greatest when injuries occurred to the left temporal lobe. Other investigators (e.g., Bach-Y-Rita, Lion, Climent, & Ervin, 1971) have reported that several months after injury persons with prominent temporal lobe injuries will often develop brief, sudden, violent or destructive outbursts of temper after minor provocations, followed by emotional distress and remorse.

Alexander (1984) has reported that postmortem computerized axial tomography (CT) studies of cerebral contusions demonstrate that they are not randomly distributed but instead show a strong predilection for the orbital frontal and inferior temporal areas of the brain. He also pointed out that frontal lobe contusions are more numerous than temporal lobe injuries and that orbital frontal lobe contusions are more commonly bilateral although often asymmetrical, while temporal lobe contusions are much more commonly unilateral. He emphasized that injury to the orbital frontal lobe produced powerful effects on personality, and on social and emotional functioning. Cummings (1985) has reported that injury to the orbital frontal regions will typically result in a pattern of disinhibition in which the individual will frequently exhibit: inappropriate social comments, inappropriate or antisocial behaviors, evidence of marked personality change, poor judgment and insight, and poor control over his or her emotions. Injury to the frontal convexity region will typically produce a pattern of apathy that is often accompanied by brief angry or aggressive outbursts. Injury to the medial regions of the frontal lobe will often typically result in an akinetic mute state, characterized by a lack of spontaneous movement, lack of verbalization, and failure to respond to orally presented commands. In general, individuals with frontal lobe disorder may be misdiagnosed as depressed or poorly motivated and are frequently sent to psychiatrists or psychologists who may not recognize their frontal lobe disorder and may

mistakenly attempt to treat them with psychotherapy and/or psychotropic medications.

Sbordone (1987) has reported that depression is very common in persons with traumatic brain injury at 6–12 months postinjury. Lezak (1987) has reported that persons with traumatic brain injury show the greatest frequency of problems with anxiety, depression, and significant relationships with others during the second half of the first post-trauma year. Numerous investigators have suggested psychological factors such as depression, anxiety, and impaired interpersonal relationships may complicate recovery following head injury (e.g., Bond, 1975). In summary, while many of individual's emotional and social problems may stem in part from such factors as coping with diminished or altered cognitive functioning and understanding the brain injury, a significant portion of emotional and social difficulties appear to be due to the site and extent of the brain injury.

EFFECT ON THE FAMILY

Traumatic brain injury typically disrupts normal family interaction patterns and creates serious adjustment problems for the family. Those who have investigated the psychological distress of family members have reported a high need for tranquilizers or sleeping tablets (Panting & Merry, 1972), high divorce rate and psychological burden on the spouse (Thomsen, 1974), breakdown in family cohesion (Bond, 1975), high emotional distress among relatives (Oddy, Humphrey, & Uttley, 1978; Panting & Merry, 1972), and feelings of being trapped (Lezak, 1978). Family members have been found to exhibit what has been described as a "command performance syndrome" while the individual with traumatic brain injury is undergoing acute rehabilitation—they tend to appear relatively "normal" and mask their emotional distress in the presence of the patient and health care professionals, often creating the erroneous impression that they are coping well and do not require psychological or psychiatric intervention (Sbordone, Kral, Gerard, & Katz, 1984).

During the first year postinjury, Romano (1974) reported that relatives exhibit a marked tendency to deny the patient's disabilities and engage in wishful fantasies regarding recovery. This most commonly involved the fantasy that the comatose patient is merely sleeping and one day will wake up and greet his or her family. Nearly all families observed tended to deny that the individual with traumatic brain injury was any different than he or she had been prior to the injury, even though such changes were obvious. Rosenbaum and Najenson (1976) found that at 1 year postinjury, the wives of severely brain-injured men experienced drastic and disturbing changes in their lives that were most pronounced in their interpersonal relationships with their brain-injured spouse, in-laws, and friends. They reported that the vast majority of the wives were described as depressed. Lezak (1978) has reported that the spouses of persons with traumatic brain injury feel trapped, isolated, have fears of being abandoned by their extended family, and are inclined to feel neglected or abused by their spouse. The spouses also lived in a social limbo since they were not able to participate in social activities with their brain-injured spouse.

Bowen (1978) has described the impact of a catastrophic event on a family as an emotional shock wave that creates a state of disequilibrium within the family, causing the family to mobilize all of its internal resources to cope with the situation. When the family remains in a chronic state of disequilibirum, it is likely to resort to such behaviors as avoidance, convergence, denial, displacement, identification, introjection, masking, postponing, projection, rationalization, repression, somatization, or transference as a means of trying to restore equilibrium. If these mechanisms are ineffective then the family may display a variety of pathological behaviors such as anger, arguing, badgering, coercion, complaining, defiance, delinquency, depression, evading, holding grudges, isolation from others, lying, nonparticipation, running away, scapegoating, school failure, silence, or emotional withholding. Many wives and mothers of persons with traumatic brain injury report feeling extremely burdened, which is frequently associated with clinically significant affective changes (e.g., anxiety and depression) in the family (Brooks, 1988).

TREATMENT OF THE CLIENT AND FAMILY

Cognitive Rehabilitation

Persons with traumatic brain injury are most likely to receive cognitive rehabilitation rather than psychotherapy, since it has been generally assumed that the emotional and social difficulties stem largely from cognitive impairments. While cognitive rehabilitation (which also includes computer-assisted cognitive rehabilitation) has been shown to improve the social and emotional functioning of brain-injured individuals (e.g., Rimmele & Hester, 1987) it may be less than adequate in producing significant behavioral, social, and emotional changes.

Behavior Modification

Recently, there has been a strong interest in applying behavior modification strategies to persons with traumatic brain injury (e.g., Wood, 1988). However, most of these approaches have focused on patients in the later stages of recovery and have not addressed common behavior management issues in acute care inpatient rehabilitation settings. Some of the reasons for this include: the patient's confusion and cognitive difficulties, the emphasis on the patient's medical rather than behavioral functioning, the typical multidisciplinary team model with its lack of integration and consistency, and the relatively few rehabilitation professionals who have received specific training in behavior modification and management techniques (Howard, 1988).

Individual Psychotherapy

Block (1987) has reported that individual psychotherapy with individuals with traumatic brain injury is often difficult and frustrating. Some of the reasons for this difficulty may stem from the individuals' cognitive deficits, which would typically include memory difficulties, problem-solving difficulties, and conceptual difficulties, as well as their failure to follow through on recommended tasks. A major obstacle for therapists working with brain-injured individuals is their frequent inadequate understanding of brain-behavior relationships. Part of the reason for this appears to stem largely from graduate training that failed to include courses in behavioral neurology. While courses in neuropsychological testing have been increasing in popularity in recent years, such courses typically focus on the administration, scoring, and interpretation of neuropsychological tests and typically provide little more than a cursory overview of brain-behavior relationships.

The traditional reliance on psychodynamic, psychoanalytic learning, and on gestalt or behavioral explanations of disordered cognitive, emotional, and social dysfunction has made it difficult for psychotherapists to view the person with traumatic brain injury within a brain-behavior perspective. For example, Sbordone and Rudd (1986) found that one third of practicing psychologists within the community failed to recognize the presence of rather salient underlying neurological disorders when they were asked to review clinical vignettes containing a description of patients with underlying neurological disorders who presented with psychological complaints. Careful analysis of the responses of these psychologists revealed that psychologists who had received psychodynamic or behavioral training were less likely to recognize the underlying neurological disorder. Failing to appreciate brain-behavior relationships, as well as the client's stage of recovery (Sbordone, 1988) following traumatic brain injury, is likely to result in treatment failures and the general unwillingness to utilize psychotherapeutic approaches with traumatically brain-injured clients even when such treatment might be warranted or even beneficial (Morris & Bleiberg, 1986).

Family Therapy

Many family members of persons with traumatic brain injury possess serious misconceptions about recovery following traumatic brain injury and frequently entertain fantasies such as that clients will awaken from coma in a state likened to sleep, or that clients can "will" themselves to make full recoveries. Recently Gouvier, Presthold, and Warner (1988) examined the attitudes and beliefs of injury and recovery in unselected adults. They reported that the most prevalent misconceptions were present in the areas of unconsciousness, amnesia, and recovery. In these areas, misconceptions were endorsed by half of the respondents. Gouvier et al. felt that, based on these findings, there was a strong need for better education of families of persons with traumatic brain injury, particularly in the domains of understanding unconsciousness, amnesia, and recovery. They also pointed out that families who hold erroneous beliefs tend to place inappropriate demands on the brain-injured individual and encourage premature return to work, school or household responsibilities, thus creating an environment designed to produce failure rather than promote successful recovery and community integration. Unfortunately, few family members receive supportive counseling or psychotherapy even though they are significantly anxious, depressed, and emotionally troubled. Families instead are likely to refer the individual with traumatic brain injury for counseling (at times when it may be inappropriate or ineffective) rather than seek therapy for themselves. The need for supportive counseling and psychotherapy for family members has been previously stressed by Lezak (1978) and Sbordone (1987, 1988).

A CONCEPTUAL MODEL OF PSYCHOTHERAPEUTIC INTERVENTION FOR PERSONS WITH TRAUMATIC BRAIN INJURY

Person-Injury-Environment-Outcome Concept

It is important for clinicians and rehabilitation professionals to understand the person-injury-environment-outcome (PIEO) interaction. This concept assumes that each person who sustains a traumatic brain injury comes into this situation with a heterogeneous background consisting of a history of prior achievements, specific intellectual skills and/or deficits, academic skills, social and behavioral skills, support system, personality style, stress management skills, and unique biological factors (e.g., age, sex, prior history of neurological insults). Brain injury is then superimposed upon these "person" variables. As was pointed out earlier the site and location of a particular brain injury has been shown by numerous investigators (e.g., Cummings, 1985) to produce specific types of neurobehavioral impairments at the cognitive, behavioral, social, and emotional levels. In addition to the site and extent of the brain injury, other injury variables also need to be considered. These variables include: the duration of coma, post-traumatic amnesia, intracranial complications, brain swelling, edema, presence of hypoxia or anoxia, post-traumatic seizures, psychotropic or anti-convulsive medications, and secondary neurological insults. When the various person and injury variables are combined, the heterogeneity and individual differences among persons with traumatic brain injury emerge.

In addition to person and injury variables, what happens to the individual following injury is of enormous significance. For example, the demands that the family and environment place on the individual with traumatic brain injury frequently determine whether he or she will succeed (i.e., attain a good outcome) or fail and become depressed, anxious, or develop significant psychiatric problems. Included within the environmental variables are such factors as the degree of structure and consistency in the brain-injured individual's environment; financial-insurance resources; community resources; the integrity of the family; vocational, academic, and household responsibilities; previous commitments; financial burdens and responsibilities; the understanding of brain-behavior relationships in significant others; and the willingness of significant others to participate in the brain-injured individual's recovery. When environmental variables place unrealistic demands on the individual with traumatic brain injury or exceed his or her capacity to meet the demands and expectations of significant others, the brain-injured individual will most likely experience a series of crippling failures (outcomes). The brain-injured individual may experience a wide variety of outcomes that could be potentially devastating to the recovery process. For example, such events as the loss of important relationships and friends, getting fired, the disintegration of the family system, a poor prognosis for recovery, suspension of driving privileges, being arrested or placed in jail, rejection, or being criticized by others are usually poorly tolerated by traumatically brain-injured individuals and their families and typically result in significant emotional problems (Sbordone, 1987, 1988).

Principle of a Conditional Neurological Lesion

Clinicians who plan on working with traumatically brain-injured clients must, in addition to understanding PIEO interactions, understand the principle of a conditional neurological lesion (Sbordone, 1987, 1988). The principle of the conditional neurological lesion argues that the behavioral manifestations of a neurological insult such as a brain injury are a function of the degree to which the individual is under stress, fatigue, emotional distress, or excessive metabolic demands. Thus, the cognitive functioning of the person with traumatic brain injury would be expected to diminish significantly when he or she becomes anxious or depressed, or is exposed to emotional stresses.

For example, a number of authors have reported that depression can exaggerate or even introduce cognitive impairment on a variety of neuropsychological tests (e.g., Fisher, Sweet, & Pfaelzer-Smith, 1986). Other authors have reported that the extent of cognitive impairment is related to the intensity and severity of the depression (e.g., Weingartner & Silberman, 1982). Since the majority of persons with traumatic brain injury become significantly depressed and anxious between 6 and 12 months postinjury (Lezak, 1987; Sbordone, 1987, 1988) it is important to design psychotherapeutic interventions to alleviate such problems in order to prevent negative emotional and social outcomes from occurring, as these may significantly interfere with the individual's recovery and functioning.

Stages of Cognitive Recovery

The person with traumatic brain injury passes through a set of qualitatively distinct stages of neurobehavioral recovery. Recognition of such stages can be invaluable for the clinician in planning psychotherapeutic intervention and management strategies since each stage requires different psychotherapeutic intervention strategies

(Sbordone, 1988). Table 10.1 presents these six stages.

During the first stage the individual typically is in coma as a result of the traumatic brain injury. The second stage begins when the individual first opens his or her eyes. The stage is characterized either by severe agitation, restlessness, confusion, or a persistent vegetative state. If the individual is not in the latter, he or she is typically disoriented to place and time, but not to person. The third stage begins when the individual becomes oriented to place, but continues to remain disoriented to time (e.g., day of the week). The most salient characteristic of this stage is the individual's marked denial of cognitive deficits. A person in the third stage, however, may complain of somatic problems, particularly if orthopedic injuries were sustained. During this stage of recovery, the individual fatigues rapidly (usually after 10–15 minutes), exhibits poor judgment, and becomes confused easily. Severe attentional deficits (particularly on tasks that involve shifting attention from one task to another), along with severe memory, social, and problem-solving difficulties are typical.

When the traumatically brain-injured individual becomes oriented to place and time, and begins to complain of cognitive deficits, he or she has entered into the fourth stage of recovery. Persons in this stage typically display mild confusion and mild to moderate attentional difficulties. Memory is typically moderately to markedly impaired, while problem-solving skills are usually severely impaired. During this stage the individual may become depressed, with frequent displays of irritability and nervousness. It is also during this stage that the individual may attempt to return to work or school (usually unsuccessfully). During this stage persons with traumatic brain injury appear relatively normal, but in spite of their "normal" appearance, they usually experience moderate to marked difficulties in their social interactions with others.

The fifth stage of recovery is characterized by an increase in the severity of the individual's depression and emotional difficulties. During this stage the individual will often make unfair comparisons to his or her preinjury functioning. For example, the individual will frequently un-

Table 10.1 Stages of recovery in traumatic brain injury

Stages of recovery	Characteristics
Stage 1	Injury In coma
Stage 2	Opens eyes Severe agitation-restlessness or vegetative state Severe confusion Disoriented to place and time
Stage 3	Oriented to place but not time Moderate confusion Denial of cognitive deficits May complain of somatic problems Fatigues very easily Poor judgment Marked to severe attention deficits Severe memory deficits Severe social difficulties Severe problem-solving difficulties
Stage 4	Oriented to place and time Becoming aware of cognitive deficits Mild confusion Mild to moderate attention difficulties Marked problem-solving difficulties Moderate to marked memory deficits Early onset of depression-nervousness Unsuccessful attempts to return to work or school Poor endurance May appear relatively normal Moderate to marked social difficulties
Stage 5	Significant depression-nervousness Mild to moderate memory deficits Mild to moderate problem-solving difficulties Frequent comparison to premorbid self Given little hope of further recovery Has returned to work or school Mild to moderate social difficulties

(continued)

Table 10.1 (*continued*)

Stages of recovery	Characteristics
Stage 6	Mild memory impairment Mild problem-solving difficulties Acceptance of residual deficits Improving social relationships Return of most premorbid responsibilities Generally positive self-image

derestimate present skills and abilities and over-estimate preinjury skills and abilities. It is usually during this stage that the individual is given little hope of further recovery. During this stage, the individual has typically returned to school or work—but he or she is frequently taking a reduced academic load or has been given reduced responsibilities or less demanding assignments. The individual also has typically withdrawn from or has been shunned by most, if not all, of his or her preinjury friends.

The sixth and final stage of recovery is characterized by the individual's gradual acceptance of his or her residual cognitive deficits. Persons in this stage have resumed most if not all of their preinjury responsibilities and have now begun forming new social relationships and friendships. It is during this stage that the traumatically brain-injured individual's self-image becomes generally positive, whereas in the previous stages it had been negative. While the individual continues to experience mild residual memory and problem-solving difficulties, he or she may have developed a number of compensatory behaviors and coping strategies (usually as a consequence of extensive rehabilitation or through the help of friends or family) that permit relatively effective functioning in his or her environment. It should be noted, however, that not all persons with traumatic brain injury reach this final stage of recovery.

DESIGNING SPECIFIC PSYCHOTHERAPEUTIC INTERVENTIONS

Designing specific psychotherapeutic interventions for clients with traumatic brain injury and their families involves an assessment of the client's cognitive-communication, emotional, and social functioning, as well as the families' psychological, emotional, and social functioning. While neuropsychological tests traditionally have been utilized to assess the traumatically brain-injured client's cognitive deficits, the conditions of formal testing, however, may mask many of the client's functional impairments (Szekeres, Ylvisaker, & Holland, 1985). Neuropsychological tests have other shortcomings as well. For example, the test items may have insufficient "ecological validity" in the sense that they do not adequately test the client in real-world situations, and may instead assess preinjury skills, abilities, or knowledge rather than cognitive functions sensitive to brain injury (e.g., intelligence). The tests may also fail to assess the client's ability to generalize newly acquired skills or compensatory behaviors from one setting to another (Sbordone, 1988).

Many neuropsychologists tend to be "test-bound" in that they only report test data and fail to obtain information from significant others or rely on behavioral observations of the client during and outside of the testing situation. Many neuropsychological reports tend to be "ahistorical" in that they frequently lack a chronological history of the client's injury and a detailed preinjury history of the client. Many neuropsychologists tend to focus on the client's deficits and presumed site of injury rather than emphasizing the client's strengths, coping strategies, and compensatory behaviors. Finally, many neuropsychologists tend to be "aprescriptive" and frequently offer little in the way of specific treatment or rehabilitation recommendations. As a consequence, the overwhelming majority of neuropsychological test reports are of little benefit in planning psychotherapeutic treatment or cognitive rehabilitation (Sbordone, 1988).

Neurobehavioral Assessment

The author strongly recommends that clinicians perform a careful neurobehavioral assessment of the traumatically brain-injured client prior to psychotherapeutic intervention. This should include obtaining a detailed history, conducting behavioral observations, and neuropsychological testing.

Historical Information The importance of obtaining a careful history cannot be overemphasized and is seen as vital in planning psychotherapeutic intervention strategies (Brooks, 1988; Prigatano & Konoff, 1988; Sbordone, 1988). In order to obtain this history it is essential that the client with traumatic brain injury be accompanied by at least one relative and/or significant other. Included within this history should be the client's childhood experiences, developmental milestones, educational and occupational achievements; the client's legal, cultural, religious, marital, sexual, medical, psychiatric, and family background; the client's current stressors; and a chronology of the client's injury and treatment. In addition, every effort should be made to review educational, medical, rehabilitation, and treatment records. One should also obtain information about the client's family, including: occupations and education of the parents and siblings; and history of possible substance abuse, criminal behavior, psychiatric problems, and/or separation or divorce.

Behavioral Observations Behavioral observations are an essential component of the neurobehavioral assessment process. Such observations should include the client's behavior under a variety of circumstances, including, but not limited to: open-ended and structured conversations, structured and unstructured settings, familiar and unfamiliar settings, and rest breaks during formal testing procedures. The client's behavior under each of these circumstances often conveys valuable information about communication skills, compensatory behaviors, motivation, cognitive abilities, emotional problems, and ability to cope with the demands of the environment. While the information obtained during behavioral observations is subjective, it should be used to cross-validate historical information and clarify neuropsychological test data.

Neuropsychological Testing Neuropsychological testing represents an important component of the neurobehavioral assessment process. Testing should permit an evaluation of basic areas of cognitive and emotional functioning. The choice of specific tests should reflect:

the client's cultural, educational, and linguistic background; the particular complaints expressed by the client and/or the family; the severity of the client's cognitive deficits; the length of time post-injury; the ability of the client to tolerate stress or fatigue; specific referral questions; the client's cooperation and motivation to perform, familiarity with specific tests, previous testing, physical disabilities, and current emotional and social factors; and the training, background, and experience of the examiner.

Psychotherapy

Once the neurobehavioral assessment process is completed, the designing of the psychotherapeutic intervention can begin. Psychotherapy can be loosely defined as a process that attempts to alleviate the client's emotional distress, as well as modify the client's behavior, and his or her perception of self, others, and the demands of the environment. Psychotherapy can also be viewed as a process that actually modifies the client's environment and teaches the client as much as possible about the nature of his or her neurobehavioral symptoms. This latter process can improve the traumatically brain-injured client's ability to cope with life's problems and to behave in a manner consistent with his or her own best interests (Prigatano & Klonoff, 1988). Included within this definition would be such treatment modalities as individual and group psychotherapy, behavior modification, family therapy, and environmental modification. The later is described next.

Environmental Modification Environmental modification refers to modifying the environment to meet the needs of the client rather than modifying the client to meet the needs of the environment. The importance of environmental modification has been stressed by a number of investigators. For example, Grimm and Bleiberg (1986), have stressed that a carefully structured environment is the treatment of choice for the severely impaired client with traumatic brain injury during the early stages of recovery and that environments can be designed to minimize some of the client's cognitive difficulties as well as to maximize the client's functioning. Environmental modification may eliminate the necessity for the severely brain-injured patient to acquire new information. For example, placing the client in a highly structured environment and on a strict routine has been shown to significantly reduce confusion and anxiety (e.g., Howard, 1988). De-Nour and Bauman (1980) have emphasized the importance of controlling the external environment during the early stages of the psychotherapeutic treatment process and focusing on the psychodynamic aspects of the client's behavior during the latter stages of the recovery process. They emphasize that these shifts in psychotherapeutic orientation require careful timing and serial neuropsychological assessment to determine the readiness of the client to accept psychodynamic interpretations of his or her behavior. Eames (1988) has recently stressed that it is essential to evaluate the stage of recovery the client has reached in deciding on the specific type of treatment or management the client should receive. He further stressed that early after injury, disturbed behavior is best managed by environmental modifications such as eliminating environmental precipitants such as pain, a full bladder or bowels, alien surroundings, or insensitive or authoritative handling of the client (Eames, 1988).

TREATMENT CONSIDERATIONS

First Stage of Recovery

During the first stage of recovery when the client is in coma, it is the family who must bear the emotional and psychological burden caused by the injury. It is during this stage that families should receive educational and family therapy to rectify their misperceptions and help them cope with their feelings of helplessness, shock, denial, and confusion.

Second and Third Stages of Recovery

Neurobehavioral assessment typically indicates that persons with traumatic brain injury, during the second and third stages of the recovery process, have severe attentional problems and are unable to comprehend environmental or social cues or are unable to organize this information. As a consequence, their behavior is poorly orga-

nized, which results in frequent rambling and incoherent conversations, and they have a poorly organized semantic base, which typically results in unusual associations. Thus individuals with traumatic brain injury lack self-awareness and are unable to monitor their behavior or recognize or correct their errors. In addition, they frequently exhibit emotional outbursts that have been described as "catastrophic reactions" (Goldstein, 1942).

It is recommended that environmental modification techniques be utilized during the second and third stages of the recovery process to minimize the client's emotional outbursts. This would include placing the client in a highly controlled and structured environment so that he or she will become accustomed to its demands and eventually learn the daily routine. Activities should be selected so that they will not exceed the client's ability to encode and process information. Consistent communication is necessary to permit orientation and integration of cognitive functioning. The structured environment may serve as an "ancillary cortex and brain stem" since it regulates the various environmental stimuli that impinge upon the client and compensates for brain injury.

It is important that the client be allowed to achieve success in this highly structured environment since with increasing successes gradual increases can be made in the environment's demand characteristics. Unfortunately, many clients with traumatic brain injury are either transferred to another program or are discharged home during these stages, which typically increases the client's confusion and precipitates catastrophic emotional behavior that may alienate the family and/or significant others. Thus, the client should not be discharged home or transferred to another program prior to entering the fourth stage of recovery—unless the home environment or new program is highly structured.

During the second and third stages of recovery, the family of the client with traumatic brain injury is frequently devastated by the enormous financial, emotional, and psychological burdens that have been placed upon it. Rather than seeking professional help or appearing depressed, family members often manifest what has been described earlier as a "command performance syndrome" in which they appear relatively composed or "normal" even though they are severely emotionally distraught. During these stages of recovery, the family typically uses denial as a means of coping with the tragedy of the client's disability. Family members are typically ill equipped or reluctant to impose a highly structured environment if the client is discharged home during these stages. Because of their massive denial and poor understanding of head injury, their demands frequently exceed the brain-injured client's ability to encode and process information, which results in considerable cognitive-communicative confusion and emotional outbursts that family members fail to comprehend or accept.

During these stages of recovery family members continue to require educational and supportive therapy, which should assist them in modifying the home environment to facilitate recovery of the client's impaired attentional and informational processing capabilities. Also, families require a great deal of supportive counseling to guide them through this very difficult process. Psychodynamic techniques may be used to alleviate the use of defense mechanisms such as avoidance, convergence, denial, displacement, projection, rationalization, repression, and somatization.

Fourth Stage of Recovery

While the client with traumatic brain injury may appear relatively "normal" during the fourth stage of recovery, neurobehavioral assessment typically reveals that the client's conceptual and problem-solving skills are markedly impaired. The ability to encode, store, and retrieve information, particularly after delays of 30 minutes or longer, is also markedly impaired. Increases in the rate of encoding, the complexity of material, or the abstractness of language is likely to produce a disproportionate number of errors of cognitive processing (Hagen, 1981). Although the client's ability to monitor his or her behavior is improved, he or she is only partially aware that errors are being made. Since the client lacks the cognitive resources to correct or rectify these

errors, he or she experiences a sense of frustration that leads to depression, catastrophic reactions, or socially inappropriate behavior. Frequently, persons with traumatic brain injury are pressured by family members to return to work, school, or household responsibilities. Unfortunately, since persons with traumatic brain injury are only minimally aware of their cognitive-communicative impairments during this fourth stage of recovery, they often attempt to return to work, school, or household responsibilities, but then are likely to fail or perform poorly. These outcomes are poorly tolerated by the client, family, and significant others. Also, traumatically brain-injured clients may receive additional pressure from their families to perform at their preinjury level of functioning at home; however, their ability to perform at this level usually falls below the families' expectations. Consequently, the client's behavior will often alienate family and friends. As a means of coping with this outcome, the client may use the disability in order to obtain attention and manipulate others (Sbordone, 1987). Recently there has been a growing awareness that clients during this stage of recovery may also develop an "atypical bipolar depression" or affective disorder characterized by rapid mood swings, irritability, grandiose thinking, impulsive and often violent behavior, pressured speech, hyperactivity, and hypersexuality, as well as exhibit behavioral manifestations of temporal lobe epilepsy (Sbordone, 1988; Shukla, Cook, Mukherjee, Godwin, & Miller, 1987), which necessitates referral for pharmacological treatment.

The treatment of clients with traumatic brain injury during the fourth stage of recovery should focus on environmental and behavioral modification. Environmental modification within this stage should focus on maximizing the traumatically brain-injured client's functioning within several relatively structured or familiar environments. Activities during this stage of recovery should be neither overwhelming nor boring. Activities should be familiar and liked by the client. Rest periods and naps are essential to reduce the client's poor endurance. Clinicians should be flexible in scheduling time with the client in order to fit in therapy when the client is alert and not fatigued. Frequent rest periods and naps, as well as keeping the demands of the client within his or her fluctuating capabilities throughout the course of the day, should be effective in preventing such outcomes as agitation, irritability, combative outbursts, lethargy, and foul language.

The use of compensatory assistive devices (e.g., notebooks, charts, calendars, watches, microcomputers, tape recorders) should be utilized to improve the client's sense of mastery over his or her environment. The use of these devices should be encouraged and rewarded by the therapist. When angry outbursts or socially inappropriate behaviors occur, the client's attention should be directed to innocuous tasks. An attempt should also be made to examine carefully the level of stimulation in the client's environment. Restraints should be kept to a minimum at all times, allowing as much freedom of movement as possible within the well-defined boundaries of the environment. In the absence of such boundaries, clients with traumatic brain injury are likely to become confused, agitated, and disoriented (Howard, 1988).

The use of behavior modification strategies during the fourth stage of recovery is highly recommended since the client's improved level of cognitive functioning permits such techniques to be utilized to decrease inappropriate behavior and increase positive behavior. During this stage, behavior modification can be utilized to increase independent ambulation (Eames & Wood, 1985) and reduce maladaptive social behavior (Burke & Lewis, 1986). Burke and Wesolowski (1988) have recommended a six-step behavior modification procedure for the traumatically brain-injured client that consists of identification of target behavior, measurement of the behavior, functional analysis of the environmental conditions, intervention, programming generalizations, and evaluation of results. Unfortunately, while behavior analysis procedures have been gaining increasing acceptance as a viable form of treatment for the client with traumatic brain injury, behavior analysis procedures are frequently misunderstood and often are applied incorrectly by many therapists (Jacobs, 1988).

During the fourth stage, the family of the client with traumatic brain injury is often dealing with problems of anger and guilt. Some members have even become martyrs. The family continues to scapegoat other members of the immediate family and becomes socially withdrawn and isolated from the community. Often families may display behaviors such as frequent arguing, coercion, lying, and running away, and may become extremely critical and demanding of the client with traumatic brain injury. During this stage of recovery the family may seek out professional help to change or eliminate the client's frequent disruptive behavioral outbursts.

Psychotherapeutic interventions during the fourth stage should consist of teaching the family to utilize behavior modification techniques to reduce the frequency of the client's inappropriate social behaviors or disruptive emotional outbursts. However, it has been this author's experience that unless family members have been receiving supportive counseling since the client's injury, they may be too emotionally distressed or "burned out" to cooperate with the therapist in setting up effective behavioral modification programs at home. The author strongly recommends that counseling be given to family members to alleviate their high levels of emotional distress. Psychodynamic techniques may be helpful to permit family members to appropriately vent their anger and feelings of frustration, and confront their unrealistic demands and expectations. Only after their emotional distress has been significantly reduced should the therapist begin to teach family members behavioral techniques to diminish the client's disruptive behaviors.

Fifth Stage of Recovery

Clients with traumatic brain injury during the fifth stage of recovery are typically characterized by mild to moderate memory, problem-solving, and emotional difficulties. They may also exhibit mild word-finding, fluency, and word-retrieval problems, as well as exhibit a number of subtle nonverbal communication problems. While their ability to self-monitor their behavior and generalize their behavior to new situations and environments has improved, it is still impaired.

During this stage, clients with traumatic brain injury become more aware of their cognitive-communicative impairments. While their ability to engage in reasoning tasks is generally good in concrete or structured settings, their reasoning skills may be poor in either stressful or unstructured settings. When presented with complex communications or material, they may become easily lost in details and fail to grasp the main idea or underlying concept. Their ability to encode and organize new information is frequently related to its rate of presentation, quantity, and complexity.

During the fifth stage of recovery clients with traumatic brain injury should continue to receive behavior modification therapy. Clients should also be considered for individual psychotherapy, which should be more task or goal oriented and supportive rather than psychodynamic. During this stage a token economy program is likely to be most effective because of improved cognitive functioning, particularly with respect to recent memory. Eames and Wood (1985) have stressed the importance of the relative preparedness of clients with traumatic brain injury when considering token economy programs. They reported that token economy programs were often ineffective when clients were placed in the program prior to reaching a sufficient level of recovery. However, when these clients were placed in the program (6–12 months later) after they had achieved a higher level of recovery, they derived considerable benefit and demonstrated significant improvement in their behavioral functioning.

During the fifth stage of recovery, families are typically depressed, and have often "given up" on the client. Marital and family problems are extremely common. The family system has usually disintegrated in that many family members have moved away (frequently to another city), and often make little effort to maintain contact with other family members. However, one member of the family (usually the client's mother) often becomes a martyr and blames him or herself for the disability. Alcohol and substance abuse problems are very common during this stage as a result of these factors. Families continue to require supportive counseling and psychotherapy. The goal of therapy during this stage should be to alleviate feelings of guilt

among family members, and to restructure the family system. In many instances, one or more members of the family will need to be referred to appropriate alcohol and/or substance abuse programs. Therapy should also focus on minimizing the use of defense mechanisms such as avoidance, denial, depression, distortions, grudges, postponing, running away, and scapegoating that have resulted in the disintegration of the family system as well as crippled the traumatically brain-injured client's support system and recovery.

Sixth Stage of Recovery

Clients with traumatic brain injury in the sixth and final stage of recovery are typically left with mild residual cognitive problems. If these clients acquired compensatory skills and strategies during the previous stages of recovery, they will often function at a relatively effective level within their environment providing it has not reinforced their disability, has not made unrealistic demands upon them, or has not been supportive of their efforts toward recovery. Many of these clients will have returned to their preinjury vocational and social responsibilities. As a consequence, their self-esteem has become generally positive. Since their social and communication skills have improved, they frequently have made new friends who may overlook some of their occasional inappropriate social and emotional behaviors. The cognitive-communicative impairments of these clients are rarely apparent to casual acquaintances; however, individuals who spend more time with them will recognize their impairments and limitations and should not make unreasonable or excessive demands. Clients with traumatic brain injury during this stage typically do not become depressed or emotional when discussing their cognitive problems (as they frequently did in stage five), but generally rely on their mastery of compensatory behaviors and strategies to cope with new situations or crises. When these clients are fatigued or placed under excessive environmental demands and stresses, they may regress and exhibit cognitive and emotional behaviors that were seen during stages four and five. When these stresses are alleviated the client's behavior will return to the level of functioning consistent with this stage.

Clients with traumatic brain injury during

stage six require a combination of individual and group counseling. These therapies should provide them with emotional support as well as continued training in the use of compensatory strategies to maximize their behavioral, cognitive, and communicative functioning. Psychodynamic and insight-oriented therapeutic approaches are appropriate during this stage since clients' insight into their problems is typically good.

During the sixth and final stage of recovery, the family now possesses a good understanding of traumatic brain injury and has generally accepted the client's residual cognitive and behavioral impairments. The family system has restructured and made a gradual return to normalcy. As a consequence, family members have become more independent and resumed community activities in which they had participated prior to the client's injury. Family members may still, however, require counseling to help them cope with the trauma that has created havoc in their lives. Certain family members may still harbor feelings of resentment or guilt that need to be resolved so that they can return to their preinjury level of social and emotional functioning.

SUMMARY

Within the past few years, there has been a growing realization that clients with traumatic brain injury are far more seriously handicapped by the behavioral, social, and emotional disturbances that accompany such injuries rather than their residual cognitive or physical disabilities. In the past, recognition of these problems has been hindered by strict reliance on psychometric test data, and failure to interview significant others and observe the client's behavior in unstructured situations. It has also been hindered by the overwhelming number of tests that are available to evaluate the client's cognitive functioning and the relative scarcity of tests available to evaluate the client's behavioral, social, and emotional functioning, particularly in real-world or unstructured settings. The failure, in the past, to interview the family and significant others of the traumatically brain-injured client has hindered an understanding of their emotional problems and contributed to a general reluctance to utilize a systems model when treating the client with brain injury.

Clients who sustain traumatic brain injury go through six discrete stages of recovery. Treatment of the client and his or her family should be determined by the stage of recovery rather than the enthusiasm of the therapist or wishes of the client or family. In this chapter, a conceptual model of psychotherapeutic intervention was proposed. This model emphasized the importance of understanding the person-injury-environment-outcome interaction. Clinicians who work with brain-injured clients must also understand the principle of a conditional neurological lesion, which argues that the behavioral manifestations of a brain injury vary as a function of the degree to which the client is under stress, fatigue, emotional distress, or excessive metabolic demands.

Neurobehavioral assessment, which includes a detailed history, behavioral observations, interviews with significant others, and neuropsychological testing, is vital in planning psychotherapeutic invention strategies for the client with traumatic brain injury and the family. Psychotherapeutic interventions should attempt to alleviate the client and family's emotional distress, modify their behavior and environment, and teach them methods of coping with others and with environmental demands.

REFERENCES

Alexander, M.P. (1982). Traumatic brain injury. In D.F. Benson & D. Blumer (Eds.), *Psychiatric aspects of neurologic disease* (Vol. II; pp. 219–250). New York: Grune & Stratton.

Alexander, M.P. (1984). Neuro-behavioral consequences of closed head injury. *Neurology and Neuro-surgery, Update Series 20*, 1–8.

Bach-Y-Rita, G., Lion, J., Climent, C., & Ervin, F.R. (1971). Episodic dyscontrol: A study of 130 violent patients. *American Journal of Psychiatry, 127*, 49–54.

Barth, J.T., Macciocchi, S.M., Giordani, B., Rimel, R., Jane, J.A., & Boll, T.J. (1983). Neuropsychological sequelae of minor head injury. *Neurosurgery, 13*, 529–533.

Baxter, R., Cohen, S.B., & Ylvisaker, M. (1985). Comprehensive cognitive assessment. In M. Ylvisaker (Ed.), *Head injury rehabilitation: Chil-*

dren and adolescents. San Diego: College-Hill Press.

Bock, S.H. (1987). Psycho-therapy of the individual with brain injury. *Brain Injury, 2*, 203–206.

Bond, M.R. (1975). Assessment of the psychosocial outcome after severe head injury. In *CIBA Foundation Symposium 34, Outcome of severe damage to the central nervous system* (pp. 141–157). Amsterdam: Elsevier/Excerpta Medica.

Bond, M.R. (1984). The psychiatry of closed head injury. In D.N. Brooks (Ed.), *Closed head injury: Psychological, social, and family consequences* (pp. 148–178). New York: Oxford University Press.

Bond, M.R. (1986). Neurobehavioral sequelae of closed head injury. In I. Grant & K.M. Adams (Eds.), *Neuropsychological assessment of neuropsychiatric disorders* (pp. 347–373). New York: Oxford University Press.

Bowen, M. (1978). *Marital therapy in clinical practice*. New York: Aronsen.

Brooks, N. (1988). Behavioral abnormalities in head injured patients. *Scandinavian Journal of Rehabilitation Medicine Supplement, 117*, 41–46.

Burke, W.H., & Lewis, F.D. (1986). Management of maladaptive social behavior in the brain-injured adult. *International Journal of Rehabilitation Research, 9*, 335–342.

Burke, W.H., & Wesolowski, M.D. (1988). Applied behavior analysis in head injury rehabilitation. *Rehabilitation Nursing, 13*(4), 186–188.

Cardenas, D.D. (1984). Antipsychotics and their use after traumatic brain injury. *Journal of Head Trauma Rehabilitation, 2*(4), 43–49.

Cooper, P.R. (1982). Epidemiology of head trauma. In P.R. Cooper (Ed.), *Head injury* (pp. 1–14). Baltimore: Williams & Wilkins.

Cummings, J.L. (1985). *Clinical neuropsychiatry*. New York: Grune & Stratton.

Deaton, A.V. (1987). Behavioral change strategies for children and adolescents with severe brain injury. *Journal of Learning Disabilities, 20*(10), 581–589.

De-Nour, A.K., & Bauman, A. (1980). Psychiatric treatment in severe brain injury. *General Hospital Psychiatry, 2*, 23–24.

Eames, P. (1988). Behavior disorders after severe head injury: Their nature and causes and strategies for management. *Journal of Head Trauma Rehabilitation, 3*(3), 1–6.

Eames, P., & Wood, R. (1985). Rehabilitation after severe brain injury: A follow-up study of a behavior modification approach. *Journal of Neurology, Neurosurgery, and Psychiatry, 48*, 613–619.

Fisher, D.G., Sweet, J.J., & Pfaelzer-Smith, E.A. (1986). Influence of depression on repeated neuropsychological testing. *International Journal of Clinical Neuropsychology, 8*, 14–18.

Goldstein, H. (1942). *After effects of brain injuries in man*. New York: Grune & Stratton.

Goldstein, H. (1952). The effect of brain damage on the personality. *Psychiatry, 15*, 245–260.

Gouvier, W.D., Presthold, P.H., & Warner, M.S. (1988). A survey of common misconceptions about head injury and recovery. *Archives of Clinical Neuropsychology, 3*, 331–343.

Graham, D.I., Hume Adams, J., & Gennarelli, T.A. (1987). Pathology of brain damage in head injury. In P.R. Cooper (Ed.), *Head injury* (pp. 72–88). Baltimore: Williams & Wilkins.

Grimm & Bleiberg. (1986). Psychological rehabilitation in traumatic brain injury. In S.B. Filskov & T.J. Boll (Eds.), *Handbook of Clinical Neuropsychology* (pp. 495–527). New York: John Wiley & Sons.

Hagen, C. (1981). Language disorders secondary to closed head injury: Diagnosis and treatment. *Topics in Language Disorders, 1*(4), 73–83.

Howard, M.E. (1988). Behavior management in the acute care rehabilitation setting. *Journal of Head Trauma Rehabilitation, 3*(3), 14–22.

Jacobs, H.E. (1988). Yes, behavioral analysis can help, but do you know how to harness it? *Brain Injury, 2*(4), 339–346.

Klonoff, H., Low, M.D., & Clark, C. (1977). Head injuries in children: A prospective five year follow-up. *Journal of Neurology, Neurosurgery, and Psychiatry, 40*, 1211–1219.

Lezak, M.D. (1978). Living with the characterologically altered brain injured patient. *Journal of Clinical Psychiatry, 39*, 592–598.

Lezak, M.D. (1987). Relationships between personality disorders, social disturbances, and physical disability following traumatic brain injury. *Journal of Head Trauma Rehabilitation, 2*(1), 57–69.

Lishman, W.A. (1968). Brain damage in relation to psychiatric disability after head injury. *British Journal of Psychiatry, 114*, 373–410.

Mandelberg, J.A., & Brooks, D.N. (1975). Cognitive recovery after severe head injury. *Journal of Neurology, Neurosurgery, and Psychiatry, 38*, 1121–1126.

Miller, H., & Stern, G. (1965). The long-term prognosis of severe head injury. *Lancet, 1*, 225–229.

Morris, J., & Bleiberg, J. (1986). Neuropsychological rehabilitation and traditional psycho-therapy. *International Journal of Clinical Neuropsychology, 8*(3), 133–134.

Oddy, M., Humphrey, M., & Uttley, D. (1978). Stresses upon the relatives of head-injured patients. *British Journal of Psychiatry, 133*, 507–513.

Panting, A., & Merry, P.H. (1972). The long-term rehabilitation of severe head injuries with particular reference for the need for social and medical support for the patient's family. *Rehabilitation, 38*, 33–37.

Prigatano, G.P., & Klonoff, P.S. (1988). Psychotherapy and neuro-psychological assessment after brain injury. *Journal of Head Trauma Rehabilitation, 3*(1), 45–56.

Rimmele, C.T., & Hester, R.K. (1987). Cognitive rehabilitation after traumatic head injury. *Archives of Clinical Neuropsychology, 2,* 353–384.

Romano, M.D. (1974). Family response to traumatic head injury. *Scandinavian Journal of Rehabilitation Medicine, 6,* 1–4.

Rosenbaum, M., & Najenson, T. (1976). Changes in life patterns and symptoms of low mood as reported by wives of severely brain injured soldiers. *Journal of Consulting and Clinical Psychology, 44*(6), 881–888.

Sbordone, R.J. (1984). Rehabilitative neuropsychological approach for severe traumatic brain-injured patients. *Professional Psychology: Research and Practice, 15,* 165–175.

Sbordone, R.J. (1985, March). *Atypical bipolar depressive disorder following right diencephalic brain injury.* Paper presented at International Conference on Traumatic Brain Injury, San José, CA.

Sbordone, R.J. (1987). A conceptual model of neuropsychologically based cognitive rehabilitation. In J.M. Williams & C.J. Long (Eds.), *The rehabilitation of cognitive disabilities* (pp. 1–25). New York: Plenum.

Sbordone, R.J. (1988). Assessment and treatment of cognitive communicative impairments in the closed-head injury patient: A neurobehavioral-systems approach. *Journal of Head Trauma Rehabilitation, 3*(2), 55–62.

Sbordone, R.J., Kral, M., Gerard, M., & Katz, J. (1984). Evidence of a "command performance syndrome" in the significant others of the victims of severe traumatic head injury. *The International Journal of Clinical Neuropsychology, 6,* 183–185.

Sbordone, R.J., & Purisch, A.D. (1987). Clinical neuropsychology: Medico-legal application (Part 2). *Trauma, 6,* 61–94.

Sbordone, R.J., & Rudd, M. (1986). Can psychologists recognize neurological disorders? *Journal of Experimental and Clinical Neuropsychology, 8*(3), 285–291.

Schacter, D.L., & Glisky, E.L. (1986). Memory remediation: Restoration alleviation and the acquisition of domain-specific knowledge. In B.P. Uzzell & Y. Gross (Eds.), *Clinical neuropsychology of intervention* (pp. 257–282). Boston: Martinus Nijhoff.

Shukla, S., Cook, B.L., Mukherjee, S., Godwin, C., & Miller, M.G. (1987). Mania following head trauma. *American Journal of Psychiatry, 144*(1), 93–96.

Smilkstein, G. (1980). The cycle of family function: Conceptual model for family medicine. *The Journal of Family Practice, 11*(2), 223–232.

Soderstrom, S., Fogelsjoo, A., Fugl-Meyer, K. S., & Stensson, S. (1988). A program for crises intervention after traumatic brain injury. *Scandinavian Journal of Rehabilitation Medicine, 17,* 47–49.

Stern, J.M. (1985). The quality of the psychotherapeutic process in brain-injured patients. *Scandinavian Journal of Rehabilitation Medicine Supplement, 12,* 42–43.

Szerkeres, S. F., Ylvisaker, M,. & Holland, A. L. (1985). Cognitive rehabilitation therapy: A framework for intervention. In M. Ylvisaker, (Ed.), *Head injury rehabilitation: Children and adolescents* (pp. 219–246). San Diego: College-Hill Press.

Thomsen, I.V. (1974). The patient with severe head injury and his family—A follow-up study of 50 patients. *Scandinavian Journal of Rehabilitation Medicine, 6,* 180–183.

Thomsen, I.V. (1981). Neuropsychological treatment and long-time follow-up in an aphasic patient with very severe head trauma. *Journal of Clinical Neuropsychology, 3*(1), 43–51.

Thomsen, I.V. (1987). Late psychosocial outcome in severe blunt head trauma. *Brain Injury, 1*(2), 131–143.

Weingartner, H., & Silberman, E. (1982). Models of cognitive impairment: Cognitive changes in depression. *Psychopharmacology Bulletin, 18,* 27–42.

Wood, R. (1988). Management of behavior disorders in a day treatment setting. *Journal of Head Trauma Rehabilitation, 3*(3), 53–61.

SECTION IV
Vocational Rehabilitation

CHAPTER 11

Vocational Memory Training

Rick Parenté and Janet K. Anderson-Parenté

Memory and cognitive impairments are perhaps the most pervasive and limiting residual effects of head injury. They not only restrict the person's ability to function socially but also reduce employment potential. In response to this problem there has been a virtual explosion of therapy techniques and computer software for memory retraining. Unfortunately, there is little in the way of systematic research to assess which of these training regimens facilitates return to work or will otherwise determine the head-injured person's success in job placement. Therefore, the major purpose of this chapter is to present a method for assessing the utility of memory therapies for vocational reentry. The discussion begins by examining the principles of generalization and transfer of learning. It is then shown how these principles can predict the effectiveness of most memory retraining therapies. The final part of the chapter describes various electronic devices and computer applications that have proven effective in the authors' prevocational training efforts.

GENERALIZATION AND THE TRANSFER OF LEARNING

The terms *generalization* and *transfer* are frequently confused. On the one hand, generalization refers to trainable skills that the person can use in a new or different context. For example, teaching a person to use memory strategies may improve his or her memory in a variety of new situations. Transferable skills, on, the other hand, are directly applicable to certain tasks but not necessarily to others. For example, the therapist may train the person to do data entry at competitive speed. This training may be useful only so long as the person eventually works in a

similar capacity. As a general rule if a person spontaneously applies what he or she learns in therapy to activities of daily living, then teaching generalizable memory strategies may be a viable cognitive rehabilitation strategy. However, if the person has lost the capacity to generalize, then training specific transferable skills may be the only viable therapy option.

Vocational memory training differs from conventional cognitive rehabilitation therapy because the therapist frequently knows in advance what the person with head injury will eventually do when he or she returns to work. Surveying the job allows the therapist to structure treatment to promote transfer of generalizable memory strategies and specific transferable skills. To the extent that the therapist is able to train memory skills that will eventually transfer to the job, then the results of therapy are predictable from well-known transfer-of-learning principles.

Ellis (1965, 1969) has comprehensively documented the basic paradigms for transfer of learning. The interventions outlined below are based on modifications of these principles. The goal of vocational memory training is simple. The therapist teaches the person with head injury to associate specific response sets (how the person learns to perform the task) to specific task elements (what the person sees, hears, and so forth while doing the task) to accomplish some measurable goal. The effects of training are predictable when the response sets and task elements are similar to those that the person will eventually encounter on the job. There are six transfer paradigms that predict the effectiveness of most vocational memory training interventions. These are described in Table 11.1.

Practically any vocational memory training procedure can be roughly divided into task ele-

Table 11.1.   Transfer paradigms

Type of transfer	Training/therapy		Employment		Amount of type of transfer
	Task element	Response set	Task element	Response set	
Positive	A	B	A	B	+ + + +
Positive	A	B	A'	B'	+ + +
Positive	A	B	C	B	+ +
Negative	A	B	A	C	– – –
Negative	A	B	A	Br	– – – –
Neutral	A	B	C	D	+

ments and response sets. The second and third columns of Table 11.1 diagram this training process. Each paradigm assumes that the person learns to associate task elements (A) with a certain response set (B). For example, training a head-injured person to be a data-entry clerk involves working with a particular computer keyboard, monitor, data forms, and so forth (A). The person must learn specific sequences of actions (B) to enter the data, and to operate the computer.

The fourth and fifth columns describe the actual job where the person will eventually work after therapy. This is also an A-B associative process although the task elements and response sets may differ from those encountered in therapy. For example, the person may have to work on a different computer (change in task elements) or learn a slightly different data-entry system (change in response set). The number of plus or minus signs in the far-right-hand column of the table indicates the amount of positive or negative transfer that each training paradigm yields.

In the first paradigm (A-B:A-B), the task elements (A) and the response sets (B) are the same from therapy to employment. Indeed, the two are literally identical. Transfer is perfect because the person's memory is unchanged when he or she eventually begins the job. However, this type of therapy is idealized and is seldom attainable in a rehabilitation facility. Usually, there are differences between the training and employment tasks, which limits the amount of transferable memory. In the second paradigm, the discrepancy between the two is abbreviated by apostrophes to the right of the A and B terms. For example, an A' indicates that the therapy and employment tasks are slightly different in terms

of their task element characteristics. Likewise, B' indicates that the way the person must respond to and organize the task will differ slightly from therapy to employment. More apostrophes indicate greater dissimilarity. Training thus becomes less and less effective because the head-injured person will have to reorganize, elaborate, or otherwise modify his or her skills upon beginning the job.

The A-B:C-B transfer in the third paradigm involves task elements that are different from those the head-injured person will eventually encounter on the job. However, the response sets are the same. For example, the person may learn data entry on one computer but may begin work with the same software package on a different computer. The computer system or screen displays may look much different (A and C) but the response sets required to operate the package are the same (B).

Vocational memory training seldom directly copies the task elements of real-world employment. If the physical environment is considerably different from training to employment, the situation is best described as an A-B:A'''-B transfer paradigm. In many cases, it is difficult to distinguish this paradigm from the A-B:C-B when the task elements are very different (e.g., A''''). However, relative to a neutral paradigm (A-B:C-D), the A-B:C-B model significantly enhances acquisition of job functions because the person's response sets are the same.

The fourth and fifth paradigms in the table inhibit transfer and should therefore be avoided. In the A-B:A-C paradigm, the task elements are similar in therapy and employment but the person's response sets are different. For example, the therapist may train a head-injured person to sort objects by size with the goal that the training will directly transfer to the job. In this example, the objects are the task elements and the response sets are how the person learns to organize the objects according to size. Unbeknownst to the therapist, the job may involve sorting the same objects by weight or color. This is, then, an A-B:A-C paradigm, which will produce negative transfer. Relative to no therapy or unrelated training, this type would actually impair job performance.

The A-B:A-Br paradigm produces massive negative transfer relative to the neutral A-B:C-D model. The lower case r after the last B indicates that the response sets are actually re-associated with the same task elements. With respect to the data-entry example, they may occur when the same response sets are reassociated with the same task elements. For example, response sets are typically the same from one date-entry system or word processor to another (e.g., search/replace, ditto rest of form); however, the same function keys may signify different operations on the various systems, thus defeating the goal of training. The A-B:A-Br negative transfer paradigm is especially important to avoid because the results are difficult to reverse or overcome. What the therapist may see as useful training may eventually lead to extreme frustration and/or a failure experience for the person with head injury.

In the sixth paradigm (A-B:C-D), the task elements (A and C) and response sets (B and D) differ from training to employment. As previously noted, this is a neutral paradigm because there are no specific aspects of training that generalize when the person with head injury begins work. There are, however, sources of transfer that result from improvements in attention/concentration, vigilance, and immediate memory (this accounts for the single + in the far-right-hand column of the table).

The advantage of this classification system is that it allows the therapist to predict whether their treatment will transfer positively to the workplace. The same paradigms are also useful for predicting the effects of learning generalizable memory strategies. Next, a discussion of how the effects of many different cognitive re-mediation procedures are predictable from this system is presented.

Stimulation Therapy

Stimulation therapy is perhaps the oldest and still the most popular model of memory training (Gross & Schutz, 1986). The goal is to enhance general cognitive capacities via cognitive exercise. Usually, computers are used to provide treatment with software that is matched to the head-injured person's specific patterns of deficits. For example, the therapist may prescribe jigsaw puzzles for a head-injured person with part/whole perceptual deficits. Generally, however, this type of training is based on the assumption that the mind is a muscle—thus, exercise or stimulation of the mental muscle will improve memory and cognitive skill. This assumption has not been consistently validated (Schacter & Glisky, 1986).

Stimulation therapy was originally proposed by Scheull, Carroll, and Street (1955), Taylor (1964), and Wepman (1951). Speech therapists still rely heavily on the stimulation therapy approach although they more commonly use paper-and-pencil materials rather than computers. Since there are no easily identifiable A-B similarities between therapy and employment, this approach is best described as an A-B:C-D memory transfer paradigm. The classification predicts that the therapy will produce only general sources of transfer.

Cognitive Skills Therapy

The goals of cognitive skills therapy go well beyond the "mental push-up" model outlined above. The purpose is to teach the head-injured person generalizable strategies or processes (Bracy, 1988) that are directly relevant to his or her activities of daily living. Parenté, Anderson, and Shaw (in press) provide an example of this type of application. In their study, persons with head injury were trained to recognize words that were presented via computer at brief durations (too fast for the eye to scan the word via muscle movements). The goal of the therapy was to force the person to process more information during the brief pauses between their saccadic eye motions. The logic was simple. If the person could learn to process more information during the eye fixations, then the training would transfer to a functional task such as reading. This was precisely the result. Training to recall letters presented with brief duration flashes increased word recognition and reading comprehension significantly relative to a group of controls who received attention/concentration training prior to the reading comprehension task.

A second example should help to clarify the point that cognitive skills training is most effective when there is a clearly transferable quality to the training. Many stimulation therapy computer packages provide "digit span" training. These programs present number strings and the head-injured person tries to recall them. The authors question the transferable quality of this type of mental exercise. However, a simple modification of the same procedure can produce marked improvement in functional memory.

Rather than remembering random number strings, the authors suggest teaching the person with head injury to remember phone numbers by grouping them into sets of 3 numbers followed by 2 groups of 2 numbers each. Specifically, the authors read phone numbers as individual digits (e.g., three, two, four, six, eight, nine, five). The head-injured person learns to organize the phone numbers into 3 groups and to recall them accordingly (e.g., three twenty-four, sixty-eight, ninety-five). The training therefore conforms to an A-B:C-B transfer paradigm because the digits (task elements) will be the same from therapy to actual-life experience. However, the grouping procedure (response set) allows the person with head injury to rehearse the digits more effectively, which improves memory.

Memory Strategies

Persons with head injury are frequently trained to use memory strategies as part of their cognitive rehabilitation therapy. The basic approach is to teach a variety of memory strategies such as mnemonics, imagery, or other forms of verbal mediation. For example, the therapist may train the person with head injury to form mental images of items on a shopping list or to imagine walking through a store and mentally locating the items on the shelves before actually going to the store. Wilson (1987) has convincingly demonstrated that these memory strategies can improve recall of word lists and text materials. Parenté and Anderson (1984) have also documented the effectiveness of these "internal" encoding skills.

Memory strategies have their roots in cognitive psychology. This literature is replete with demonstrations that memory strategies can boost the memory capacity of "normals" to incredible new heights (Bower, 1970). The assumption is that they can also increase a head-injured person's memory capacity to at least average levels. The challenge is to get the person with head injury to use the strategies spontaneously.

The authors have found that training to use mnemonic devices as a prevocational therapy is seldom effective unless the devices are context specific. For example, mnemonic training may emphasize rote memorization of specific rhymes that the person with head injury can use to mediate retrieval of important job-related information. Motivation to learn the rhymes is increased because the person can see immediate relevance to the job. However, mnemonic or imagery training that is unrelated to the job may improve memory for word lists or other contrived materials but will seldom generalize to the head-injured person's work or activities of daily living.

According the principles of memory transfer outlined above, training the head-injured person to use context-specific mnemonic strategies conforms to an A-B:C-B paradigm. The task elements differ from therapy to the actual job but the response set is the same. For example, the goal may be to train the person to spell by teaching rhymes for remembering spelling or grammar rules (e.g., "i before e except after c"). This type of therapy has been useful for those who have eventually gone on to work in a clerical capacity. Training seldom includes all of the words or phrases the person with head injury will eventually encounter on the job. However, the response of using the mnemonic device to mediate the correct spelling will be the same whenever the person encounters a particular word or phrase where he or she can apply it. Many times, the therapist will have to create the rhymes for the head-injured person. The therapist must study the job and create a rhyme that integrates relevant information, then train the person to use the rhyme. The following clarifies the process.

Case # 1

Paul was a lab technician prior to his automobile accident. After a year of cognitive skills therapy he returned to work but was unable to figure simple fractional amounts in his head. Although he usually used a calculator, there were many times when his hands were occupied and he had to do mental calculations that included manipulation of fractions. Paul and the authors developed the following rhyme to do fractional manipulations correctly.

> Multiply straight across
> To divide, first invert
> To add or subtract, you must be alert to the common denominator.
> Keep in mind the proper sign
> Don't stop until the bottom and top are reduced and refined.

This rhyme cued Paul to multiple numerators by numerators and denominators by denominators. When dividing fractions, he had to invert the denominator before he multiplied the fractions. When adding or subtracting, he had to first find a common denominator. It was always necessary to label the fraction with the correct positive or negative sign. He had to reduce the fraction to its lowest terms and if necessary, refine the result by converting to a mixed number. This rhyme was sufficient to solve his problem at work.

Academic Therapy

A second class of vocational memory remediation procedures involves relearning functional academic skills. This type of therapy includes remediation of reading, spelling, quantitative skills, grammar, and written communication. Computers are frequently used due to an extensive and growing software base. The assumption is that the basic academic skills are relearnable or that the person can learn them anew to functional levels. It also assumes that the person with head injury has transcended the stage where basic attention training is necessary.

Academic therapy is usually included as part of a comprehensive training program that will eventually return the person with head injury to work. If the head-injured person's academic skills are too low for effective performance in a particular job, then directed treatment may improve his or her level of functioning in a short time. If the person does not have a high school diploma, then training may also target a goal such as obtaining a G.E.D. (general equivalency degree) certificate.

Academic therapy is effective because it restores older functional memories and procedural skills. The training conforms to an A-B:C-B transfer paradigm because these skills (response sets) are applicable in a variety of new situations. For example, training a head-injured person to do column addition involves relearning a procedure that he or she can invoke with each new column of numbers. Before training, the person with head injury would simply look at the numbers and wonder what to do. Once he or she learns to organize the task by carrying numbers from one column to the next, then the response set can be used with any set of numbers.

Simulation

Simulation training is designed to replicate the eventual employment environment as closely as possible. It is popular in the Soviet Union (R.J. Spordone, personal communication) and has only recently been discussed in the Western literature (Schacter & Glisky (1986). The goal is to train a head-injured person to perform a specific task and to continue training until he or she reaches competitive levels of performance. To the extent that the training matches the actual task, then the person can begin work with a minimum of adjustment.

Simulations have been used by the military for years. They are effective because the training conforms to an A-B:A'-B' paradigm, which promotes rapid learning. Simulation as a therapy tool also facilitates rapid acquisition of job skills. The only disadvantage is that it is often difficult to develop a reasonable facsimile of the job. In addition, the person with head injury may become a robot, trained to do only one thing. Despite these drawbacks, it is perhaps the most expedient form of prevocational training.

The following examples of actual placements should help to illustrate how the transfer of learning models outlined above have been applied to facilitate vocational placement and adaptation in the workplace.

Case # 2

Bob worked for Blue Cross and Blue Shield as a claims examiner prior to his automobile accident. He was comatose for several months and was unable to return to his former job for 2 years after the injury. Bob's attention/concentration was deficient for several months after he emerged from coma. He therefore began a daily regimen of cognitive skills training using conventional computer software. After 6 months of training, his attention had returned to low average levels.

At this point Bob began working in a simulation that was designed to retrain his former job skills according to the A-B:A'-B' format outlined previously. The simulation differed from the actual job because the computer terminal was different and Bob was actually inputting different information. Bob trained on an Apple II computer at the Maryland Rehabilitation Center (MRC) whereas he eventually worked at a work station at Blue Cross. He practiced inputting old center records at MRC whereas he input actual claims forms at Blue Cross.

The therapists structured Bob's preemployment training so that the task elements and response sets would be similar to his job at Blue Cross (A-B:A'-B'). This feature predicts positive transfer. Moreover, care was taken to limit reassociation of task elements and response sets. This feature avoided negative transfer (A-B:A-Br). In fact, after 3 months of training in the simulation, Bob returned to work in his former capacity and remains employed after 2½ years.

Case # 3

Alice is a 27-year-old woman who was employed by a law firm as a legal secretary. She sustained a head injury in an automobile accident and was comatose for 2 months. After a year she was unable to return to her job due to memory and cognitive deficiencies. Cognitive skills training was initiated with software written by the authors. Alice worked on the programs for 6

months and her attention/concentration improved markedly. Eventually, she felt ready to begin work.

Alice returned to work in the law firm in a different capacity. She controlled a typing pool and was responsible for distributing jobs from the lawyers to the various word-processing personnel. She also had to proofread reports before giving them to the lawyers. Alice's therapy included writing a computer simulation of her job that she could practice after work. The software was a modification of the popular game "Air Traffic Controller." The program was rewritten so that Alice had to keep in mind a changing set of input reports, assign them to different word processors, then file them for pickup by the lawyers. The set of input and the finished reports were always changing, which required a high level of mental control. The program used the actual names of the lawyers and word-processing personnel with whom she worked at the law firm.

The purpose of the program was to provide training that would directly transfer to the workplace. Alice worked on the program for 1 hour each day. She also practiced using a specially constructed checklist so that she would have a written record of which word processor received which lawyer's reports. She used this form to keep track of which reports had been picked up. The program kept track of her errors and gave her feedback concerning her accuracy. Since Alice had to proofread, academic therapy software for related functional skills such as grammar, punctuation, and spelling was also provided. She memorized various rhyming mnemonics to improve her spelling and grammar. Alice worked on these skills for an hour each day in addition to the hour she spent on the simulator. The combination of these therapies worked quite well. Alice is still employed full time at the law firm and she has not reported problems doing the job.

PROSTHETIC MEMORY DEVICES

The above discussion concerned training to overcome memory and cognitive impairments prior to returning to work. The chapter now turns to a discussion of various devices that can be used to obviate memory problems. These devices allow head-injured persons to perform tasks they once did without them. This type of memory training does not conform directly to the paradigms outlined earlier because the devices actually store and encode information for the head-injured person. Moreover, the mechanics of the therapy differ from those methods previously outlined. The therapist teaches the person with head injury to use an external device that, in turn, eliminates the memory or intellectual problem.

Electronic Cuing Devices

Many persons with head injury forget telephone numbers or have difficulty dialing them correctly. To remedy the problem, the authors train head-injured persons to use electronic phone dialers that store phone numbers electronically. Thereafter, the head-injured person simply calls the number up on the screen and puts the phone dialer up to the receiver. After pressing the button on the side of the phone dialer, the device dials the number for them. These devices can store as many as 200 phone numbers plus a variety of personal information. The smaller ones are about the size of a credit card and fits conveniently into a purse, shirt pocket, or wallet. They usually cost less than $40.

The best approach to using the phone dialers is to solicit a list of names and phone numbers from family members. The therapist then inputs these into the dialer and teaches the person with head injury how to operate it. If possible, a family member can also learn to enter additional phone numbers when necessary. Training to use the phone dialer seldom takes more than 3 hours.

Casio and Seiko have developed a line of "data bank" watches that store phone numbers and message reminders. The head-injured person can enter dates, times, and various reminder messages into the watch, which makes an audible alarm and presents the message on the display at the appropriate time. The watch can hold as many as 50 message alarms, which is sufficient to accommodate most schedules. The Casio data bank series is especially easy to use. The authors recommend the DB-30 model because it is waterproof. The head-injured person can

shower with it on and literally never has to take it off. The various models in this series cost less than $50.

Dictation Tape Recorders

Small microcassette recorders are generally available for less than $50. These devices are effective for several purposes. After a person with head injury has been placed in a job, he or she may not have time to write down instructions or to refer to notes. The dictation tape recorder allows the individual to record instructions and to play them back when convenient. This takes less time because speaking into a recorder is usually faster than writing a note. The smaller executive microcassettes are the easiest to use. They fit easily into a shirt or coat pocket or a purse. The cassettes have 60-minute tapes, short enough to limit rewinding time yet long enough to hold extensive messages. The head-injured person can set the data bank cuing watch to beep on the hour, which serves as a reminder to rewind the cassette and review the messages. This combined procedure ensures several rehearsals during the day, which greatly improves retention.

Dictation recorders also permit the person with head injury to record phone messages. The individual simply holds the recorder to the earpiece while talking and records the conversation. Afterward, the head-injured person can take additional notes or simply review the message. This eliminates the embarrassment of having to constantly ask the other party to repeat the message. Verbal instructions or lectures can also be recorded. In general, the combination of the cuing watch and the dictation recorder can eliminate many of the head-injured person's functional memory problems.

Dialing Telephones

Dialing telephones are especially useful for those head-injured persons who work in a clerical capacity. Although the data bank watches and phone dialers improve accuracy and speed of dialing numbers, these phones accomplish the same task with the push of a single button. The phones will retain as many as 200 names and associated codes. When dialing, the head-injured person simply pushes the abbreviated code that in turn dials the desired number. The procedure is quick and accurate and greatly facilitates efficiency on the job. The authors recommend installing this type of phone at the head-injured person's desk and putting a chart with the appropriate names and dialing codes immediately above the phone for easy reference.

Signaling Devices

Head-injured persons frequently lose or misplace important items such as keys, wallets, or appointment calendars. Several companies make small electronic sounding devices that affix to commonly misplaced items. At the sound of a whistle or a hand clap, the device produces an audible alarm that makes it easy to locate the misplaced item.

There are several devices available for this purpose. Most sell for under $20. Sonica produces the device with the highest quality sound. It comes with a small pad that is about half the size of a credit card. When the item is misplaced, the person with head injury simply presses the pad and the alarm goes off. Other versions require whistling at a certain frequency or clapping hands at a particular rhythm. They are harder to activate and are somewhat unreliable. The best approach is to encourage the person with head injury to purchase a half dozen of the Sonica devices and to affix one to each important thing he or she regularly carries. The press pads may be positioned strategically in the home, car, or anywhere else the head-injured person would usually lose the article.

Car Finders

For those persons with head injury who drive, a common problem is losing a car in the parking lot. The situation may be dangerous at night if the car is parked in a secluded area. DAK sells an electronic device that mounts under the dashboard and connects to the car's battery. The head-injured person carries a small signaling device on a keychain that activates the car's lights and horn from as much as 100 meters away. If there is an emergency, the device will also sound a loud alarm to frighten off potential muggers.

Checklists

Many jobs can be reduced to a series of procedures that are performed the same way each time. These operations are easily summarized as a checklist. Kreutzer, Wehman, Morton, and Stonnington (1988) have long extolled the value of checklists as a compensatory aid. They are simple to generate and easy to fill out. There are two major advantages to checklists. First, they ensure that a job is completed consistently and completely. Second, they reduce obsessive/compulsive behavior that results when the head-injured person forgets doing something and must repeat the action over and over again. This can be especially frustrating, embarrassing, and time consuming.

The following example shows how these devices are effective in a vocational context.

Case # 4

Jane was a nurse in an intensive care unit before her automobile accident. After several months of intensive cognitive skills training she tried to return to work and found that it was still too difficult for her. She forgot to give patients their medications and could not recall the various services she had to perform on her rounds in the emergency room. She was frequently late for work because she misplaced her keys. She also worked in a dangerous section of Baltimore and had to leave the hospital late at night and would spend considerable time searching for her car in a multi-level parking garage.

The authors were able to reduce most of what Jane did in the intensive care unit to a checklist. After 1 month of testing and refining different prototypes, a finalized version of the checklist was developed that was convenient to use and complete. The checklist was sufficient to allow Jane to return to work in the intensive care unit and to work effectively. It is interesting to note that other nurses on her unit adopted her checklist once they realized how it eliminated needless repetition and checking.

However, other problems persisted. The biggest problem was with memory for instructions that the physicians would give her during her shift. They were annoyed with her memory deficit and she was embarrassed to ask for repetition. The authors constructed a wooden clipboard for Jane so that she could carry her patient checklists conveniently. Under the clipboard was a slot for her to keep her dictation recorder. It was out of sight and easily activated. Thereafter, when the physicians gave her instructions she used the cassette recorder to tape them. This combination of devices allowed her to return to work in her former capacity. She became proficient with the devices after 5 hours of training.

Jane also purchased several sounding devices and a car finder. Thereafter, she no longer misplaced her keys and other important items. She was also able to find her car in the parking garage with minimum effort. The total cost of solving all of Jane's problems was less than $200.

COGNITIVE ORTHOTIC DEVICES

The use of cognitive orthotic devices is a relatively unknown area of cognitive rehabilitation therapy. The logic is simple. Rather than retrain a person with head injury to perform cognitively the way he or she did before the injury, the therapist writes a computer program that performs the same task and then trains the individual to operate the program. Again, the purpose of the therapy is to obviate the problem rather than to alter the deficit.

One easy-to-use cognitive orthotic device is the "expert system shell" (Harmon & King, 1985). This is an artificial intelligence development tool that is designed to allow the novice computer user to develop software that performs an intelligent decision-making activity. No prior knowledge of programming is necessary. The user operates the software by formulating a set of rules for making certain decisions, then provides these rules to the shell program. The shell program then develops a rule structure for implementing the decisions so that literally anyone can answer complex work-related questions using the program.

Expert system shells have been popular in business and government for years. Previously, high-priced experts were hired to diagnose problems. But with the development of expert system shell technology, those experts' "knowledge bases" were stored in shell programs as a set of rules. Literally anyone could then consult the computer for an immediate solution to problems. This approach was found to be considerably cheaper than keeping human experts on retainer.

The authors have found that expert system shells are quite easy to use and provide an inexpensive and rapid solution to some vocational reentry problems. The general procedure involves going to the job and examining exactly what the head-injured person previously did or will do. The next step is to reduce the job to a set of rules or decisions. These rules are subsequently inputted into the expert system shell along with advice to the person with head injury concerning any of the various situations that may arise on the job. The therapist then provides the head-injured person with a computer at work and training to use the expert system. Ideally, this will be a "laptop" computer that the person with head injury can carry to and from work or a desktop model that is available exclusively to him or her during the day. The therapist trains the head-injured person to use the software and continues modifying the rule structure until the individual can perform the job with at least the same level of accuracy as before the injury.

However, expert system shells do not fit every job application. The job may be too difficult to structure as a set of rules or too simple to warrant expert system shell development. In many situations, a simple computer program may fill the need.

Case # 5

Lois was a 54-year-old woman who had a stroke, previously employed as a dispatcher for a trucking firm. She had worked for the firm for 25 years and her services and dependability were highly valued by the company. Her job included keeping in mind a variety of different delivery schedules and price rates that she would convey to customers. In essence, Lois acted as a consultant, informing customers of the cheapest and fastest way to ship their freight.

After her stroke, Lois could not mentally

retrieve the schedules or pricing information she needed to provide rapid and accurate estimates for customers. Although the company valued her skills, they placed her on temporary disability. Fortunately, however, her job could be reduced to a set of decision rules. The situation was therefore ideal for an expert system shell application.

After examining the job, the authors constructed 100 rules and inputted them into an expert system shell program. The entire operation took approximately 5 hours. The program posed questions that Lois would ask the customers. It also provided the correct pricing, time, and the least to most expensive shipping method for each customer, given specific needs. Lois simply talked to the customer over the phone, and asked the sequence of questions the computer presented on the screen. She answered the program's queries, then gave the customer the advice the expert system related at the end of the conversation.

After the software was developed, the company agreed to purchase a laptop computer that Lois could take to and from work each day. This machine was available to her at all times during the workday. Lois took the computer to work each morning, set it up on her desk next to phone, and used it continuously throughout the day. Her accuracy and speed improved to acceptable levels and she was returned to full-time employment within 1 year after her stroke. It took approximately 2 months to study the job, develop the software, and train Lois to use it.

Case # 6

Ted's memory impairment resulted from an automobile accident. After a 3-month coma and 1 year of therapy, he tried, unsuccessfully, to return to his previous job as a teacher. He then tried several jobs but was usually fired because he could not manage complex tasks accurately or in a timely fashion. He was eventually hired by a sheltered workshop and given the responsibility of tallying jobs completed by the various workers throughout the day. He could do the job but it was stressful and his work was error prone.

The authors wrote a simple computer program for Ted that would accept the various data and tabulate them for him. He took his work home at night and used the computer to perform his calculations. The program printed out all of the necessary information so that he could simply turn in the printout the next day. He could save the data, update them, correct them, and regenerate previous days' work summaries. The program was written in a standard BASIC language and took approximately 5 hours to prepare and debug. Ted learned to use the program in less than 1 hour.

The preceding case examples illustrate the value and potential of cognitive orthotic devices. The person with head injury is able to return to work with them but could not without them. The training time necessary to learn to use the computer software is always less than would be needed in conventional therapy to enable a head-injured person to return to work. Advances in computer software and hardware have made this type of vocational reentry cost-effective and feasible, and have greatly expanded the range of potential applications (Bowling, 1988).

SUMMARY AND EVALUATION

Various memory and cognitive retraining procedures that have proven effective in vocational settings were discussed in this chapter. A systematic method for predicting the success of various memory retraining procedures and several rules for planning vocational memory training interventions were introduced. First, training will facilitate employment potential to the extent that the head-injured person's mental organization of the job is similar to what was learned in therapy. Ideally, memory training conforms to an A-B:A'-B' paradigm where the task elements (A) and response sets (B) in training are similar to those that will be encountered on the job. Second, if it is impossible to recreate the job as an A-B:A-B or A-B:A'-B' simulated training paradigm, then it is important to train transferable response sets. The training then conforms to an A-B:C-B model, which also predicts positive transfer. Third, the therapist must avoid training that will eventually force the person with head injury to associate new response sets to the same task elements. It is especially important to avoid training where the same response sets are reassociated or mismatched with the same task elements. Both of the latter training environments will produce negative generalization and job failure. The effects of most conventional memory training procedures are quite predictable using this method. The authors recommend that therapists use it to evaluate a planned therapy before implementing it.

Since stimulation therapy and cognitive skills training are most frequently used in prevocational training, it is important to evaluate their advantages and disadvantages. Despite the criticisms against stimulation therapy (Schacter & Glisky, 1986), the authors have found that it is a valuable prevocational adjunct therapy. A major advantage is that computer software is generally available and there are a variety of paper-and-pencil materials as well. The therapy is extremely cost-effective, which is one reason for its rapid assimilation into the therapeutic community. Often it is the only long-term treatment that is feasible on an in-home basis. It also provides a respite for the family members or therapists while the head-injured person is doing the therapy. If the therapist can specify the nature of the outcome task, then cognitive skills training can conform to an A-B:A'-B' paradigm and will yield substantial generalization. Sanford (1988) has outlined other benefits from computer-based therapy approaches.

Perhaps the biggest disadvantage of stimulation training is that the materials have only face validity and there have been few validation studies to document their usefulness relative to other therapies. For example, it is unclear exactly how much job-related generalization occurred in the two cases presented earlier. What has become clear to the authors over the years is that these cognitive skills training materials improved the head-injured person's attention to the point where more complex therapies were possible. Indeed, during the initial stages of treatment, they were perhaps the only exercises the head-injured person could perform without experiencing severe frustration.

The practice of training persons with head injury to use memory strategies and mnemonic devices was also discussed. Although persons with head injury may be able to use memory strategies to improve performance on standardized tests or word lists, they typically will not use them spontaneously on the job. In the authors' experience, training the person with head injury to use memory strategies is useful so long as the strategy is context specific. That is, the therapist must show how the strategy is directly applicable to activities of employment or daily living. Frequently rhymes or other organizational schemes can be used that are unique to the head-injured person's job.

Academic therapy is an important part of any cognitive rehabilitation program. The skills generalize readily and the training is usually effective because it retrains old skills rather than establishing new ones. Head-injured persons see the relevance of the training and invest in it. There are several journals and periodicals that disseminate new information in this field, and there are a variety of software and training materials available. In short, the disadvantages of using academic therapy for prevocational training with head-injured persons are few. Perhaps the only problem is the lack of research to document which academic therapy approaches work best with persons with head injury.

Several prosthetic memory devices were also discussed that have been helpful in a variety of situations. These do not solve the head-injured person's memory problems but they do obviate them. They also provide immediate solutions to nagging problems. The authors recommend that the reader contact the following vendors to obtain information about the devices discussed in this chapter:

Solutions Inc. (1-800-342-9988)
Impact (1-800-345-4422)
Danmark (1-800-533-3379)
Sharper Image (1-800-344-4444)
Hammacher/Schlemmer (1-800-543-3666)
Synctronics (1-800-972-5855)

Expert system shell programs are especially useful cognitive orthotic devices. These programs allow the therapist to develop software that performs an intelligent decision-making function. Rather than improve the head-injured person's job-related memory and intellectual skills, the therapist trains the individual to use the expert system to do the job. The obvious advantage of this and other cognitive orthotic devices is that they allow the person with head injury to return directly to a job armed with an electronic brain. This immediate return to work is attractive to persons with head injury as well as to insurance agencies and employers. With the cost of computers decreasing each year, total therapy costs will be considerably reduced. If the software is written correctly, thoroughly debugged, and tested, then the head-injured person can actually perform *better* on the job after their return to work postinjury. Expert systems are ideally suitable when the task involves a specific set of rules that the therapist can isolate. They are less useful when the job involves abstraction or human judgment, or the rule base is prone to exceptions. In Case # 5, the total training time and cost was clearly less than would have been accumulated with traditional therapy. However,

the entire process may be very expensive in some situations. Despite these drawbacks, the potential of expert system development tools for vocational training far outweighs the disadvantages.

Cognitive orthotic devices have additional limitations, however. The person with head injury is literally trained in a domain-specific operation, often to the exclusion of other types of therapy. The head-injured person also becomes dependent upon the computer and software to function in the job. If the computer "crashes," if it is left at home, or if it is otherwise unavailable, then the individual's skills are limited. Also, the therapist must first assume that a significant portion of the job can be performed by the computer program, and the employer must be willing to let the person with head injury use a computer to do the job. Finally, the person with head injury must become proficient with the software to the point where he or she can work at competitive levels.

REFERENCES

Bower, G.H. (1970). Organizational factors in memory. *Cognitive Psychology, 1,* 18–46.

Bowling, C. (1988). *Principles and elements of thought construction, artificial intelligence, and cognitive robotics.* Houston: CYS Publishers.

Bracy, O. (1988, September). *A process approach to cognitive rehabilitation.* Cognitive Rehabilitation: Community Re-entry Through Scientifically Based Practice Conference, Richmond, VA.

Ellis, H.C. (1965). *The transfer of training.* New York: Macmillan.

Ellis, H.C. (1969). Transfer and retention. In M.H. Marx (Ed.), *Learning processes* (pp. 381–478). New York: Macmillan.

Gross, Y., & Schutz, L. (1986). Intervention models in neuropsychology. In B. Uzzell & Y. Gross (Eds.), *Clinical neuropsychology of intervention* (pp. 179–204). Boston: Martinus Nijhoff.

Harmon, P., & King, D. (1985). *Expert systems.* New York: John Wiley & Sons.

Kreutzer, J.S., Wehman, P., Morton, M.V., & Stonnington, H.H. (1988). Supported employment and compensatory strategies for enhancing vocational outcome following traumatic brain injury. *Brain Injury, 2*(3), 205–223.

Parenté, F.J., & Anderson, J.K. (1984). Techniques for improving cognitive rehabilitation: Teaching or-

ganization and encoding skills. *Cognitive Rehabilitation, 1*(4), 20–23.

Parenté, F.J., Anderson, J.K., & Shaw, B. (1989). Retraining the mind's eye. *Journal of Head Trauma Rehabilitation.*

Sanford, J. (1988, September). *Software development for cognitive rehabilitation.* Paper presented at the Cognitive Rehabilitation: Community Re-entry Through Scientifically Based Practice Conference, Richmond, VA.

Schacter, D., & Glisky, E. (1986). Memory remediation, restoration, alleviation, and the acquisition of domain specific knowledge. In B. Uzzell & Y. Gross (Eds.), *Clinical neuropsychology of intervention* (pp. 257–282). Boston: Martinus Nijhoff.

Schuell, H.M., Carroll, V., & Street, B.S. (1955). Clinical treatment of aphasia. *Journal of Speech and Hearing Disorders, 20,* 43–53.

Taylor, M.T. (1964). Language therapy. In H.G. Burn (Ed.), *The aphasic adult: Evaluation and rehabilitation* (pp. 156–200). Charlottesville, VA: Wayside Press.

Wepman, J.M. (1951). *Recovery from aphasia.* New York: Ronald Press.

Wilson, B.A. (1987). *Rehabilitation of memory.* New York: Guilford Press.

CHAPTER 12

Vocational Rehabilitation Counseling

Robert T. Fraser, David C. Clemmons, and Brian T. McMahon

Vocational rehabilitation counseling as a profession has been in existence since the early 1950s. Much of the impetus for the development of the profession has been: 1) the need on the part of state vocational rehabilitation agencies for counselors to deal with clients having chronic disabilities and 2) funding targeted to institutions of higher education to develop these professionals, through legislation passed in 1954. (PL 83-565). Szymanski (1985) offers the following definition of rehabilitation counseling:

> Rehabilitation counseling is a profession that assists individuals with disabilities in adapting to the environment, assists environments in accommodating the needs of the individual, and works toward full participation of persons with disabilities in all aspects of society, especially in work. (p. 3)

As a profession, these rehabilitation counseling personnel may lack a full understanding of some of the behavioral technologies that can be very assistive in aiding clients with chronic disabilities such as traumatic brain injury into competitive employment. For example, there is still frequently much to be understood among these personnel about the different supported employment models. Rehabilitation counselors, however, have a number of critical skills that they can apply to the task of assisting individuals with traumatic brain injury back into the work force. Among these skills are the following: 1) assessment skills that take into account the needs of the "whole person"; 2) an understanding of the world of work to include types of jobs, levels of complexity, and transferable skills; 3) an appreciation of clients' work values as they relate to job choices; and 4) a counseling practicum in which they have had to utilize a number of different counseling strategies to include behavioral approaches.

In a recent study by Fraser, Dikmen, McLean, Temkin, and Miller (1988), a review of the work backgrounds of 48 individuals receiving acute care for traumatic brain injury at a major trauma center indicated that 92% of these individuals had been working in skilled or semi-skilled jobs at the time of injury. Only 8% were involved in unskilled occupations. Since vocational rehabilitation counselors have the best understanding of the labor market among allied health professionals, it becomes crucial to include this type of professional as part of the rehabilitation team. Since a major issue in successful vocational rehabilitation of persons with traumatic brain injury is the initial job matching, the utilization of these personnel becomes an important consideration.

The vocational rehabilitation process tends to follow a standard sequence that includes intake and screening in which an eligibility decision is made, evaluation, counseling and planning, choice of a job placement approach and implementation, and postemployment services. This sequence is still followed in traumatic brain injury vocational rehabilitation. The process that is offered within this chapter, however, is expanded and involves more elaborate tracking than is generally the case for individuals with other chronic disabilities. In consideration of the current state of the art of vocational rehabilitation in traumatic brain injury, it becomes obvious that one cannot be locked into one model of service delivery. One must compare and contrast the effectiveness of different service delivery models and make modifications accordingly.

BASIC INFORMATION
FOR THE INTERVENTION

In order to make a successful intervention in traumatic brain injury vocational rehabilitation, certain areas of information must be covered. These include a medical history that provides indices of the injury's severity (e.g., Glasgow Coma Scale Score, length of coma or time to follow command, and period of post-traumatic amnesia), the course of hospital and current medical treatment, diagnostic exam results, and other system injuries. It is very common that an individual with a severe head injury could have a hemiparesis, be treated for an actual seizure condition or be taking anticonvulsants prophylactically, have a shunt requiring medical management, or have some other type of complication. Traditional demographic information is also gathered on each client to include specific information on education and training, behavioral dispositions, social/recreational activity, and health background (e.g., alcohol, drug, or psychiatric history). Information relative to current level of functioning is very important. Specifically, it is important to understand financial status and support sources, level of independence at home and in the community, review of current organizational involvement and use of free time, level of community mobility, and other functionally oriented information.

Social support needs to be assessed very carefully. It is common for an individual with traumatic brain injury to experience divorce and loss of contact with previously close friends. It is important to determine which significant others still exist for the client within the community and the level of support that they can provide. If significant others do not exist or those who do exist are dysfunctional and not supportive of the client's progress, it becomes important to determine how the client's case can be managed. Since an addiction history is common for brain-injured clients and could be a cause of the traumatic injury, it becomes important to establish the type of social support that is assistive in framing a new life-style for the client.

If a rehabilitation team has provided services to the client, data from the discharge summary can be most helpful in securing the basic information for intervention with a client. If the client was served not by a team, but by a group of allied health professionals, this information can still be secured (although often not as completely) through these professionals. It is important to make contact with individuals who serve the client during the postacute period, because they tend to have a full appreciation of the client's needs and level of functioning and the quality of social support that may be available.

SPECIFIC
ASSESSMENT CONSIDERATIONS

Vocational Interest
and Values Assessment

It can very important that an individual's vocational interests are assessed carefully as part of the vocational rehabilitation process. Due to the severity of the injury, many individuals cannot go back to a prior position or even a related area of work. Consequently, as part of a basic vocational assessment a client's vocational interests are often assessed by use of traditional paper-and-pencil inventories (the Career Assessment Inventory, the Gordon Occupational Checklist, the Strong-Campbell, etc.) and computer-assisted approaches such as the Valpar Guide to Occupational Exploration. Within the University of Washington Department of Neurological Surgery's Vocational Services, some of the better placements evolved from careful review of occupational interest themes using these inventories and then brainstorming job options by using the *Guide for Occupational Exploration* (U.S. Department of Labor, 1979) or the *Dictionary of Occupational Codes* (Gottfredson, Holland, & Ogawa, 1982). Review of a client's vocational and avocational activities can also be helpful in identifying which jobs may be optimal within different job groupings. For example, it was through utilization of this process that a job goal of prosthetics/orthotics technician was identified for a college graduate with severe receptive language deficits. The job was of interest to the individual and met the individual's work values, which involved clean and pleasant working conditions, helping others, and an interest in fine craft work.

There are a number of work values common among clients seen both at the University of Washington Department of Neurological Surgery and at Community Re-entry Services of Washington (CRS-Washington; a New Medico postacute residential center). Some of these work values include: regular working hours; reasonable salary, job security, and good fringe benefits; some prestige or recognition associated with the position; varied job activities; the opportunity to interact with others; the opportunity for self-expression; physical mobility (not having to stand or sit in one position for prolonged periods of time); outdoor or indoor work; the opportunity to work with males, females, or both of a certain age grouping; substantial physical exertion; the opportunity to participate in teamwork; the opportunity for advancement; and available supervision. It is obvious that achieving work with a number of these characteristics will be difficult or sometimes impossible for a number of clients with traumatic brain injury. Nevertheless, the initial job match will be more successful if the job identified has as many of the reinforcing characteristics as possible that have been identified as desirable by the client.

Utilizing Neuropsychological Data for Vocational Planning

The multiplicity of brain-related problems that are likely to be present in a person with traumatic brain injury complicates the process of vocational planning. Moderate to severe deficits in sensory/motor functioning aspects of memory, attentional abilities, problem solving, and ability to pursue a task in the presence of distracters are frequent among individuals who have suffered any significant head trauma. Disruptions in language ability, spatial ability, and overall cognitive efficiency may also be present. Problems in some of these areas, particularly when pronounced, may be evident to the casual observer. It is sometimes the case, however, that the presence and magnitude of brain-related deficits may be overlooked or underestimated even by a skilled counselor. For this reason, the use of neuropsychological testing can be quite assistive. In

requesting neuropsychological testing, it is important to seek a psychologist who is qualified in the area of neuropsychology. The Twelfth Institute on Rehabilitation Issues (TIRI, 1985) recommended that the counselor should seek an individual who is a diplomate of the American Board of Clinical Neuropsychology, a board-eligible Ph.D. with 1 year of supervised experience, or a Ph.D. or Ed.D. with 2 years or more of supervised experience in clinical neuropsychology. If the counselor has difficulty in identifying this type of professional, the National Head Injury Foundation, a state psychological association, or local universities and hospitals can provide assistance.

In requesting neuropsychological assessment, it is most helpful to utilize a standardized neuropsychological battery such as the Halstead-Reitan Neuropsychological Test Battery (Reitan & Wolfson, 1985), the Luria-Nebraska Neuropsychological Battery (Golden, Hammeke, & Purisch, 1980), or some other type of standardized battery as a basis for planning interventions. This is not to say that additional testing should not be used to supplement the battery and more closely examine upper or lower ranges of abilities or areas of deficit. By utilizing a specific battery versus a hypothesis testing approach in requesting neuropsychological evaluations, the counselor is often better able to identify assets and develop expertise in planning by being able to compare one client to another relative to the effectiveness of an intervention. It should be understood that actual performance on a work sample or situational work experience is generally the best provider of functional performance information, but neuropsychological testing can be very useful in the planning of even the basic vocational assessment steps. The identification and measurement of specific abilities on a neuropsychological evaluation may over time save significant effort and frustration on the part of both the client and the counselor. Successful rehabilitation of persons with traumatic brain injury generally requires a clear understanding of their residual neuropsychological abilities before proceeding into a vocational evaluation sequence. Many global measures of ability traditionally used in vocational assessment (e.g., the

Wide Range Achievement Test [Guidance Associates, 1965], the Weschler Adult Intelligence Scale–Revised [Psychological Corporation, 1981], the General Aptitude Test Battery [United States Department of Labor, 1970]) can provide a distorted picture of a client's vocational abilities unless used in connection with neuropsychological test results. It is not uncommon clinically to see individuals with essentially "normal" standardized aptitude profiles who nevertheless demonstrate impairment on neuropsychological measures that are barriers to successful job procurement or maintenance.

During the first 6 months or year following the injury, many individuals with moderate to severe brain injuries will make dramatic gains cognitively, which results in fluctuating neuropsychological test results. However, battery results obtained relatively early in the rehabilitation process can still be helpful because these results provide a frame of reference relative to functioning within the context of a norm group. Additionally, work at the University of Washington indicates that early test results may reflect the impact of the injury on employment perhaps more clearly than medical indicators (Fraser, Dimken, McLean, & Temkin, 1988).

In requesting neuropsychological testing, the vocational counselor should provide the neuropsychologist with a cover letter framing the reasons for the referral relative to vocational needs. When working with available neuropsychological data, it may be necessary to contact the clinician who generated the report or to enlist the aid of an available neuropsychologist in order to extract the useful vocational information from the test scores. Whenever possible, job analysis data should be included relative to the client's job goal in order to orient the neuropsychologist to some of the potential areas of concern. In general, the following areas should be addressed by a neuropsychologist who is providing data for vocational planning purposes (TIRI, 1985):

1. Identification of the individual's areas of asset and deficit.
2. Comment on the individual's ability to engage in a task and remain focused on the task activities.
3. Comment on the individual's ability to per-

form simple through complex levels of task activity with accuracy and speed.
4. If the individual makes an error, is he or she able to identify the error and make the correction?
5. What level of supervision will be required for the individual to perform competently?
6. Comment on the individual's motivation for the testing sequence and stamina while involved in the testing activity.
7. Comment on the individual's self-awareness of areas of neuropsychological strength and deficit.
8. If training is a consideration for a client, comment on the type of training (formal academic or on-the-job training) that may be most appropriate.

Psychosocial Assessment

A thorough psychosocial assessment of the client with traumatic brain injury is also essential to vocational planning. The presence of any significant brain impairment is likely to compound the effect of premorbid emotional or characterological difficulties, family or environmental stressors, and other preexisting social or psychological concerns. Due to a decrease in problem-solving ability, frustration tolerance, and general cognitive flexibility, concerns that were manageable preinjury may become overwhelming postinjury. In addition to these concerns, the amount of social disruption and isolation related to an individual's losing his or her job, the loss of contact with familiar social and friendship networks, and the impact of an ambiguous "new role" in the community may be considerable. Finally, the demographic profile of persons who receive significant head injuries is similar to that of individuals who are involved in other catastrophic events, such as spinal cord injuries. Young males with drug and alcohol abuse problems with a high tolerance for physical risk taking tend to be overrepresented in this population. Both prexisting and accident-related psychosocial concerns may be compounded by organic factors. Persons who have suffered brain injuries may have difficulty inhibiting or moderating inappropriate responses, including those related to anger and frustration. Other concerns can commonly involve a lessened empathy for other persons' concerns, a flat or altered affect, alterations in sexual drive and performance, and a decrease in self-initiated behaviors. These factors can have a significant effect on the client's social interpersonal environment, which may lead to a disruption of family and other social support networks. Unlike recovery from other types of injuries, recovery from a significant brain injury may never be complete in the area of emotional and personality function.

Because clients with intact social support networks tend to enter or reenter employment at a higher rate than those without such networks, psychosocial assessment of the client's significant other and community support networks are critical concerns. When possible, family members and significant others should not only be informed of, but involved in the development of rehabilitation plans. They will add not only to the quality of planning in the client's behalf, but their investment in and cooperation with the rehabilitation plan may be key factors in the plan's success. Parents who have reservations about a plan or have a different agenda for their son or daughter will not contribute and in fact may be detrimental to the plan's success. In a number of instances, dysfunctional family members or individuals who have a self-investment in the client's litigation outcome may jeopardize the plan and need to be excluded from alliance with the rehabilitation counselor or team. One or more visits to the client's living situation, before or during the initial phases of rehabilitation planning can be very useful in assessing the degree of social support, in building rapport with the family, and in engaging the client in the rehabilitation process.

For purposes of assessment, a number of instruments may be useful in assessing psychosocial factors in tramatic brain injury vocational rehabilitation. The Minnesota Multiphasic Personality Inventory (MMPI) (Hathaway & McKinley, 1951) can be a useful instrument in assessment. Since the inventory is relatively long (400–566 items), it is sometimes difficult to complete for individuals with low frustration thresholds or those having difficulties with attention span and so forth. Nevertheless, clients who have the requisite reading ability tolerate this inventory fairly well. For some clients, it may be desirable to use the tape version of the inventory due to the reading or attentional deficits. Scale elevations on the MMPI cannot be interpreted as literally as they would be for psychiatric patients, due to the endorsement of items related to the head injury experience. If the inventory is valid, however, it can still provide very useful information for rehabilitation planning. Assessment, of course, should not be based solely on a personality inventory and needs to be complemented with data from the clinical evaluation process. The Millon Clinical Multiaxial Inventory (MCMI) may also be useful in psychosocial assessment of clients with head injury (Millon, 1982). Similar in content to the MMPI, it provides an index of emotional status and an overview of characterological functioning, but in a manner that is more directly linked to the *Diagnostic and Statistical Manual of Mental Disorders–III–Revised (DSM-IIIR,* American Psychiatric Association, 1987). It is a shorter inventory (175 questions), and is also viewed as being more long-term "trait" oriented, rather than "state" oriented as is the MMPI. Thus, the MCMI may be more helpful in providing an index of premorbid personality propensities. A third inventory that can be helpful in assessment is the Washington Psychosocial Seizure Inventory (Dodrill, Batzel, Queisser, & Temkin, 1980), which was developed to rapidly assess areas of psychosocial functioning with particular relevance to clients having a seizure condition. The emphasis is on assessing psychosocial functioning across eight areas of adjustment: family background, emotional adjustment, interpersonal adjustment, vocational adjustment, financial adjustment, adjustment to seizures, medicine and medical management, and overall psychosocial functioning. Preliminary work at the authors' center (Fraser, Trejo, Clemmons, & Freelove, 1987) suggests that psychosocial functioning as assessed by this inventory was a better predictor of program dropouts than were tested abilities or other demographic variables.

COUNSELING AND INTERACTION STYLE CONSIDERATIONS

Providing vocationally supportive counseling for clients with traumatic brain injury can be a difficult and challenging task. Cognitively, it is likely that some impairment will be experienced related to memory, problem solving, language use, and general cognitive efficiency that can impose special considerations on counseling style. The counselor should keep in mind that there are no "cookbook" counseling approaches that are likely to be satisfactory for every client with head injury. Most traumatic brain-injured clients seeking vocational assistance tend to have difficulties with memory functioning. While verbal or visual/spatial memory may be differentially affected, depending upon the location or severity of the injury, difficulties with recent memory functioning (and the ability to learn new material) are common. The degree of memory impairment is frequently underestimated by clients and counseling sessions may be more effective by providing clients with a written review of major points covered, agreements reached, and other pertinent information. The most useful memory device tends to be some type of daily log, schedule book, diary, or similar device. It is ordinarily useful to review briefly the main points of a previous counseling session before proceeding with a new session. Actively involving the client by having him or her paraphrase understandings and their main points can also be an effective memory aid. Depending upon the quality of an individual client's memory, initial planning may have to proceed relatively slowly, especially when building rapport. At this point in the vocational rehabilitation process, several meetings per week as opposed to once a week can be quite useful. Frequently persons with significant head injuries experience problems related to problem-solving deficits. These deficits also impose limitations on the counseling interaction. Clients with traumatic brain injury have increased difficulties in choosing from an array of options—the challenge for the skillful counselor is to limit options while maximizing the client's rehabilitation potential. A counselor working with a client whose neuropsychological assessment indicates the desirability of a semiskilled manual job activity might limit the discussion to two or three specific occupations that are in line with the client's interests and work skills.

In working with clients who perseverate on unfeasible job goals or have difficulty accepting change, a negotiating style with counseling support is recommended. Many clients with traumatic brain injury display decreased problem-solving abilities and a loss of cognitive flexibility, with a concomitant tendency to perseverate on an idea. A common difficulty counselors may have in such a case is that of polarizing the counseling situation by offering logical arguments against a particular client goal or objective. A more useful strategy might be to negotiate a series of steps that would, if successfully completed, result in the attainment of the desired goal. For example, the development of a series of entry-level warehouse positions within a client's range of ability might be offered as logical steps for someone seeking to later earn a supervisory role. The client then receives feedback from environmental experiences, the counselor, and on-site employees relative to performance over time. This approach has the advantage of leaving much of the decision-making power with the client and provides the counselor with environmental aids in working with the client toward acceptance of limitations. It is often not reasonable to expect clients who previously performed high-level work to easily accept the fact that they are unlikely to be able to perform at that level postjury. As with any other loss or grieving process, much is to be gained by providing ongoing support and acceptance of a client's position. The client's denial or defensiveness relative to limitations can be confronted steadily over time with the counselor being assisted by the environmental input of supervisors and coworkers.

Some common brain-related syndromes merit specific discussion relative to counseling style. Individuals with frontal lobe involvement can have a number of difficulties, including tangential and anecdotal speech patterns, social disinhibition resulting in inappropriate behavior, difficulty in planning and in anticipating consequences, and general euphoric moods or disinterested attitudes. These concerns are generally exacerbated with bilateral involvement. Walsh (1978) provides a comprehensive discussion of frontal lobe syndrome. Because these clients can still have reasonable or above average IQ scores and be quite conversationally pleasant, they may encourage the counselor to unrealistically expect an ability to carry-through on tasks. Conversely, these clients often do better in highly structured situations that do not demand their initiative or decision making. Counseling issues for these individuals are often focused on behavioral management, initiating task activity, and follow-through issues. In some cases, a specific behavioral management consultation is recommended and in others, behavioral shaping can be done on the job site through the utilization of a job coach. Minor forms of difficulties manifested by these clients include rambling, anecdotal speech, odd forms of humor, and inappropriate social/sexual comments or approach behavior toward members of the opposite sex.

Because the vast majority of people are left brain dominant for language, injuries that affect the left temporal area frequently interfere with expressive or receptive language capabilities. For persons with even mild language-related abilities, particularly receptive, the use of visual aids such as graphs, charts, and pictures may be highly desirable. The use of simple bar or line graphs may be used to discuss the length of rehabilitation program, segments of rehabilitation activity to be supported by a job coach, and so forth. Simple graphic or pictorial material is also useful to send home with a client as a memory aid between counseling sessions.

In conclusion, there are a number of other basic considerations that can be kept in mind when interacting with brain-injured clients. These include the following (Cicerone, 1989; Fraser, McMahon, & Vogenthaler, 1988; Prigatano, 1989):

1. In general, be very concrete and use simpler sentence structures when interacting with individuals having language-related deficits.
2. Review neuropsychological information and recommendations in order to identify the best interactive modality; for example, utilizing charts and figures may be more helpful in making a point in verbal interchange when dealing with a client having

language deficiencies. Use the most relevant cues.
3. At times, it may be helpful to prepare for meetings with clients having organically mediated emotional imbalances by attempting to release any personal negative emotions through discussing the upcoming meeting with a colleague or using another outlet in order to maintain one's emotional balance in the upcoming meeting.
4. If a client is particularly frustrated, angry, or otherwise out of balance, present an issue that may be volatile when the client is calmer, or in a more comfortable discussion point during the session.
5. Allow clients time to reframe their self-concept or mourn the implications of their loss of brain-related abilities, while gradually supporting them in proactive steps.
6. Improve the client's capability to handle difficult feedback by anticipating his or her response in your verbalization (e.g., "As I explain this to you it may be saddening, but. . . .").
7. Continually accentuate the positive. When presenting information that can be construed negatively by the client, it can be helpful to wedge the information between two positively reinforcing statements ("sandwich technique"—see Prigatano, 1989).
8. Always strive to provide accurate information to the client, specifically about their brain-related assets and areas of deficit, using a consulting neuropsychologist whenever necessary.

It should be emphasized that these strategies are very assistive in working with individuals who have cognitive deficits. Some of these can also be assistive in working with clients with characterological disorders that include distrustfulness, social deceptiveness, obsessiveness, dependency, and oppositional characteristics (Cicerone, 1989). However, traumatic brain injuries can exacerbate some of the client's previous personality difficulties. The emotional sequelae of the injury can include anxiety, depression, anger, social withdrawal, and so forth. Similarly, a client's prognosis for vocational outcome is worsened if he or she was also emotionally maladjusted prior to the accident. A number of such clients will profit by referral for ongoing counseling and psychotherapy. In order to improve generalization, group forms of psychotherapy and behavioral treatment are recommended. Due to these clients' range of cognitive difficulty the use of videotaping is very helpful as both a feedback mechanism and a tool to assessing change. Traumatically brain-injured clients tend to profit more from therapy styles that are more directive to include cognitive behavioral, rational-emotive, and reality therapy types of approaches. Consultation with and plan implementation by behavioral psychologists or consultants will often be of great assistance.

ISSUES IN COGNITIVE REMEDIATION

Kreutzer, Gordon, and Wehman (1989, p. 118) have defined cognitive remediation as "a set of strategies intended to improve the intellectual, perceptual, psychomotor, and behavioral skills of persons with brain dysfunction." As further discussed by these authors, cognitive remediation has been used to describe a number of different interventions, including: comprehensive day rehabilitation programs, practice sessions using computer software, compensatory strategies for memory improvement, social skills training, driving training programs, and others. An agency vocational rehabilitation counselor is often asked to provide cognitive remediation services for a client—within the context of the diverse services being offered and a wide range of costs, it is difficult to make a choice or support these types of services unless outcomes can be more functionally described.

In considering the purchase of these services, it is helpful to focus on some of the issues identified by Kreutzer et al. (1989) in their review. They emphasize that there should be a prioritization of the problem(s) to be treated. Treatment should be linked to an important functional outcome goal, and to the likelihood of success. The problem area should be carefully defined in terms that can be measured relative to duration, change, and a description of environments in which the problem occurs. The treatment itself

should be delineated carefully and in a manner that can be clearly recorded for purposes of documentation and replication. As Kreutzer et al. point out, problems of generalization can be minimized by providing treatment in the environment in which the problem to be treated (e.g., a difficulty in fully scanning a warehouse shelf) is most likely to occur (i.e., in a warehouse setting). In their review article, Kreutzer et al. provide examples of functionally oriented cognitive remediation such as perceptual training for improved driving performance, supported employment interventions, and compensatory techniques to improve daily living.

Mikula (1984) has also established some guidelines for the provision of cognitive remediation services. He emphasizes the importance of a neuropsychological battery indicating a range of cognitive strengths and weaknesses before embarking on a specific cognitive remediation plan. Also, the criteria for advancement to more difficult levels of a program should be clearly described, and criteria for completion of the cognitive remediation services should be similarly well delineated. The reader is referred to the recent work by Kreutzer et al. (1989), and the TIRI (1985) monograph for further information.

VOCATIONAL EVALUATION SEQUENCE

Whether a client is involved in an outpatient or a residential program, the vocational evaluation sequence is basically the same. There is always a period of initial data collection. If an individual's work goal is to return to a prior position or a preexisting skill-relevant area, a number of steps are taken in which information is secured from a prior employer, relevant work samples are utilized, and so forth. If a client performs well on prior work-relevant samples, the evaluation may proceed to an on-site intermediate level evaluation that actually involves paid or nonpaid work experience. If prior work experience does not provide for a job goal, this individual must be cycled through a basic evaluation process. Individuals with no prior work experience will also be cycled through a basic evaluation process. It appears that the initial job matching can be critical to the success of the entire rehabilitation plan. The authors are advocating, therefore, a quality evaluation program, but also a relatively efficient one. For example, within the University of Washington Vocational Re-entry Program the majority of clients have been involved in an actual paid work experience (being either an intermediate level evaluation or a terminal job) by 3–4 months from intake. The basic level evaluation is completed within 3–4 weeks within either the University of Washington program or Community Re-entry Services of Washington. Table 12.1 overviews the sequence of activities within the vocational evaluation process specific to the CRS-Washington program.

There are two other issues related to the evaluation process that need to be emphasized. The first is that a decision has to be made relative to the primary individual who will manage the case. In some cases, this can be done by the vocational rehabilitation counselor, while in others this will require contracting with a community case manager, utilizing a key family member or significant other as the case manager, utilizing a sympathetic employer in the case management process, or some combination of the above. If the rehabilitation counselor is working with a rehabilitation team, this decision can be made within the team context. In other cases, the rehabilitation counselor will need to examine the community support structure and identify an optimal case management plan.

The second issue is that of planning evaluation steps toward job placement. As part of the intermediate evaluation, what is actually being described is a continuum to placement. The client will have been evaluated utilizing some work samples and, based upon the goal, the sequential steps involving in vivo work experience evaluations may be paid or not paid. Unpaid evaluations can be conducted within nonprofit institutions or organizations and within U.S. government agencies under the work experience program. Examples of nonprofit work experiences include medical stores clerk, mail clerk, or print shop worker within a local hospital. Any number of evaluation opportunities exist within federal agencies based upon

the size of an urban area. Within the area of Seattle, Washington, federal agencies have been very helpful in establishing work experience sites for work activities such as photograph development specialist, scientific program manager, data entry operator, home loan processing clerk, retail clerk, and other positions. Large metropolitan areas offer numerous opportunities for evaluating clients within diverse job activities. In any of these intermediate level evaluation efforts, evaluation protocols can be utilized that are specific to concerns about a client's functioning (cognitive, sensory, behavioral, or physical functioning).

In the state of Washington, a client can be evaluated within the private sector for up to 120 hours if he or she is a client of the State Vocational Rehabilitation Agency. This continues to be a national pilot project and Washington is the only state in which this agreement between the U.S. Department of Labor and the State Division of Vocational Rehabilitation exists. In a residential program setting such as CRS-Washington, clients can also be hired through a nonprofit organization (i.e., Vocational Opportunities of Washington) and leased to the facility to do work on the grounds (landscaping, kitchen work activity, maintenance work, etc.) or leased to employers in the community for temporary work activity. This is an example of affirmative industry programming and it appears to be a necessary step for residential postacute traumatic brain injury programs. Discussion of this type of programming and its implications follows.

Affirmative Industries

Although supported employment does not require that participants are job ready, some traumatically brain-injured individuals are still too cognitively and/or behaviorally impaired for the rigors of supported job arrangements. This is particularly true in remote, rural communities (in which many residential traumatic brain injury rehabilitation programs are found) that lack the level of commercial activity that lends itself to supported employment programming. As a transitional step toward a supported jobs situation, seriously disabled candidates with traumatic

Table 12.1.   Vocational evaluation procedures, Community Re-entry Services of Washington   (CRS-Washington)

Initial Steps in the Evaluation Process:

1. Completion of comprehensive intake form to include extensive demographic, social, education/training, and work history.
2. Identification of individual's employment objectives, information being secured from the client and significant others.
3. Review of salient team evaluation data relative to neuropsychological, physical, communicative, independent living, and other various areas of life functioning.
4. Evaluate the effects of return to work on the client's financial benefits and litigation status.
5. Following synthesis of all relevant information at 3 to 4 weeks from intake, identify job goals and specific barriers to achieving these goals.

If Return to Prior Work or Preexisting Skill-Relevant Area:

1. Secure prior job description and conduct job analysis, securing competitive standards data relative to productivity and work accuracy.
2. Utilize relevant work sample specific to return-to-work goal.
3. Based upon level of performance, contact former employer with client's permission to establish the feasibility of:
    a. Client returns to work performing the same job with the same employer.
    b. Client returns to the same company with a modified job or different position.
    c. Client returns to work utilizing prior work skills with a new employer.
4. Decide on method of employment reentry (selective placement, on-the-job training, a supported employment approach, etc.).
5. Depending upon goal, the client may need an *Intermediate level assessment.*
6. If client needs an entirely new job goal, a *basic evaluation* is initiated.

Basic Evaluation (Clients with no substantial work histories or those requiring a new job goal):

1. Review evaluation data from rehabilitation team members and client's significant others.
2. Review neuropsychological report, including intellectual functioning, pattern of cognitive assets and limitations, and client's emotional/personality functioning.
3. Utilize vocational interest assessment in addition to client's professed interests (utilizing the Career Assessment Inventory, the Strong-Campbell, Valpar Guide to Occupational Exploration, or the Gordon Occupational Checklist).
4. Utilize McCarron-Dial Neuropsychometric Battery to complement neuropsychological evaluation and refine job goals (used in selective cases).
5. Review speech pathologist's report to establish functional communication skills, functional academic skills, and interpersonal pragmatics.
6. Use Worker Performance Assessment (WPA) tool, as developed at the Arkansas R & T Center, when concerns about client work behaviors are an issue.
7. Review occupational therapy evaluation for information relative to independent living skills and need for assistive devices.
8. Utilizing neuropsychological and other team evaluation data, establish an individual's best learning approaches for specific job tasks.
9. Establish initial job goal or goals (realizing these goals may have to be reformulated several times).
10. Utilize University of Wisconsin–Stout Work Samples keyed to high-frequency jobs in the national economy, or utilize specific work samples based on return to an area of prior work or other desired private sector work samples for which competitive work norms are available.
11. Refer for formal academic or technical training when appropriate.
12. Refer for job information–seeking activity, with the aid of a vocational staff member or other team member as necessary.
13. Refer for *intermediate level evaluation.*

Intermediate Level Evaluation (Clients with actual paid or nonpaid work experience):

1. Vocational counselor provides input to rehabilitation team or subgroup of team specialists in order to establish the questions that need to be answered through the job station experience and the type of data that needs to be collected during this experience.

(continued)

Table 12.1. *(continued)*

2. Work experience site is identified and may involve one of the following options based upon a client's individual needs:
    a. Vocational Opportunities of Washington job experience.
    b. Federal agency work experience.
    c. Community nonprofit work experience.
    d. A 120-hour job tryout in the private sector (Washington State residents only)—based upon special U.S. Department of Labor and Division of Vocational Rehabilitation Agreement in the state of Washington.
3. A vocational counselor, job coach, site supervisor, or other team member is assigned data-taking responsibilities relative to work production, accuracy, specific behavioral activity, or other types of information that need to be recorded on an individualized protocol. In some cases a specific behavioral plan will be implemented on the job site in order to improve either work or interpersonal functioning.
4. Goals of the evaluation are established relative to a transition point when the vocational emphasis would move to placement activity and the choice of a best method for approaching placement needs to be made (secured through outside vendor).
5. With rehabilitation team input, a work schedule is established, an evaluation meeting scheduled (biweekly, weekly, etc.) in order that information can be shared with the client. The assigned team member resolves any supervision, physical access, transportation, safety, or other work-related issues involving the client.
6. The client is referred to CRS-Washington Job-Seeking Skills Sequence, in order to complement his or her work experience sequence of activity.
7. A choice of placement approach is made following the review of the evaluation findings. CRS-Washington then refers for placement services. If a competitive job-placement goal is targeted, the approach to placement can later involve a selective placement, on-the-job training, a supported employment approach, or selective worker certification (a U.S. Department of Labor procedure in which a client can be paid less than minimum wage based upon productivity). If noncompetitive in nature, a sheltered workshop position or a volunteer job station slot is targeted.

brain injury may find an affirmative industry program helpful. Affirmative industries are businesses that make an assertive effort to provide realistic employment opportunities to severely disabled workers. More specifically, an affirmative industry is a corporate (nonprofit) entity that provides employment opportunities for adults and young adults who have handicapping conditions which prevent them from competing successfully in the open job market.

Unlike sheltered workshop situations, affirmative industry employees perform real work for real wages and are held to performance standards that are as competitive as is feasible given their specific vocational impairments. As in other models of supported employment, placement is immediate and precedes the provision of all other services, similar supports are provided, work tasks are varied, work settings are integrated, and employees are paid for services rendered. Unlike other models of supported employment, affirmative industry arrangements are intended to be short term and transitional to more rigorous supported employment arrangements,

particularly the supported jobs model. When used in this fashion, affirmative industries may be viewed as a variation of supported employment that extends its reach to include more severely disabled individuals with traumatic brain injury. When viewed in isolation from other placement options, however, or if poorly planned or managed, affirmative industries are marginally distinguishable from sheltered workshops, and share many of their disadvantages.

There is an additional advantage of the affirmative industries approach in that many such programs have developed an employee leasing feature. Under this option, the affirmative industry functions as a valuable resource to community-based employers to meet their needs for temporary labor during peak periods. Alternately, the community-based employer who manifests reluctance to enter into a supported jobs arrangement directly with the disabled worker and sponsoring rehabilitation facility may agree to lease the same rehabilitant from an affirmative industry that absorbs the full legal responsibility for the worker's productivity, safety, benefits, and insurance coverages. Thus many supported jobs arrangements may be negotiated only because an affirmative industry (structured as an employee leasing service) is available to "broker" the clients' services.

The employee leasing feature is fast becoming an integral part of vocational programming in remote residential traumatic brain injury rehabilitation facilities. Many such facilities are for-profit businesses that cannot or will not employ their own residents to perform both necessary and therapeutic work tasks due to legal, regulatory, or marketing constraints. By leasing the services of their own resident-workers through a separate nonprofit affirmative industry, however, real work for real wages becomes possible in the absence of a neighboring commercial district. Furthermore, as no preconceived limits exist on the design of available jobs, a resident's own rehabilitation program can be construed as his or her job and wages paid for compliance and performance therein. Consequently, a powerful motivational and normalizing twist to an otherwise routine regimen of therapies becomes possible.

To maximize the face validity of the affirmative industry experience, and to legitimize this approach as a variation of supported employment, it is imperative that resident-workers be involved at all levels of project planning, implementation, and monitoring. These include understanding the nature of business, staff needs and capabilities; ascertaining potential markets and potential financial resources; developing a sound business plan with goals, objectives, and timetables; determining an organizational structure; developing actual products/services for which a legitimate demand exists; and developing an effective marketing strategy, financial management, and an evaluation component.

It is worth noting that preliminary reports from project managers of affirmative industry programs listed the following characteristics of the sponsoring rehabilitation facility as essential to their own success: strong support from the highest levels of management, a clinical program with behavioral underpinnings, modest capital, and an entrepreneurial focus. When asked to subjectively describe characteristics of clients with traumatic brain injury who succeed

in the affirmative industry program (i.e., eventually transition to community-based supported jobs arrangements), the project managers listed initiation; acceptance of verbal instruction; the ability to communicate in a reasonable manner while working; and willingness not only to participate, but also willingness to implement the strategies learned in other therapies at the workplace (e.g., memory aids).

It is also worth noting that the process of job procurement in the affirmative industry, while facilitated by rehabilitation specialists, is competitive and realistic. It includes procuring and completing job applications and other employment forms, a series of interviews, follow-up contacts, and negotiation of the terms and conditions of work. All of this is carefully monitored and evaluated by the resident's case manager and the project manager of the affirmative industry, who must take special care to arrange for medical clearance and sponsor/payer approval of the affirmative industry arrangement.

At the New Mexico Rehabilitation Center of Wisconsin, formerly directed by B. McMahon, for adults with traumatic brain injury, workers are employed at the minimum wage or higher in a variety of positions. These include woodworking, horticulture, auto and building maintenance, painting, landscaping, concession operation, and housekeeping. Between 7 and 25 residents are employed weekly. Table 12.2 describes the vocational status of 148 discharged residents during a 30-month study period, the first 30 months of this affirmative industry project. The first clear conclusion is that more residents were able to participate in combination of supported jobs/affirmative industry experiences than in supported jobs alone. Thus the intention to extend the reach of the supported employment experience appears to have been realized. Second, it is clear that the highest percentage of subjects who were discharged into paid employment were in the "used individual supported jobs model." Forty-five percent who used the affirmative industry program as a bridge to supported jobs, however, also found paid employment and an additional 13% were gainfully active. The authors hasten to add, however, that job retention is more challenging than job pro-

Table 12.2. Vocational model participation and discharge status of residents ($n = 148$) discharged between June 5, 1986 and December 2, 1988 (New Medico Rehabilitation Center of Wisconsin)

	Used individual supported jobs model	Used affirmative industry as bridge to jobs model	Used affirmative industry model only	Nonparticipants in any supported employment model
Discharge status				
Medical disability	6	6	9	18
Unemployed	5	11	10	28
Paid—competitive	18	12	0	2
Paid—supported	0	6	0	0
Sheltered workshop	1	1	0	3
Student	1	2	1	0
Volunteer	2	2	1	2
Homemaker	0	0	0	0
Total number per model	33	40	21	54
Percentage of group	22%	27%	14%	36%
Summary:				
% gainfully active (last six statuses)	67	58	10	15
% paid employment (competitive and supported)	55	45	0	4

curement with traumatically brain-injured individuals, and so such preliminary data as these must be interpreted with caution.

Choosing a Placement Model

In a recent article (Fraser, 1989) the development of a decision tree was explicated for choosing job placement approaches in traumatic brain injury vocational rehabilitation. This model requires consideration of a number of salient client variables (neuropsychological, job-related, financial, and emotional/interpersonal) before choosing a placement approach and a level of necessary employer involvement. In early work at the University of Washington Epilepsy Center, the approaches to placement were felt to be relatively linear (Fraser, 1989, p. 181). In other words, if an individual had a mild degree of neuropsychological impairment, it was thought that he or she could be simply coached in order to return to work or move into the job market effectively. On the severe end of the impairment range, it was felt that an individual would have to be "job coached" and have significant employer support with a subsidy occasionally being provided to the employer.

Over the years, the clinical experience of Fraser, Clemmons, and McMahon indicate that

the placement directions taken need to be highly individualized. For example, an individual may have an overall mild range of neuropsychological impairment, but have specific deficits in areas such as memory or off-task behaviors that still require some type of job coaching. The authors have also experienced placing individuals with relatively severe neuropsychological impairment who do not need a job coach because the work activity did not require a great deal of decision making, the client had performed the sequence of work tasks for years and the tasks were very well learned, or there was a great amount of environmental support. Financial variables have also influenced the placement goal because some individuals probably could work full time, but their level of impairment would provide them access to jobs with insufficient salaries for supporting themselves and their family members. In consideration of the present federal subsidy structure, these individuals are at less risk financially if they work on a reduced or part-time basis and secure volunteer work activity to aid in their daily time structuring. Figure 12.1 provides an overview of a job placement decision tree. It should be noted that other client variables are considered in choosing a placement approach, but the variables identified in the deci-

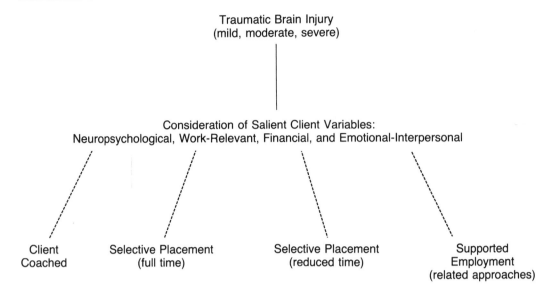

Figure 12.1. Job placement tree for vocational rehabilitation of persons with traumatic brain injury.

sion tree deserve consideration in every client's case.

It should further be noted that when a supported employment approach is indicated that there are a number of forms of supported employment that can be considered. A recent article by Nisbet and Hagner (1988) suggests a reconceptualization of supported employment approaches. It, of course, references the traditional supported jobs or job coach model, but also presents a number of alternative models of job support. These include a mentor approach in which a supervisor or co-worker assumes the role of a mentor to the trainee. A rehabilitation agency employee or other community training representative acting as a training consultant is another model. These authors also discuss job sharing and use of an attendant as a provider of job support in their discussion of other support methods.

Table 12.3 reviews the job placement models used within the demonstration grant "Vocational Re-entry of Traumatic Brain Injury" supported by the National Institute of Disability and Rehabilitation Research within the University of Washington Departments of Neurological Surgery and Rehabilitation Medicine. This demonstration project involves a 6-month intensive vocational intervention that includes vocational and neuropsychological assessment, personal

Table 12.3. Clients working competitively and placement strategy[a]

Client	Placement strategy	Support
C.W.	Direct placement	R.C. training consultant
D.S.	Direct placement	Training consultant
M.B. (1,2)	Direct placement/ OJT	Mentor
S.D. (2)	Direct placement/ OJT	Mentor
D.K. (2)	Direct placement	Mentor
M.M. (1)	Direct placement/ OJT	Mentor
A.B. (1,2)	Direct placement/ OJT	Job coach/ mentor
T.F. (2)	Direct placement	Job coach
K.P.	Direct placement— two	Job coach
L.E. (2)	Direct placement	None
L.F.	Direct placement	None
T.S.	Self-placement	None
P.D.	Self-placement	None

[a]Data obtained from demonstration project titled "Vocational Re-entry of Traumatic Brain Injury," supported by the National Institute of Disability and Rehabilitation Research, Office of Special Education and Rehabilitative Services, Grant award number G00 872 0108-89, within the University of Washington Departments of Neurological Surgery and Rehabilitation Medicine.

(1) = 120-hour job tryout.

(2) = job station.

OJT = on-the-job training subsidy.

R.C. = rehabilitation counselor.

and group counseling, job-specific compensatory training, paid and nonpaid job tryouts, placement assistance, and job coaching. At 18 months into the program, 24 clients have completed the intervention with 13 securing competitive employment (Fraser, Clemmons, Andrechak, & Dicks, 1989). Eleven of those securing jobs were still working at 18 months into the project with a range from 1 week to 8 months. Three were working with some on-the-job training subsidy from state vocational rehabilitation, but there was no indication that these jobs might not convert to permanent employment. The mean salary for those working was $5.64 per hour; standard deviation was $1.44 at the time of hire.

A model that is being used within this demonstration project with growing frequency involves employers assuming the role of training mentor and receiving on-the-job training subsidy for their efforts. The basis for utilization of the model is a very careful client-to-job/employer match. Since most of the clients entering the University of Washington project were involved in semiskilled or skilled types of work at the time of injury, use of this model is very reasonable. It can be difficult to find job

coaches to train welders, finish carpenters, and other types of skilled workers. The job coach, however, can still be very helpful in the initial implementation of the training program and in educating the employer as to how to utilize compensatory strategies and deal with maladaptive interpersonal and work behaviors. It will be of interest to determine which model seems most beneficial for which type of client over the life of the project, in terms of such considerations as job retention.

CONCLUSIONS

Some of the client-specific and programmatic considerations have been reviewed in the effort to improve vocational rehabilitation services for clients with traumatic brain injury. It is conceded that we continue to be at the "frontier" in service delivery within this field, but it is felt that major gains will be made over the next few years through the continuing efforts of vocational rehabilitation and other allied health professionals. The challenge continues to be long-term vocational stabilization of clients with traumatic brain injury within the community.

REFERENCES

American Psychiatric Association. (1987). *Diagnostic and statistical manual of mental disorders* (3rd ed., rev.). Washington, DC: Author.

Cicerone, K.D. (1989). Psychotherapeutic interventions with traumatically brain injured patients. *Rehabilitation Psychology, 2,* 105–114.

Dodrill, C.B., Batzel, L.W., Queisser, H.R., & Temkin, N.R. (1980). An objective method for the assessment of psychological and social problems among epileptics. *Epilepsia, 21,* 123–135.

Fraser, R.T. (1989). Refinement of a decision tree in traumatic brain injury job placement. *Journal of Rehabilitation Education, 2,* 179–184.

Fraser, R.T., Clemmons, D.C., Andrechak, D.A., & Dicks, M.B. (1989, August). *Vocational re-entry of the traumatic brain injured: A demonstration project.* Paper presented at the American Psychological Association Conference, New Orleans.

Fraser, R.T., Dimken, S., McLean, A., & Temkin, N. (1988). Employability of head injured survivors; The first year post-injury. *Rehabilitation Counseling Bulletin, 31,* 278–288.

Fraser, R.T., McMahon, B.T., & Vogenthaler, D. (1988). Specific considerations for vocational re-

habilitation with the head injured. In S. Rubin & N. Rubin (Eds.), *Contemporary challenges to the rehabilitation profession* (pp. 217–242). Baltimore: Paul H. Brookes Publishing Co.

Fraser, R.T., Trejo, W., Clemmons, D.C., & Freelove, C. (1987, November). *Psychosocial adjustment of the early dropouts compared to competitive placements.* Paper presented at the American Epilepsy Society Meeting, San Francisco.

Golden, C.J., Hammeke, T., & Purisch, A. (1980). *The Luria-Nebraska Neuropsychological Battery: Manual* (rev. ed.). Los Angeles: Western Psychological Service.

Gottfredson, G.D., Holland, J.L., & Ogawa, D.K. (1982). *Dictionary of occupational codes.* Palo Alto, CA: Consulting Psychologists Press.

Guidance Associates. (1965). *The Wide Range Achievement Test.* Wilmington, DE: Author.

Hathaway, S.R., & McKinley, J.C. (1951). *The Minnesota Multiphasic Personality Inventory.* New York: Psychological Corporation.

Kreutzer, J.S., Gordon, W.A., & Wehman, P. (1989). Cognitive remediation following traumatic brain injury. *Rehabilitation Psychology, 2,* 117–130.

Mikula, J., (1984, December). Standards for cognitive rehabilitation. In J. Mikula (Chair, Subcommittee on cognitive rehabilitation standards), *Proceedings of the Meeting of the American Congress of Rehabilitation Medicine,* Boston.

Millon, T. (1982). *Millon Clinical Multiaxial Inventory.* Minneapolis: Interpretive Scoring Systems, A Division of National Computer Systems.

Nisbet, J., & Hagner, D. (1988). Natural supports in the workplace.: A reexamination of supported employment. *Journal of The Association for Persons with Severe Handicaps, 13,* 260–267.

Prigatano, G.P. (1989). Bringing it up in milieu: Toward effective traumatic brain injury rehabilitation interaction. *Rehabilitation Psychology, 2,* 135–144.

Psychological Corporation. (1981). *Manual for the Weschler Adult Intelligence Scale–Revised.* New York: Author.

Reitan, R.M., & Wolfson, D. (1985). *The Halstead-Reitan Neuropsychological Test Battery.* Tucson, AZ: Neuropsychology Press.

Szymanksi, E.M. (1985). Rehabilitation counseling: A profession with a vision, an identity, and a future. *Rehabilitation Counseling Bulletin, 29,* 2–5.

Twelfth Institute on Rehabilitation Issues. (1985). *Rehabilitation of traumatic brain injury.* Menomonie: University of Wisconsin–Stout, Research and Training Center.

United States Department of Labor. (1970). *Manual for the United States Employment Service General Aptitude Test Battery.* Washington, DC: Authors.

United States Department of Labor. (1979). *Guide for occupational exploration.* Washington, DC: U.S. Government Printing Office.

Walsh, K.W. (1978). *Neuropsychology, a clinical approach.* London: Churchill Livingstone.

CHAPTER 13

Supported Employment
Model Implementation and Evaluation
Paul Wehman

Returning to meaningful paid employment has proven to be difficult for many persons recovering from traumatic brain injury. Brooks and associates (1987), for example, found that within the first 7 years postinjury only 29% of a sample of 98 persons were employed, compared to a preinjury rate of 86%. Jacobs (1988), in a comprehensive survey of 142 head-injured clients in Los Angeles, found that wages were the primary source of income for 78% of respondents preinjury compared with only 26.7% postinjury. These two major studies and many other reports by Stapleton (1986), Weddell, Oddy, and Jenkins (1980), Dresser (1973), Ben-Yishay et al. (1987), and MacKenzie (1987) all support the apparent disappointing long-term vocational outcome for persons who have experienced a severe head injury. Notably, efforts to assess pre- versus postinjury vocational outcome have used either a survey or structured interview format.

Several approaches have been used to improve vocational outcome. Prigatano (1986) presents a cognitive training program that focuses on improving cognitive and social deficits. Ben-Yishay and his associates (1987) have developed a comprehensive program of holistic cognitive remediation and occupational trials. Unfortunately, with both of these approaches there has been little evidence of skill generalization and maintenance. Because of these problems Fawber and Wachter (1987) argue for more structured job placement and case management. Similarly Burke, Wesolowski, and Guth (1988) present an intensive behavioral program within a 24-hour residential center as a means for im- proving long-term community reentry. Wehman and his colleagues (in press) have presented a supported employment model to help place and retain difficult-to-place individuals with severe disabilities. This approach focuses not only on structured job placement and case management but heavily on job retention and generalization as well.

The supported employment approach, which has been described earlier by Kreutzer and Morton (1988) and Kreutzer et al. (1988), has the advantage of providing direct professional staff support at the point of placement in the work environment. An employment specialist, also known as a job coach, focuses exclusively on one client at the workplace. Training and counseling support are provided over a number of weeks or months until the individual's performance is stabilized. At that time the employment specialist "fades" his or her time from the job site. Clients are usually accepted only if they have failed with other rehabilitation approaches to placement and have been consistently unable to gain or hold any competitive job.

This chapter is divided into two major parts. The first part provides a presentation of the different supported employment models currently in practice, with the advantages and disadvantages of each model. The second part of the chapter provides for an analysis of the employment outcomes associated with a major supported employment program for persons with traumatic brain injury that has been underway for 2 years at the Medical College of Virginia in Richmond.

REVIEW OF SUPPORTED EMPLOYMENT MODELS

The concept of supported employment has evolved within recent years as an alternative for persons with severe disabilities who cannot get a job or hold a job without *permanent* follow-along support placement. Supported employment provides opportunities to work for the first time for many people who are at substantial risk of not gaining and maintaining employment. It may involve a host of different arrangements within industry or outside of industry, in different occupations, and with different staffing patterns. Major characteristics of supported employment are:

Real pay for real work—not work experience or volunteer work

Integration with and around nonhandicapped co-workers

Permanent ongoing or intermittent support through the life of employment

Emphasis on people with severe disability who cannot hold employment without ongoing support

Tangible outcome—not a process-service activity

Supported employment was included in Title VI(c) of the Rehabilitation Act Amendments of 1986 for the first time as a major rehabilitation outcome. It has been defined as:

> . . . competitive work in integrated work settings (a) for individuals for whom competitive employment has not traditionally occurred. . . . Services available, but not limited to are provision of skilled job trainers, on-the-job training, systematic training, job development, follow-up services. . . . (p. 8911, October 2, 1986)

In this law is the provision of funds for supported employment activity and state planning development. Furthermore, funds are made available for major state-level discretionary projects to change day program systems for adult activity centers to industry-based employment. In 1985, 10 states were funded for this activity and in 1986 another 17 states were funded (both years for a 5-year period), all by the Rehabilitation Services Administration, Office of Special Education and Rehabilitative Services (OSERS), U.S. Department of Education. If the effort at systemic change is successful within these states, transition-age youth will likely have better employment opportunities after school.

Common Characteristics

Paid Employment

Supported employment is paid employment that cannot exist without a regular opportunity to work. The federal government has suggested that an individual should be considered to meet the paid employment aspect of supported employment if he or she engages in paid work for at least an average of 4 hours each day, 5 days per week, or another schedule offering at least 20 hours of work per week. This standard does not establish a minimum wage or productivity level for supported employment.

The amount of hours worked should not be viewed as the only criterion for supported employment, because some people (such as adolescents with severe handicaps) may choose to work only 15 hours a week. The stipulation of number of hours worked, however, does convey the seriousness and impact that paid employment may have on the young person with disabilities.

Community Integration

Work is integrated when it provides frequent daily social interactions with people without disabilities who are not paid caregivers. The federal government has suggested that integration in supported employment programs be defined in terms of a place where: 1) no more than eight people with disabilities work together, which is not immediately adjacent to another program serving persons with disabilities; and 2) persons without disabilities who are not paid caregivers are present in the work setting or immediate vicinity.

For example, an individual with severe cerebral palsy who works in a local bank creating microfilm records of transactions clearly meets the integration criteria for supported employment. Other examples include: four individuals with severe emotional disorders who work together in an enclave within a manufacturing plant, a mobile janitorial crew that employs five persons with moderate mental retardation in community worksites, and a small bakery that employs persons with and without disabilities.

Ongoing Support

Supported employment exists only when ongoing support is provided. In contrast to time-limited support, such as transitional employment, which may only be provided for a few months, ongoing support continues as long as the client is employed. An individual should be considered to be receiving ongoing support when public funds are available on an ongoing basis to an individual or service provider who is responsible for providing employment support and when these funds are used for specialized assistance directly related to sustaining employment. It is this aspect of supported employment that distinguishes the model significantly from other models. Such a characteristic positively influences the concerns of parents and employers.

Severe Disability

Supported employment exists when the persons served require ongoing support; it is inappropriate for persons who would be better served in time-limited preparation programs leading to independent employment. The most significant way to describe who should receive supported employment is to assess how much an individual is at risk of not gaining and maintaining employment. Youths who are highly likely to lose jobs shortly after placement because of their disability may be prime candidates for supported employment. Individuals labeled as autistic, moderately, severely or profoundly mentally retarded, and multiply handicapped would thus constitute the principal target groups for this approach. These individuals would not be able to hold jobs without permanent, long-term follow-along at the job site.

Final Thoughts

Since supported employment has become such a widespread mode of employment in recent years, it is essential that service providers under-

stand the above four characteristics. There can be a significant lack of understanding by service providers in these points.

Specific descriptions of several emerging supported employment models follow in the next sections. These models are among the principle models currently receiving attention in the field and are among the most likely placement alternatives of individuals with traumatic brain injury.

Supported Competitive Employment Model

A supported work approach to competitive job placement requires specialized assistance in locating an appropriate job, intensive job-site training for clients who are usually not "job ready," and permanent, ongoing follow-along. A qualified staff person essentially establishes a one-to-one relationship with a client in need of individual employment services and provides placement and ongoing training right at the job site. *The person is employed immediately with wages paid by the employer.* Follow-along is differentiated from follow-up in that there is daily and weekly on-site evaluation of how the client is performing while follow-up suggests only periodic checking at established intervals of time. Competitive employment is defined here as a real job providing the federal minimum wage in a work area with predominantly nonhandicapped workers. Table 13.1 presents the characteristics of this model.

Supported competitive employment is contrasted with traditional placement into competitive employment in that the latter is time limited. That is, once the client has been placed and trained at the job site to the satisfaction of the employer, the service is terminated. With supported employment there is a permanent commitment for follow-along services provided by professional staff. An approach that has worked well in Virginia has been for the Virginia Department of Rehabilitative Services to fund the initial job placement and intensive job-site training costs through case service funds. The permanent follow-along component is paid for through local and state mental health/mental retardation

Table 13.1.   Characteristics of supported competitive employment

Integration: Moderate to high
Staff-to-consumer ratio: 1 staff : 1 consumer
Economic cost to society: Limited, especially over long term
Economic benefit to society: High
Placement: Selective
Job-site training: Intensive
Postemployment services: Ongoing follow-along
Service provision: Ongoing
Wages to consumers: Minimum wage or above
Type of work: Service industry–related positions
Service provision locations: Community based
Fringe benefits: Equivalent to co-workers

funds. This interagency shared responsibility is now happening in at least four areas of Virginia (Hill et al., 1987).

Mobile Work Crews and Enclaves

Mobile work crews and enclaves are employment options for adults with disabilities that have existed for many years (McGee, 1975), but have recently received renewed attention within the supported employment initiative (Mank, Rhodes, & Bellamy, 1986). Enclaves and work crews both allow individuals previously served in sheltered employment alternatives an opportunity for meaningful employment in more integrated community-based settings. In both options, individuals with severe disabilities are provided continuous ongoing support by a human services professional to enable them to succeed in more challenging employment settings. Workers are paid based on performance and wages are commensurate with those paid to nonhandicapped workers performing the same duties. While similarities exist between the two models, each is discussed separately to differentiate the array of alternative approaches used to implement enclave and work crew options.

Mobile Work Crews

Mobile work crews or work-force teams comprise four to six individuals with severe disabilities who spend their day away from a center-based rehabilitation facility or adult vocational program performing service jobs in community settings. Mobile work crews may operate inde-

pendently as private, not-for-profit corporations, or may be a component of a large array of employment options operated by a rehabilitation or adult services agency. Whatever the organizational structure, the sponsoring agency contracts with community businesses or individuals to perform groundskeeping, janitorial, home maintenance, or similar tasks. Workers are generally paid by the sponsoring agency based upon productivity. A training supervisor or manager accompanies the crew on a full-time basis and is responsible for training work crew members, providing ongoing supervision to maintain productivity and quality control, and guaranteeing that the contracted work is completed to required standards.

The work crew is staffed by a single supervisor or manager. The supervisor is responsible for all aspects of the operation, including securing and negotiating contracts, training and supervising crew members, and maintaining program records. While the small size of the crew allows for intense supervision and the inclusion of individuals with significant learning and production problems, the reliance on a single staff member makes the operation of the crew challenging. Since the crew functions away from the service agency or rehabilitation facility, the manager is often isolated from other professionals. Also, the need to provide continuous supervision to crew members often makes it difficult for the supervisor to perform the required contract-procurement and administrative activities. In larger communities, establishing a number of crews may be one way in which direct service and management functions may be shared to maximize total program effectiveness.

The flexibility of the work crew, both in terms of the type of work performed and the make-up of the crew, allows the model to accommodate the needs of individuals with a wide array of disabilities. The majority of work performed is in the area of buildings and grounds maintenance, although housecleaning in suburban areas, farm work in rural areas, and motel room cleaning in areas with large tourist industries have also been identified as successful alternatives. A crew may have contracts with a number of different agencies and may perform

Table 13.2. Characteristics of mobile work crews

Integration: Moderate
Staff-to-consumer ratio: 1 staff : 3–6 consumers
Economic cost to society: Moderately high
Economic benefit to society: Moderately high
Placement: Selective
Job-site training: Moderate to intensive
Postemployment services: Ongoing follow-along
Service provision: Ongoing
Wages to consumers: Paid by sponsoring agency based on consumer productivity
Type of work: Groundskeeping, janitorial, home maintenance, etc.
Service provision location: Community based: multiple contracts with businesses in the local community
Fringe benefits: Usually very limited

work in a large number of settings in the course of a week. While work crews have been successful in areas with high unemployment rates, securing enough contracts to provide work during all standard work hours is frequently a problem. Table 13.2 provides an overview of the features of work crews.

The use of mobile crews is an option that may have particular applicability in small communities and rural areas. Service agencies in rural areas attempting to provide supported employment alternatives to persons with severe disabilities face a unique set of challenges. Many rural areas often have a relatively high unemployment rate. With little or no industrial base, service agencies encounter serious problems accessing an adequate amount of work. The small number of individuals to be served within a large geographical area creates severe logistical problems for the agency. In addition, it is often difficult for the areas to identify and recruit highly trained staff with the skills necessary to implement supported employment alternatives. A major strength of the mobile work crew model is its ability to provide stable employment for a small number of workers with severe disabilities in the types of work found in a local area.

Enclaves

Enclaves are employment options in which small groups of workers with disabilities (generally six to eight) are employed and supervised among nonhandicapped workers in a business or industry. Continuous, long-term, on-site supervision is provided by a trained human services professional or host company employee. Workers may be employed directly by the business or industry, or remain employees of the not-for-profit organization that provides support to the individuals. Enclave members work alongside others performing the same work, although in some situations workers with disabilities may be grouped together to facilitate training and supervision.

Enclaves provide an excellent potential to both supported competitive employment and traditional sheltered employment. The model provides intensive on-site supervision designed to maximize worker productivity and prevent job termination. This will allow access to community-based employment settings for workers with substantial handicaps who might otherwise be unsuccessful when daily training and supervision are faded during the follow-along stage of supported competitive employment. At the same time, enclaves provide extended employment in an integrated community setting for individuals who traditionally have been served exclusively in segregated workshops or work activity centers. The model may also be contrasted with the mobile work crew approach. Within mobile work crews, workers will generally move to different work settings on a daily basis, or may work at several different sites in the course of a single day. Enclave employees are able to work in a single setting for a prolonged period of time. Additionally, enclave employees in some instances are paid wages and receive benefits directly from the company, whereas work crew members remain employees of the sponsoring service agency indefinitely. In one demonstration (Rhodes & Valenta, 1985), workers who had reached 65% of standard productivity were hired as employees of the host company at a competitive rate and with full fringe benefits.

The critical feature of the enclave model is the extended training and supervision provided to address low worker productivity and difficulties in adapting to changing work demands. Systematic intervention is necessary to allow workers to acquire all needed skills and produce at an acceptable rate. This extra support may in some

Table 13.3. Characteristics of enclaves

Integration: Moderate to high, depending on type
  of enclave
Staff-to-consumer ratio: 1 staff : 6–8 consumers
Economic cost to society: Moderately high
Economic benefit to society: Moderately high
Placement: Selective
Job-site training: Moderate to intensive
Postemployment services: Ongoing   follow-
  along
Service provision: Ongoing
Wages to consumers: Workers are paid based on
  productivity; wages are often commensurate
  with those paid to nonhandicapped workers
Type of work: Assembly work for a host company
Service provision location: Community based: in
  a host company
Fringe benefits: Limited

cases be provided by the host company, but in most instances is the responsibility of the sponsoring service agency. The enclave supervisor is the key to providing this support. It is a major commitment for the company to hire a group of workers with severe disabilities and allow the involvement of an outside service organization. The enclave supervisor must be highly skilled in effective instruction and supervision techniques while also being sensitive to the production demands and concerns of the host company. Table 13.3 presents a summary of enclave characteristics.

Major Outcomes Associated with Mobile Work Crews and Enclaves

Major positive outcomes associated with mobile work crews and sheltered enclaves are the physical and social integration of individuals with severe disabilities in natural work settings and opportunities to earn significant wages. Wages paid to work crew and enclave members are based upon productivity, with members earning a percentage of the standard hourly wage for individuals performing similar work. Since the workers in most instances are clients of a not-for-profit agency, fringe benefits are generally not provided. Mank, Rhodes, and Bellamy (1986) report data from two mobile work crew agencies in which individuals earned from $130 to $185 per month. Rhodes and Valenta (1985) report wages of $295 after 8 months of employment for

six individuals in an enclave. Public costs are required to make up the excess costs incurred in both models due to low worker productivity and the need for intense, continuous supervision. While these figures may not seem particularly high, they are quite significant when compared to earnings of clients in sheltered employment alternatives (Noble, 1986). For example, in the enclave described by Rhodes and Valenta, the individuals involved had averaged less than $40 per month prior to placement in the enclave.

The outcomes associated with the work crew and enclave options must be evaluated in the context of the individuals served by these models. In most cases workers are not making minimum wage or only a percentage of the prevailing competitive wage, and public costs for the programs are not significantly reduced from the costs of traditional workshop programs. In spite of this, the models are very justifiable on the grounds that they provide employment in integrated settings for individuals who traditionally would have no opportunity for such work. Individuals who may have medical conditions such as seizure disorders or severe diabetes, or individuals who may exhibit significant maladaptive behaviors such as stereotypic or inappropriate behavior may at long last have an opportunity to secure and maintain employment in a natural work setting.

Small Business Option

Another type of possible employment option has been the small business alternative. This option usually reflects a manufacturing, production, or assembly operation that occurs in a building located in the community. Two major characteristics of this option are: 1) smallness (i.e., 8–10 as the maximum number of disabled persons with small numbers of nonhandicapped employees), and 2) homogeneity of the business (e.g., printing, electronics, or micrographics). Bellamy, Horner, and Inman (1979) have been leaders in this type of vocational alternative, which has been devoted to persons with the most handicaps. Generally persons who work in these settings are in continual need of behavior training and production training. Table 13.4 briefly summarizes this model.

Table 13.4.   Characteristics of small businesses

Integration: Low to none
Staff-to-consumer ratio: 1 staff : 8 consumers
Economic cost to society: High
Economic benefit to society: Usually limited
Placement: Selective
Job-site training: Moderate to intensive
Postemployment services: Ongoing follow-along
Service provision: Ongoing
Wages to consumers: Subminimum, based on consumer productivity
Type of work: Printing, electronics, bakeries, micrographics, etc.
Service provision location: Center based, usually within an industrial park
Fringe benefits: Very limited

Deciding Which Model to Choose

Deciding which vocational alternative is best is difficult at times. Obviously, each job situation in each unique industry will vary. The mobile work crew program may be excellent because of special government contracts, but the amount of 40-hour work weeks may be limited by seasonal constraints. Movement out of restricted enclaves into a more dispersed arrangement may be excellent or poor depending on the management's philosophy toward integration.

What is most important for families and consumers is to push hard for having multiple choices in their community. The more options one has, the greater the likelihood of finding job satisfaction and developing long-term employment histories. It is a positive statement on the progress made in adult services that there are increasingly multiple vocational choices being made available in more and more communities. Ultimately, it will be best if vocational arrangements are offered in multiple industries, not only in food service or benchwork assembly. This type of job development will depend directly on the economic conditions of the local community and the creativity and ingenuity of the vocational professionals.

INDIVIDUAL PLACEMENT MODEL OF SUPPORTED EMPLOYMENT

An individual placement model of supported employment has been used for approximately 2 years at the Medical College of Virginia, and data are reported for this effort herein. In order to fully asses the meaning of vocational outcomes postinjury it is critical to determine the preinjury occupational status of a client. Therefore, the preinjury work history, postinjury work history, and supported employment work performance of individuals with traumatic brain injury who have been placed into competitive employment is presented. Competitive employment is defined as: 1) wages equal to or greater than the federal minimum wage of $3.35 per hour, and 2) employment in work environments with people who are not labeled as being handicapped.

Client Profile

All clients are under medical supervision of a physiatrist upon referral to the supported employment program. A total of 41 clients have been referred from physicians, psychologists, rehabilitation counselors, and families for supported employment services. Virtually all have been initially accepted for potential placement provided they are between 18 and 64 years of age, have a history of severe head injury, and are not active substance abusers. There are no exclusion criteria based on cognitive, physical, or social limitations. However, there must also be a very strong indication that the person *cannot* work successfully without ongoing job support. This indication is determined by: 1) documented previous employment failures, postinjury; or 2) reports from the family, physician, referring rehabilitation counselor, or client indicating concern about independent work ability.

Table 13.5 presents a brief description of the persons placed to date and selected demographic information along with the major presenting vocational problems. The mean age at injury was 22.2 years, with the current age of each person placed being 29.9. Time in coma averaged 65 days with a range of 3 days to 233 days. A total of 92.1% have received some form of financial aid. A total of 90% of all persons experienced head injuries as a result of motor vehicle accidents. It should also be noted, consistent with the findings of Ben-Yishay et al. (1987) and Brooks et al. (1987), that 12 of the 20 persons (60%) experienced memory problems;

Table 13.5. Client demographic profiles

Client no.	Gender	Age at injury (years)	Cause of injury	Length of coma (days)	Current age (years)	Preinjury educational level	Current residential status	Major presenting vocational problem areas
1.	M	12	Auto accident	35	31	Elementary student	Independent	Nervousness, restlessness, anxiety, memory
2.	M	48	Fall in home	Unknown	50	Some college courses	Independent	Complex reasoning, stress tolerance, memory
3.	M	21	Auto accident	53	27	College graduate	Parents' home	Motor/coordination, strength
4.	F	23	Struck by auto	92	27	Some college courses	Parents' home	Short-term memory, fine motor coordination, compliance
5.	M	30	Auto accident	60	33	High school graduate	Shares home	Motor/ambulation, fine motor coordination, strength
6.	M	24	Auto accident	21	31	High school graduate	Parents' home	Short-term memory, following instructions
7.	M	34	Auto accident	92	39	Some college courses	Parents' home	Vision, memory, ambulation, speech, fine motor coordination
8.	M	19	Auto accident	60	27	High school graduate	Supervised apt.	Ambulation, memory, wandering, argumentative
9.	M	15	Motorcycle accident	92	30	Some college courses	Independent	Temper, argumentative

#	Sex	Age	Cause			Education	Residence	Impairments
10.	M	23	Auto accident	233	31	Some high school	Parents' home	Ambulation, fine motor coordination
11.	M	16	Gunshot wound	3	18	Some college courses	Parents' home	Ambulation, seizures, memory, vision
12.	M	9	Auto accident	138	20	Elementary student	Parents' home	Work speed, compliance with instructions
13.	M	27	Motorcycle accident	59	29	High school graduate	Parents' home	Vision, coordination, communication
14.	M	20	Auto accident	153	33	College student	Supervised apt.	Short-term memory, thinking, motor/coordination
15.	M	16	Auto accident	10	37	High school student	Independent	Seizures, attention span, memory
16.	F	24	Auto accident	1	26	High school graduate	Independent	Motor strength, coordination, concentration
17.	M	20	Auto accident	62	26	Some high school	Supervised apt.	Memory, strength, extended standing or walking
18.	M	14	Auto accident	120	31	Some college courses	Supervised apt.	Vision, motivation, memory, coordination
19.	M	27	Struck by auto	5	28	Some college courses	Independent	Speech, thinking and organization skills
20.	M	22	Motorcycle accident	11	25	High school graduate	Supervised apt.	Vision, memory, depression, coordination
Means =		22.2		65.0	29.9			

10 persons (50%) presented serious motor and/or ambulation limitations.

An effort is made to complete a neuropsychological and psychiatric examination on each person referred for supported employment. Measures of intellectual, cognitive, and psychomotor ability include the Galveston Orientation Amnesia Test (GOAT) as well as portions of the Wechsler Adult Intelligence Scale–Revised, the Wide Range Achievement Test–Revised (WRAT), and the Halstead-Reitan. On most of the subtests of the battery of tests, scores were below the 50th percentile relative to the normal population with a range of 10% to 59%.

Data Management System

Data are collected on a number of key outcome measures. The data are collected at initial intake, and then after placement data are recorded weekly by employment specialists in the program. These data are then stored in the university mainframe computer.

Employment Data Management System

The employment data management system allows evaluation to occur at the individual, program, and system levels. Numerous client-related job performance factors are evaluated, such as wages earned and hours worked weekly as well as direct behavioral observation of work performance. Additionally, employers are asked to fill out a five-point Likert scale form periodically on the work habits of the placed clients.

Monthly Employment Ratio

A key outcome indicator used to assess return-to-work capacity is the monthly employment ratio. This index of assessing vocational outcome was developed because of the difficulty in capturing vocational progress and retention presented by many postacute severely head-injured individuals. The strength of this index is that it *directly* measures over time the actual work behavior exhibited by the individual.

The employment ratio is derived by dividing the number of months the client was employed during an employment phase by the total possible months that he or she would have had an

opportunity to be employed. For determining the month of first employability for the employment phases, the following protocol was used:

1. If the client was injured as a child or teenager, the 20th birthday was used as the date of first employability for the postinjury phase, unless the client's work history also began prior to the 20th birthday. In those cases the start date of the client's first job was used as the beginning of employability for the preinjury phase.
2. For those clients injured as adults, the 20th birthday was used as the month of first employability for the preinjury phase. The start date of the postinjury phase was determined to be the date of hospital discharge.
3. If the date of hospital discharge was unknown, a date of first employability was derived by adding 6 months to the end of the period the client was comatose.
4. The supported employment phase is initiated by the date of first placement and continues either to the current date or to a date of final discharge from the program.

Major Components of Supported Employment Program Model

Screening and Job Placement

When clients are referred to the supported employment program for placement they are individually interviewed, previous vocational histories are reviewed, and home visits are made for the purpose of determining the nature of employment and work situation by the client. No standardized or formal vocational evaluation testing is performed. However, an in-depth analysis of potential job sites is undertaken by the employment specialist. Each person is rated by the employment specialist on 28 items ranging from transportation, willingness to work part time versus full time, endurance required in a specific job, and so forth, as different potential job opportunities arise. This form, which is presented in Form 13.1, provides an ecological analysis of the assets and liabilities of the client and, even more, a profile of what types of work conditions will be acceptable and not acceptable.

CONSUMER SCREENING FORM

Date of screening (month/day/year): ____/____/____

Type of screening: Initial ____ Ongoing/Employed ____ Ongoing/Unemployed ____

<u>Total</u> number of hours per week presently working: ____ Months per year: ____

General Directions: PLEASE DO NOT LEAVE ANY ITEM UNANSWERED!

Indicate the most appropriate response for each item based on observations of the consumer and interviews with individuals who know the consumer (i.e., family members, adult service-providers, school personnel, employers).

---

1. Availability: (Circle Yes or No for each item)

Will Work Weekends	Will Work Evenings	Will Work Part Time	Will Work Full Time
Yes No	Yes No	Yes No	Yes No

Specifics/Comments:

---

2. Transportation: (Circle Yes or No for each item)

Transportation Available	Access to Specialized Travel Services	Lives on Bus Route	Family Will Transport	Provides Own Transportation (Bike, Car, Walks, etc.)
Yes No	Yes No	Yes No	Yes No	Yes No

Specifics/Comments:

---

3. Strength; Lifting and Carrying:

Poor (<10 lbs.)	Fair (10–20 lbs.)	Average (30–40 lbs.)	Strong (>50 lbs.)
____	____	____	____

Specifics/Comments:

---

4. Endurance: (Without Break)

Works <2 Hours ____	Works 2–3 Hours ____	Works 3–4 Hours ____	Works >4 Hours ____

Specifics/Comments:

---

5. Orienting:

Small Area Only ____	One Room ____	Several Rooms ____	Building Wide ____	Building and Grounds ____

Specifics/Comments:

---

6. Physical Mobility:

Sit/Stand in One Area ____	Fair Ambulation ____	Stairs/Minor Obstacles ____	Full Physical Abilities ____

Specifics/Comments:

---

7. Independent Work Rate: (No Prompts)

Slow Pace ____	Steady/Average Pace ____	Above Average/Sometimes Fast Pace ____	Continual Fast Pace ____

Specifics/Comments:

---

8. Appearance:

Unkempt/Poor Hygiene ____	Unkempt/Clean ____	Neat/Clean but Clothing Unmatched ____	Neat/Clean and Clothing Matched ____

Specifics/Comments:

---

9. Communication:

Uses Sounds/ Gestures ____	Uses Key Words/Signs ____	Speaks Unclearly ____	Communicates Clearly, Intelligible to Strangers

Specifics/Comments:

(continued)

10. Appropriate Social Interactions:	Rarely Interacts Appropriately ⎯⎯	Polite, Responses Appropriate ⎯⎯	Initiates Social Interactions Infrequently ⎯⎯	Initiates Social Interactions Frequently ⎯⎯

Specifics/Comments:

11. Unusual Behavior:	Many Unusual Behaviors ⎯⎯		Few Unusual Behaviors ⎯⎯	No Unusual Behaviors ⎯⎯

Specifics/Comments:

12. Attention to Task/Perseverance:	Frequent Prompts Required ⎯⎯	Intermittent Prompts/High Supervision Required ⎯⎯	Intermittent Prompts/Low Supervision Required ⎯⎯	Infrequent Prompts/Low Supervision Required ⎯⎯

Specifics/Comments:

13. Independent Sequencing of Job Duties:	Cannot Perform Tasks in Sequence ⎯⎯	Performs 2–3 Tasks in Sequence ⎯⎯	Performs 4–6 Tasks in Sequence ⎯⎯	Performs 7 or More Tasks in Sequence ⎯⎯

Specifics/Comments:

14. Initiative/Motivation:	Always Seeks Work ⎯⎯	Sometimes Volunteers ⎯⎯	Waits for Directions ⎯⎯	Avoids Next Task ⎯⎯

Specifics/Comments:

15. Adapting to Change:	Adapts to Change ⎯⎯	Adapts to Change With Some Difficulty ⎯⎯	Adapts to Change With Great Difficulty ⎯⎯	Rigid Routine Required ⎯⎯

Specifics/Comments:

16. Reinforcement Needs:	Frequent Required ⎯⎯	Intermittent (daily) Sufficient ⎯⎯	Infrequent (weekly) Sufficient ⎯⎯	Pay Check Sufficient ⎯⎯

Specifics/Comments:

17. Family Support:	Very Supportive of Work ⎯⎯	Supportive of Work With Reservations ⎯⎯	Indifferent About Work ⎯⎯	Negative About Work ⎯⎯

Specifics/Comments:

18. Consumer's Financial Situation:	Financial Ramifications No Obstacle ⎯⎯	Requires Job With Benefits ⎯⎯	Reduction of Financial Aid Is a Concern ⎯⎯	Unwilling to Give Up Financial Aid ⎯⎯

Specifics/Comments:

19. Discrimination Skills:	Cannot Distinguish between Work Supplies ⎯⎯		Distinguishes between Work Supplies with an External Cue ⎯⎯	Distinguishes between Work Supplies ⎯⎯

Specifics/Comments:

FORM 13.1
(*continued*)

20. Time Awareness:	Unaware of Time and Clock Function ____	Identifies Breaks and Lunch ____	Can Tell Time to the Hour ____	Can Tell Time in Hours and Minutes ____

Specifics/Comments:

21. Functional Reading:	None ____	Sight Words/ Symbols ____	Simple Reading ____	Fluent Reading ____

Specifics/Comments:

22. Functional Math:	None ____	Simple Counting ____	Simple Addition/ Subtraction ____	Computational Skills ____

Specifics/Comments:

23. Independent Street Crossing:	None ____	Crosses Two-Lane Street with Light ____	Crosses Two-Lane Street without Light ____	Crosses Four-Lane Street with Light ____	Crosses Four-Lane Street without Light ____

Specifics/Comments:

24. Handling Criticism/Stress:	Resistive/ Argumentative ____	Withdraws into Silence ____	Accepts Criticism/Does Not Change Behavior ____	Accepts Criticism/ Changes Behavior ____

Specifics/Comments:

25. Acts/Speaks Aggressively:	Hourly ____	Daily ____	Weekly ____	Monthly ____	Never ____

Specifics/Comments:

26. Travel Skills: (Circle Yes or No for each item)	Requires Bus Training Yes No	Uses Bus Independently/ No Transfer Yes No	Uses Bus Independently/ Makes Transfer Yes No	Able to Make Own Travel Arrangements Yes No

Specifics/Comments:

27. Benefits consumer needs (Circle Yes or No for each choice):
Yes No 0 = None
Yes No 1 = Sick Leave
Yes No 2 = Medical/Health Benefits
Yes No 3 = Paid Vacation/Annual Leave
Yes No 4 = Dental Benefits
Yes No 5 = Employee Discounts
Yes No 6 = Free or Reduced Meals
Yes No 7 = Other (specify): _____

28. CHECK ALL THAT CONSUMER HAS PERFORMED:

Bus Tables ____	Sweeping ____	Dish Machine Use ____	"Keeping Busy" ____
Food Prep. ____	Assembly ____	Mopping (Indust.) ____	Clerical ____
Buffing ____	Vacuuming ____	Food Line Supply ____	Pot Scrubbing ____
Dusting ____	Restroom Cleaning ____	Trash Disposal ____	Other _____
Stocking ____	Washing Equipment ____	Food Serving ____	_____

Medications? _____

(*continued*)

Medical Complications/Conditions? _____

_____

Additional Comments: _____

_____

_____

As stated above, each job opportunity is similarly analyzed in terms of working conditions and necessary employee characteristics. Items on the Consumer Screening Form are then compared with identical items on the Job Screening Form, thus providing employment specialists with an instrument for matching supported employment clients with available jobs.

Screening takes place for all referred clients while employment specialists are doing job development and contacting businesses for possible jobs. With the use of a detailed job analysis, staff go to businesses and are able to analyze extensively the most salient aspects of a given job. Jobs are selected for analysis in many different fields, such as child care, manufacturing, food service, and so forth. Client interests and previous employment are key elements in determining the general area of occupational interest that employment specialists investigate.

Job-Site Training and Compensatory Strategies

At the point of initial placement and employment, the employment specialist accompanies the client to the job site and stays for as long a period as is reasonably expected to stabilize job performance. Stabilization has been defined previously in individual placement of supported employment programs as the point at which the client requires 20% or less of the employment specialist's time at the job site (Hill et al., 1987). This can take weeks or even months of daily intervention. Behavioral training, skill training, social adjustment, cognitive training strategies, and physical adaptations are among the types of interventions utilized at the job site. Often the employment specialist will have to help in completion of the job. Considerations that are accounted for in choosing a particular

cognitive compensatory strategy include: 1) the general cognitive level of the individual and how he or she learns best, 2) the individual's degree of short-term memory loss, 3) the individual's effective self-selected strategies, 4) the individual's problem-solving ability, and 5) the opportunity to use compensatory skills in a functional setting. One primary consideration in the selection of effective compensatory strategies is the participation of the client in planning.

Job Retention

As the client becomes increasingly competent at work, the amount of staff time required at the job site for support will be reduced. Gradual removal of the job coach from the job site is usually completed by several strategies. These include: 1) unobtrusive observation of the client's performance, 2) frequent phone communication with the supervisor or immediate intervention (if warranted) at the job site when it appears that the person is at risk of losing the job, 3) ongoing efforts to help the person with psychosocial adjustment in the work environment, and 4) helping arrange whatever community services are necessary to deal with nonvocational problems that may arise. Taking a proactive and anticipatory position toward job retention is an essential aspect of the supported employment model.

Staffing

Employment specialists who provided services in the program at the Medical College of Virginia had either bachelor's or master's degrees in counseling, adult education, or psychology. The work expectations for them were: 1) job placement skills; 2) ability to train head-injured clients at a job site; 3) counseling skills with the employer, family, and client; and 4) skill in travel training and other aspects of arranging em-

Table 13.6. Client work histories

Client no.	Preinjury					Postinjury					Supported employment				
	Number of jobs[a]	Industrial category	Mean wage[a]	Mean hrs./wk.[a]	Employment ratio[b]	Number of jobs	Industrial category	Mean wage[c]	Mean hrs./wk.[c]	Employment ratio[b]	Number of jobs	Industrial category	Mean wage	Mean hrs./wk.	Employment ratio[b]
1.	NA	NA	NA	NA	NA	14	Laborer	4.31	27.9	.7967	2[d]	Unskilled	4.40	30.5	1.0000
2.	2	Retail sales	5.21	40	.7207	0	NA	NA	NA	.0000	2[e]	Food service	3.98	20	.8213
3.	5	Retail sales	4.18	24	.8710	2	Clerical	5.57	20	.1367	2[e]	Retail sales	4.15	22	.8555
4.	3	Clerical	5.07	18.7	1.0000	0	NA	NA	NA	.0000	1	Office aide	5.16	30	1.0000
5.	3	Maintenance	5.08	40	.3566	0	NA	NA	NA	.0000	1	Office worker	5.00	39	1.0000
6.	1	Sportswriter	6.25	40	.4363	2	Clerical	3.35	40	.1310	1	Human services	3.55	20	1.0000
7.	5	Retail sales	6.12	34.4	.9747	0	NA	NA	NA	.0000	1	Office aide	4.93	20	.2708
8.	1	Construction	5.00	40	1.0000	1	Workshop	.58	30	.1017	1	Warehouse	3.35	30	1.0000
9.	NA	NA	NA	NA	NA	3	Clerk	3.45	25	.4621	1	Warehouse	3.90	30	.2500
10.	2	Printing	3.60	38.5	.6286	1	Workshop	1.40	37	.5639	1	Maintenance	3.60	39	1.0000
11.	1	Stock clerk	3.35	5	1.0000	0	NA	NA	NA	.0000	1	Bagger	3.75	25	.3333
12.	NA	NA	NA	NA	NA	3	Retail sales	3.78	21.3	.2530	2[e]	Retail sales	3.80	24	1.0000
13.	3	Construction	5.67	40	1.0000	2	Custodial	2.19	18.4	.2587	1	Retail sales	3.60	40	1.0000
14.	1	Human services	2.81	40	1.0000	0	NA	NA	NA	.0000	1	Human services	4.00	15	1.0000
15.	NA	NA	NA	NA	NA	17	Food service	3.42	27	.8287	1	Food service	4.50	40	1.0000
16.	3	Food service	4.15	40	.6098	1	Food service	4.50	40	.5000	1	Food service	4.50	40	1.0000
17.	1	Construction	3.35	40	1.0000	1	Food service	3.35	25	.0187	1	Unskilled	4.50	25	1.0000
18.	NA	NA	NA	NA	NA	0	NA	NA	NA	.0000	1	Food service	4.05	32	1.0000
19.	1	Commercial	11.45	40	1.0000	1	Recreation	4.00	18	.2857	1	Commercial	11.45	25	1.0000
20.	3	Construction	5.50	40	1.0000	1	Construction	5.00	30	.1818	1	Maintenance	4.15	38	1.0000
Means =	2.3		5.11	34.7	.8398	2.5		3.45	27.7	.2245	1.2		4.52	29.2	.8765
Standard deviation =	1.4		2.05	10.5	.2287	4.6		1.39	7.6	.2687	.37		1.70	8.0	.2602

[a] Participants whose injuries occurred prior to their 20th birthday were coded NA, and not included in mean computation.

[b] Employment ratio = Actual months employed during the period ÷ potential months of employment.

[c] Participants who had no postinjury employment history were coded NA, and not included in mean computation.

[d] Jobs are concurrent.

[e] Jobs are sequential.

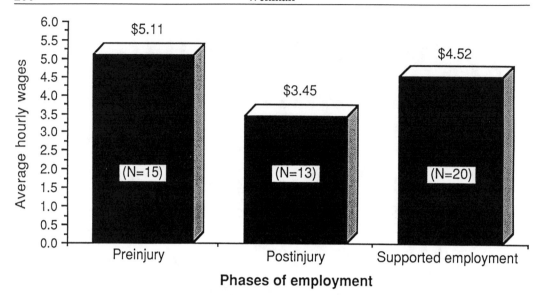

Figure 13.1.   Average hourly wages.

ployment. A total of 4.0 employment specialists have been involved in the placements reported in this chapter to date.

Results

Preinjury, postinjury, and supported employment work histories for each client are presented in Table 13.6 including the number of known positions, the type of job last held, mean wages and hours per week, and the monthly em-

ployment ratio during each phase of employment. Figures 13.1, 13.2, and 13.3 display in graphic form the mean values for hourly wages, work hours per week, and employment ratios by employment phase.

Preinjury Work Histories

Five of the 20 clients were injured prior to their 20th birthday and were therefore not included in the preinjury analyses of the dependent vari-

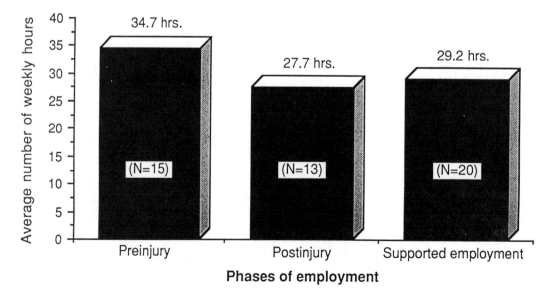

Figure 13.2.   Mean hours worked per week.

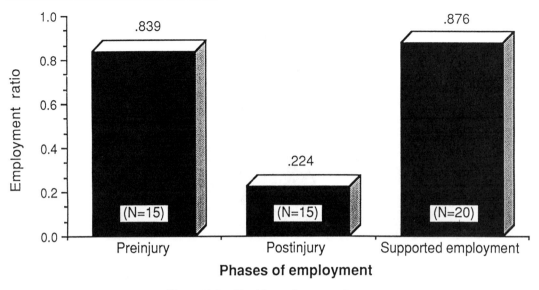

Figure 13.3. Monthly employment ratios.

ables. Of the remainder, ten (66.7%) were full-time employees at the time of injury. Seven (46.7%) had been employed continuously from their date of first employability and were assigned monthly employment ratios of 1.0. This was the modal value for the preinjury employment ratio.

Postinjury Work Histories

Seven of the participants were unable to get any type of employment postinjury and therefore were not included in analyses of work hours or wages, but were assigned monthly employment ratios of zero. Three of the participants (client numbers 8, 10, and 13) had worked in sheltered workshops postinjury, accounting for their low mean hourly wages. Two participants (client numbers 1 and 15) had acquired and then separated from a considerable number of jobs (14 and 17, respectively), thus scoring relatively large monthly employment ratios but not exhibiting job stability.

Only one participant (client number 16) was employed at the time that supported employment services began. She had returned to her preinjury job but was in danger of termination.

Supported Employment

A review of Figure 13.4 indicates the business supervisors' perceptions of the placed individuals. A mean score of 5 would indicate that the supervisor strongly agreed with statements related to positive work habits (i.e., attendance and attitude exhibited on the job). A mean score of 1 would indicate strong disagreement. Currently employed persons showed higher scores across the time intervals than those who have been separated from employment.

The mean number of hours per person for supported employment intervention is 278 hours. This computes to a cost of $7,483 per placement at the state vocational rehabilitation negotiated rate of $26.92 per hour, paid to the Medical College of Virginia by the Virginia Department of Rehabilitative Services.

Statistical Analyses

One-way analysis of variance revealed no significant differences at the .05 alpha level in the number of jobs held ($F = 1.21$, $p = .3073$) or client work hours per week ($F = 2.62$, $p = .0841$) across the three phases of employment. Differences were found in hourly wages ($F = $

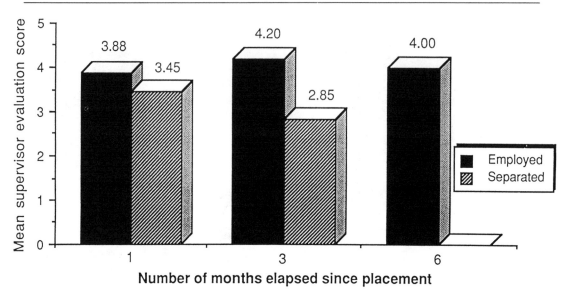

Figure 13.4. Mean supervisor evaluation scores.

3.22, $p = .0491$) and employment ratios ($F = 39.59, p < .0001$). Scheffe multiple comparison procedures revealed that monthly employment ratios preinjury and during supported employment were comparable. The postinjury employment ratio was significantly different from both preinjury and supported employment ratios. Scheffe procedures also revealed that preinjury and postinjury wages were significantly different, but supported employment wages were not significantly different from either of these two phases. The results of the statistical analyses are summarized in Table 13.7.

DISCUSSION

The purpose of this chapter has been: 1) to present an overview of supported employment models, and 2) to provide a prospective analysis of the impact of a supported employment program on the vocational outcomes of postacute traumatically brain-injured persons. Although descriptive and preliminary in nature, the program data provide some evidence for considering the use of supported employment as a rehabilitation intervention. Work histories were reconstructed for preinjury and postinjury levels to the highest degree of accuracy that was possible. The outcomes that resulted from these occupational histories were then compared with supported employment outcomes. Salient measures of vocational success included wages earned, hours worked, total months of actual work performed, and consecutive months of employment. Also, supervisors at the business were regularly queried to assess their satisfaction with traumatically brain-injured workers.

The data reported in this chapter suggest

Table 13.7. Summary of statistical analyses

| | Analysis of variance | | Scheffe groupings | | |
| | | | | | Supported |
Variable	F-value	p	Preinjury	Postinjury	employment
Jobs	1.21	.3073	—	—	—
Work hours per week	2.62	.0841	—	—	—
Hourly wage	3.22	.0491[a]	A	B	A,B
Employment ratio	39.59	.0001[a]	A	B	A

[a]Statistical significance ($\alpha = .05$)

that supported employment can help improve the vocational capacity of severely head-injured individuals. All of these persons were consistently resistant to vocational placement and had been considered poor prospects for vocational rehabilitation. As noted in Figures 13.1, 13.2, and 13.3, however, in most cases the placed group as an aggregate has been able to approach its collective preinjury level of vocational capacity. As noted earlier, a supported employment approach is especially useful in helping a person stay employed once a job is located. The data in Figure 13.3 related to months worked support this notion. Hence, not only has supported employment been helpful in facilitating work reentry, but, for the most part, individuals have returned to levels and stability of employment comparable to their preinjury status.

The overall positive reaction of employers in business and industry to the work habits and general work performances of the individuals employed is noteworthy. The comments on the supervisor evaluation sheets, as well as checked marks on the scale, support the positive view of employers (see Figure 13.4). While almost all employees with traumatic brain injury experienced significant problems at work at one time or the other, the presence of or access to a supported employment specialist seemed to be a major factor in promoting job retention. Employers were quick to pick up the telephone and seek specialized intervention assistance from employment specialists.

There are at least two major methodological limitations to the report presented in this chapter. The first is that there was no randomized assignment of clients to a supported employment group and to an a priori control group. Obviously, this is a serious limitation that prevents inferences about the efficacy of supported employment. It is known, however, that most of the persons who were placed from the overall referral group were highly comparable in terms of age, severity of injury, postacute status, neuropsychological status, and education status. Furthermore, it is also known that the placed persons actually served as their own controls during the postinjury phase and while they were on the waiting list for supported employment services.

The other major limitation in generalizing from present findings inherent in this study is that it only provides a "snapshot" in time of the effectiveness of supported employment. It was not the focus of this study to report in-depth cumulative data, costs, or benefits associated with this study.

Several concluding observations can be made about the vocational behavior of the individuals discussed in this study. For the most part, each person exhibited at least serious cognitive dysfunction, psychiatric instability, or physical deficit while employed as well as prior to employment. These were problems that the employment specialist was faced with managing at the job site as they occurred. Some persons showed more than one of these categories of problems. Often they occurred as a result of a job change, change in management at the company, home difficulties, or socialization problems away from work. Such problems mandated an ongoing case management approach and also made imperative a willingness by the employment specialist to provide intervention directly at the job site.

Furthermore, a team approach to problem solving and planning is absolutely essential. The problems are so complex and multidimensional that frequent input from experts, with the overall case managed by the physician, is critical. It is clear that persons who have experienced severe head injury will probably need very structured job placement with access to systematic and ongoing intervention as needed. There are a myriad of problems that are almost continually present and that vary as a function of the type of work, social ecology of the workplace, and present home environment in which the person with traumatic brain injury is living.

REFERENCES

Bellamy, G.T., Horner, R., & Inman, D.(1979). *Vocational habilitation of severely retarded adults*. Baltimore: University Park Press.

Ben-Yishay, Y., Silver, S.M., Piasetsky, E., & Raltok, J. (1987). Relationship between employability and vocational outcome after intensive holistic cognitive rehabilitation. *Journal of Head Trauma Rehabilitation, 2*(1), 35–48.

Brooks, N., McKinlay, W., Symington, C., Beattie, A., & Campsie, L. (1987). Return to work within the first seven years after head injury. *Brain Injury, 1*, 5–19.

Burke, W., Wesolowski, M., & Guth, M. (1988). Comprehensive head injury rehabilitation: An outcome evaluation. *Brain Injury, 2*(4), 313–322.

Dresser, A.C. (1973). Work status following head injury: The late effects of head injury. *Psychological Medicine, 12*, 286–294.

Fawber, H.L., & Wachter, J.F. (1987). Job placement as a treatment component of the vocational rehabilitation process. *Journal of Head Trauma Rehabilitation, 2*, 27–33.

Federal Register. (1987, August 14). Final Regulations. Vol. 52 (157), pp. 30546–30552. Washington, DC: U.S. Government Printing Office.

Hill, M., Hill, J., Wehman, P., Revell, W.G., Dickerson, A., & Noble, J. (1987). Supported employment: An interagency funding model for persons with severe disabilities. *Journal of Rehabilitation, 53*(3), 13–21.

Jacobs, H. (1988). The Los Angeles Head Injury Survey: Procedures and initial findings. *Archives of Physical Medicine and Rehabilitation, 69*, 425–430.

Kreutzer, J., & Morton, M.S. (1988). Supported employment for persons with head injury. In P. Wehman & M.S. Moon (Eds.), *Vocational rehabilitation and supported employment* (pp. 291–311). Baltimore: Paul H. Brookes Publishing Co.

Kreutzer, J., Wehman, P., Morton, M.V., et al. (1988). Supported employment and compensatory strategies for enhancing vocational outcome following traumatic brain injury. *Brain Injury, 2*(3), 205–233.

MacKenzie, E.J., Shapiro, S., Smith, R.T., Siegel, J., Moody, M. & Pitt, A. (1987). Factors influencing return to work following hospitalization for traumatic injury. *American Journal of Public Health, 77*(3), 329–334.

Mank, D., Rhodes, L., & Bellamy, G.T., (1986). Four supported employment alternatives. In W. Kiernan & J. Stark (Eds.), *Pathways to employment.* Baltimore: University Park Press.

Noble, J. (1986, June). Seminar on benefits and costs associated with transitional employment at Virginia Commonwealth University. Seminar on supported employment, Richmond.

Prigatano, G.P. (1986). *Neuropsychological rehabilitation after brain injury.* Baltimore: Johns Hopkins University Press.

Rhodes, L., & Valenta, L. (1985). Industry based supported employment: An enclave approach. *Journal of The Association for Persons with Severe Handicaps, 10*, 12–20.

Stapleton, M.C. (1986). Maryland rehabilitation center closed head injury study: A retrospective survey. *Cognitive Rehabilitation, 4*(5), 34–42.

Weddell, R., Oddy, M., & Jenkins, D. (1980). Social adjustments after rehabilitation: A two-year follow-up of patients with severe head injury. *Psychological Medicine, 10*, 257–263.

Wehman, P., Kreutzer, J., Stonnington, H.H., Wood, W., Diambra, J., & Morton, M. (1989, February). Supported work model for persons with traumatic brain injury: Three case studies. *Archives of Physical Medicine and Rehabilitation, 70*, 109–114.

SECTION V
Family Role in Community Reentry

CHAPTER 14

Family Outcome following Adult Traumatic Brain Injury
A Critical Review of the Literature

Patricia Stiles Camplair,
Jeffrey S. Kreutzer, and Kathleen R. Doherty

Professionals who participate in community re-entry should be knowledgeable about family reactions and functioning following the head injury of a relative. This is essential since relatives so often assume primary caregiving responsibilities for years after the injury. Family members also suffer emotionally as a result of the trauma. If the injured person has been characterologically altered, relatives often experience grief over the lost relationship. The family's ability to cope in the face of these stressors influences the quality of support they can provide to the head-injured person. Rehabilitation professionals require accurate information regarding family reactions and functioning in order to better understand and respond to the needs of families. Information about family outcome is also essential in order to develop programs and services that facilitate the family's, and therefore the injured person's, adjustment to disability following traumatic brain injury.

This chapter first presents research pertaining to the reactions and functioning of relatives following the head injury of a loved one. Second, the few studies that have addressed family needs during the head-injured individual's initial hospitalization or long-term rehabilitation are reviewed. A summary of major research findings, discussion of methodological limitations, and recommendations for further research are included within each section.

RESEARCH PERTAINING TO FAMILY REACTIONS

Although studies that examined family reactions to head injury appeared during the 1970s, considerable attention to the family was not apparent until the 1980s. The recent interest in families parallels the greatly increased attention to head injury rehabilitation during the 1980s. Researchers have begun to address several aspects of family reactions. First, the relative's sense of burden and emotional distress has been explored. The ability of family members to function in their psychosocial roles has been addressed as another aspect of the relative's status. Second, researchers have attempted to identify the major correlates of burden, emotional distress, and impaired psychosocial functioning. Investigators have primarily focused on client characteristics, such as injury severity and residual deficits, as potential predictors of relatives' reactions. The following studies have called attention to several important aspects of the family's response to traumatic brain injury. However, they represent only an initial step in the empirical exploration of family reactions to head injury and subsequent disability.

Panting and Merry (1972) were among the first researchers to investigate family reactions. They obtained follow-up information for a sample of 30 severely head-injured Britons who had

This work was partly supported by Grants #H133B80029 and #G0087C0219 from the National Institute on Disability and Rehabilitation Research, United States Department of Education.

been hospitalized on a rehabilitation unit during a 5-year period. Based on family interviews, they concluded that the injury had been a "great strain" on all relatives. Nearly two thirds of the relatives had received treatment with tranquilizers or sleeping pills, whereas none had required these medications before the injury. Additionally, these authors suggested that relationships between parents and their injured children were more stable than relationships between wives (or husbands) and their injured spouses. Panting and Merry believed that the greater strain on marriages stemmed from the fact that parents were able to share the burden of caring for their family member, whereas spouses were alone with this responsibility. However, they did not provide quantitative information to support the conclusion that marital relationships were more adversely affected than parental relationships.

Another early study was conducted by Thomsen (1974) on a group of 50 very severely injured Danes who ranged from 12 to 70 months postinjury (mean of 30 months). Following unstructured interviews with family members, Thomsen concluded that relatives were disturbed more by intellectual than by physical deficits. Personality changes, which presented the greatest difficulties in daily living, were reported for 42 of the 50 patients. These changes included irritability, anger outbursts, aspontaneity, restlessness, emotional regression, lability, and stubbornness. Consistent with the findings reported by Panting and Merry (1972), Thomsen (1974) observed that relationships between single adult patients and their mothers were better than those between married patients and their spouses. This was attributed to the greater role changes and guilt about circumstances of the injuries among spouses. At 10–15 years postinjury, Thomsen (1984) again concluded that the most difficult changes for relatives to cope with were alterations in the injured person's personality.

Romano (1974), based on extensive contact with 13 families of severely head-injured patients, was most impressed by the "very persistent family denial" of problems during the acute phase of the individual's recovery. She argued that denial was evidenced by several tendencies on the part of family members. These included: 1) *common fantasies,* such as expectations that the individual would suddenly "wake up" and return to his or her preinjury self, or perceptions of measurable improvement when the staff could see none; 2) *verbal refusals,* such as statements indicating that the individual had not changed despite staff perceptions of obvious change, or a focus on physical abilities to the exclusion of apparent cognitive problems; and 3) *inappropriate responses,* such as refusing to set necessary limits on the individual's behaviors, and holding unrealistic expectations for the individual. Romano observed that these responses adversely affected the severely head-injured person's rehabilitation.

Rosenbaum and Najenson (1976) investigated spouse reports of depression and changes in family life following head injury. They surveyed wives of 10 brain-injured Israeli veterans (8 sustained penetrating missile wounds, 2 had closed head injuries), 6 persons with spinal cord injury, and 14 noninjured veterans. At 1 year postinjury, wives of men with brain injury were significantly more depressed than those of men with spinal cord injury or those of noninjured veterans. Although the number of subjects per group was small, group differences were noted for depressed affect, irritability, and total "low mood" scores on a 22-item mood scale (Rosenbaum & Najenson asserted that the scale was similar to the Beck Depression Inventory; Beck, 1972). Across all subjects, total low mood scores were significantly correlated with ratings of changes in family activities, especially the extent to which these changes were perceived as disturbing.

Alterations in family life were assessed via a questionnaire developed by Rosenbaum and Najenson (1976). The extent of familial changes differed significantly among the three groups, particularly in the areas of sexual activities, child care, leisure time, visits with in-laws, and social life. Furthermore, groups were distinguishable by negative descriptions of family circumstances, including: husband's childlike dependency, husband's self-orientation, wife's assumption of the man's role, husband's sexual difficulties, wife's dislike of physical contact with her husband, children's dependency on the mother, children's fear of the father, wife's closeness to her in-laws, friends' desertion of the family, and husband's social handicap. Wives of men with brain injury provided the strongest negative ratings to the preceding items, followed by wives of men with spinal cord injury and then by wives of noninjured veterans. The only exception to this pattern was that the wives of spinal cord–injured veterans were most likely to report that their husbands experienced sexual difficulties. Despite this finding, spouses of brain-injured veterans were more likely to endorse the item "wife dislikes physical contact with her husband."

Rosenbaum and Najenson (1976) further investigated changes in family roles by presenting spouses with 10 randomly ordered roles that wives have typically fulfilled in the family (Hurwitz, 1960). Spouses rank ordered the importance of these roles for actual (current) and ideal (if both partners were functioning normally) circumstances. Ideal roles were ranked similarly for wives of brain-injured, spinal cord–injured, and noninjured veterans. Wives of both injured groups indicated that the role of handling family matters outside the home had gained in importance. Only wives of men with brain injury reported that being a sexual partner to their husbands had lost importance. Compared to the other two groups, spouses of brain-injured veterans reported the greatest increase in assuming the man's role and the greatest decrease in sharing child-care responsibilities.

Like Thomsen (1974), Lezak (1978, 1986, 1988) has suggested that characteriological alterations create the greatest disruption in family relationships after head injury. She has observed that families can accommodate to or compensate for mild personality changes. However, family members and particularly primary caregivers clearly suffer in the face of significant alterations, such as when the head-injured individual becomes "dependent, demanding, irresponsible, foolish, ill-mannered, or frankly dangerous" (Lezak, 1978, p. 593).

Lezak (1986) discussed family reactions as they relate to different phases of rehabilitation.

She suggested that initially relatives will experience anxious bewilderment as they become aware of changes in their family member. As the family attempts to help the head-injured individual return to premorbid activities, problems such as poor judgment and social inappropriateness become clear. Caregivers can become deeply conflicted between feelings of responsibility, anger, and frustration, and their hopes for the individual's recovery, making them prone to depression. A significant degree of emotional freedom does not occur until the caregiver acknowledges the permanence of characterological changes and recognizes that he or she is not responsible for the family's emotional distress. Detachment from and reorientation to the individual with brain injury are viewed as necessary conditions for the resumption of a relatively normal life-style. In many families this process is believed to culminate in separation, divorce, or placement of the head-injured family member in an extended care facility.

Head injury presents unique stressors to parents versus spouses of survivors (Lezak, 1988). Although the strain imposed on parents may vary depending on whether the child with head injury was a minor or an independent adult, the parents' hopes for the child's future are commonly destroyed. In contrast with a family's normal evolution toward the independence of children, these parents are faced with carrying major responsibility for neurologically impaired children throughout their lives. The extra demands created by a child's disability may strain marital relationships, and lead to conflict over how to care for the child.

Spouses of persons with brain injury may suffer the loss of a relationship that satisfies even the most basic expectations of marriage (Lezak, 1988). If there is significant impairment, the healthy spouse will typically have responsibility for running the household, caring for children, and dealing with medical, insurance, or social agencies, in addition to providing care or supervision for the injured spouse. Feelings of responsibility or past gratitude to the spouse, along with guilt and fears of social rejection, may make it exceedingly difficult to initiate a separation or divorce. Finally, the caregiving spouse is likely to receive the brunt of the head-injured individual's frustration, anger, and fear, not uncommonly resulting in verbal or physical abuse.

Lezak's (1978, 1986, 1988) observations paint a picture of terrific burden for the relatives of brain-injured persons. However, because her observations were drawn primarily from work with families in a support group setting, they may not generalize to other families. In addition, Lezak's descriptions of family reactions were based on clinical impressions rather than quantified indices of psychological distress or family functioning.

A group of British researchers systematically explored family reactions to traumatic brain injury. Oddy, Humphrey, and Uttley (1978a) evaluated relatives of 54 moderately to severely head-injured British adults. Approximately half the persons with head injury demonstrated 1–7 days duration of post-traumatic amnesia (PTA), and half had more than 7 days of PTA. Parents and spouses, who had lived with the head-injured individuals for at least 6 months, were interviewed at 1, 6, and 12 months postinjury. Family stressors were examined at the 6- and 12-month intervals. More than half of the relatives reported that they were experiencing significant stress in response to the family member's head injury. Forty percent of parents and spouses identified the major source of stress as some aspect of the head-injured person's condition, such as poorly controlled behavior, fear of epilepsy, or the physical stress of caring for a disabled family member. Twelve percent of all relatives identified the major source of stress as concern for the head-injured person's future. Included in this category were fears that the individual would sustain another injury, concern about eventual recovery, and questions about long-term care.

Oddy and his colleagues (1978a) additionally employed standardized measures to evaluate the emotional distress reported by relatives. Utilizing a cutoff score on the Wakefield Depression Scale (Snaith, Ahmed, Mehta, & Hamilton, 1971), 39% of significant others were considered depressed at 1 month postinjury, dropping off to about 25% at 6 and 12 months postinjury. There were no significant differences in depression scores between parents and spouses. Greater depression levels were associated with whether the person with head injury returned to work, and with two factors suggestive of personality change on the Katz Adjustment Scale (Katz & Lyerly, 1963), termed "confusion" and "verbal expansiveness." Depression was also associated with the number of the head-injured person's physical, cognitive, and behavioral problems reported by relatives at 6 months, and the strength of this correlation increased at 12 months. The relatives' depression was not associated with the duration of post-traumatic amnesia, length of hospitalization, the head-injured person's social involvement, or problems reported by the person with head injury.

In a related study, Oddy, Humphrey, and Uttley (1978b) investigated friction in families of persons with head injury compared to families of persons with traumatic limb fractures, matched by age and socioeconomic status to the former group. These researchers used a semistructured interview to assess family conflict. No significant increase in the friction between head-injured persons and their parents or siblings was noted during the first year postinjury. However, there was a tendency for families of both persons with head injury and persons with limb fracture to report increased friction over time. Employing essentially the same sample and methodology at 12 months postinjury, Oddy and Humphrey (1980) reported that communication was diminished between persons with head injury and siblings, but not between persons with head injury and parents. Adverse personality changes were associated with strained family relationships, especially when siblings were present in the home. Poorer relations were also associated with a greater number of problems of the head-injured individual, particularly when the relatives' perceptions were considered. At 2 years postinjury, these investigators generally found that persons with head injury were getting along with their families. Neither patients nor parents in the head injury group rated their relationships more negatively than patients and parents in the limb fracture control group. Finally, Weddell, Oddy, and Jenkins (1980) compared ratings from relatives of the most severely injured persons in their series to retrospective "preinjury" ratings obtained at 1 month postinjury from relatives of a similar group of individuals. Family friction was significantly greater for the postinjury sample than for the preinjury comparison group. Extreme friction was noted in about 20% of families following severe head injury.

The British research group further investigated family reactions at approximately 7 years postinjury (Oddy, Coughlan, Tyerman, & Jenkins, 1985). Relatives completed an adjective checklist designed to assess emotional distress. Seventeen percent of the family members reported clinically significant levels of depression or anxiety. However, this percentage was similar to that found within the general British population when employing the same checklist. These researchers did not evaluate long-term stressors or family friction at this late interval.

Mauss-Clum and Ryan (1981) investigated caregiver reports of distress for an American population of persons with neurological impairment. They compared survey responses from wives and mothers of 30 postacute head injury, stroke, or degenerative disease patients. Ninety percent of mothers and wives combined reported personality changes within their children or spouses. Nearly half of the wives agreed with the statement "I'm married but don't have a husband" and one third said they were "married to a stranger." Over half of both mothers and spouses reported that they experienced significant frustration and irritability. Approximately half of each group indicated that they felt trapped in their caregiving situations. One quarter of the wives and one third of the mothers described the patients as verbally abusive. One fifth of the caregivers reported that the patients had threatened them with physical violence. Overall, more wives reported negative emotional reactions and life changes than mothers. Wives were more likely to report depression, anger, guilt, decreased time for self, decreased social contacts, and financial insecurity. However, differences between mothers and wives in this study may be attributable to differences in the patient's age,

injury type, or injury severity between the two groups.

Researchers in Glasgow, Scotland, have published several studies investigating relatives' perceptions of burden, emotional distress, and psychosocial functioning following head injury. In their initial report, McKinlay, Brooks, Bond, Martinage, and Marshall (1981) examined caregiver burden for 55 severely head-injured adults, with duration of post-traumatic amnesia averaging 21 days. The relative with primary caregiving responsibility was interviewed at 3, 6, and 12 months postinjury. Objective and subjective burdens were defined in line with prior research on families of chronically mentally ill persons (e.g., Grad & Sainsbury, 1963; Hoenig & Hamilton, 1967). Objective burden was defined as the head-injured person's residual problems and was assessed with a 90-item problem checklist targeting physical functioning, language, emotional functioning, dependence, subjective complaints, memory, and disturbed behavior. Subjective burden was defined as the amount of psychological strain attributable to patient changes and was assessed with a 7-point rating scale ranging from (1) "I feel no strain as a result of the changes in my spouse/relative" to (7) "I feel severe strain as a result of the changes in my spouse/relative."

McKinlay et al. (1981) reported that the mean subjective burden rating for relatives in their sample was 3.5 at each follow-up visit, with 70% reporting medium (3–4) or high (5–7) burden. Subjective burden was significantly related to length of post-traumatic amnesia at the 3-month assessment, but not at 12 months postinjury. Subjective burden was significantly associated with emotional problems, subjective complaints, and disturbed behavior at all assessments. Burden ratings were significantly associated with the number of memory problems at 3 and 6 months postinjury, and the head-injured individual's level of dependency at 6 and 12 months postinjury. Language functioning and physical problems were not related to burden ratings at any time point.

Brooks and McKinlay (1983) further investigated links between personality changes and relatives' burden for the above sample. Care-

givers were asked to rate persons with head injury on a Likert-type personality scale at 3-, 6-,
and 12-month assessments. The relationship between adverse personality changes and subjective burden was significant and increased over
the first year postinjury. However, relatives did
not report significantly more problems across
assessment points. Brooks and McKinlay therefore concluded that caregivers were less able to
tolerate personality changes over time.

Caregiver burden was evaluated by the
Glasgow researchers (Brooks, Campsie, Symington, Beattie, & McKinlay, 1986) at 5 years
postinjury for many of the relatives included in
previous reports. They reported that the percentage of relatives who indicated high burden levels
increased from 24% at 1 year to 56% at 5 years.
The proportion reporting low burden decreased
from 43% to 10%. Subjective burden was significantly associated with disturbed behavior and,
to a lesser degree, other problem categories at 5
years postinjury. In addition, burden ratings
were significantly associated with injury severity
at this late assessment.

In another report, Brooks, Campsie, Symington, Beattie, and McKinlay (1987) evaluated
subjective burden employing cross-sectional
data obtained from 134 relatives. Relatives were
divided into four groups based on time postinjury (0–3 years, 3–4 years, 5 years, and 5–7
years). Subjective burden ratings were similar
across groups. Pooled together, 89% of the relatives reported either medium or high subjective
burden. These researchers concluded that relatives of persons with shorter lengths of post-
traumatic amnesia reported either low, medium,
or high burden, but that relatives of the persons
most severely injured consistently reported high
subjective burden. A significant relationship between subjective burden and the number of problems in all categories except physical problems
was reported for this large, cross-sectional
group. This association was most pronounced
for the emotional and disturbed behavior categories. Finally, relatives' characteristics that might
be related to subjective burden were investigated. Burden ratings were significantly associated
with the perceived accessibility of help. However, half of the relatives in the high burden cate-

gory did not report a need for help. The presence
or absence of a confidant did not predict burden
ratings. Finally, no clear differences were found
between parents and spouses, or mothers and
wives, regarding the proportion of each group
reporting low, medium, or high burden.

In addition to perceptions of burden, the
Glasgow research group addressed relatives'
emotional distress and impaired psychosocial
functioning. Livingston, Brooks, and Bond
(1985b) compared distress reported by caregivers of severely head-injured persons to that
reported by caregivers of mildly head-injured
persons. At 3 months postinjury, both groups
were administered the General Health Questionnaire (GHQ; Goldberg, 1978), the Leeds scales
(Snaith, Bridge, & Hamilton, 1976), the Social
Adjustment Scale—Self-Report (Weissman &
Bothwell, 1976), and the Perceived Burden scale
developed by Livingston et al. (1985b) (items
targeted patient problems and the negative effects of problems on caregivers/ families). Caregivers of persons with severe head injury were
significantly more anxious than the comparison
group, and reported greater burden. In addition,
they were significantly more impaired in their
marital and family roles. Interestingly, caregivers of persons with severe head injury were
not more depressed than caregivers of persons
with mild head injury.

Livingston, Brooks, and Bond (1985a) additionally conducted 6- and 12-month assessments with severely head-injured persons and
their relatives. Significant anxiety was reported
by more than one third of relatives at 3, 6, and 12
months postinjury. One fifth to one fourth of
caregivers were significantly depressed at each
interval. Perceived burden scores did not change
appreciably across follow-up visits. Consequently, Livington et al. (1985a) concluded that
the high level of emotional distress experienced
by relatives does not change significantly during
the first year postinjury. However, a decline in
psychosocial functioning was observed over
time. Social functioning in general, and marital
functioning specifically, declined between 3 and
6 months postinjury and remained impaired at 12
months.

Finally, Livingston et al. (1985a) examined

whether injury-related factors were associated with the caregivers' status. The number of complaints reported by the head-injured individual accounted for the most variance on measures of anxiety and psychosocial functioning. Length of post-traumatic amnesia, Glasgow Coma Scale (Teasdale & Jennett, 1974) scores, dependence in activities of daily living, and personality changes were not significant predictors of family reactions once the number of a head-injured person's complaints was considered. Mothers and wives did not differ regarding their emotional distress or psychosocial functioning. Livingston (1987) examined associations between anxiety or impaired psychosocial functioning and the relative's social class, age, prior psychiatric and medical status, and work before and after the injury. This researcher concluded that the major correlate of relatives' postinjury adjustment was their previous psychiatric and medical history.

Although few American researchers have investigated family reactions, the extent to which families assume the burden of care for head-injured relatives in the United States has been addressed. For example, Kozloff (1987) conducted initial and follow-up interviews with 37 severely head-injured persons and their families. She found that the head-injured person's social network decreased in size over time following his or her injury. The circle of people who remained involved with the head-injured individual increasingly included family members. Relatives attempted to compensate for the head-injured individual's loss of relationships by expanding the nature of their involvement with the head-injured person. For example, relatives not only provided financial and practical support, they also assumed responsibility for meeting the head-injured individual's social and recreational needs.

The extent of family burden was further underscored by Jacobs (1988), who surveyed 142 families of severely head-injured individuals in the Los Angeles area. Families identified themselves as the primary long-term providers of care and rehabilitative therapies for their head-injured relative. They assumed roles as caregivers and therapists despite the virtual absence of formal training that might have assisted them in these roles. Jacobs commented that the wide range of the head-injured individual's long-term needs and the unavailability of needed services often impaired or destroyed the family unit.

Summary of Family Reactions to Head Injury

Research conducted primarily in the United Kingdom suggests that psychological distress is common among relatives of individuals with head injury. Brooks and his colleagues in Scotland found that during the first year postinjury, more than two thirds of relatives felt moderately to severely burdened by the changes in their family member (McKinlay et al., 1981). Moreover, the family's sense of burden increased rather than dissipated over the years. Five years after the injury, 90% of relatives reported moderate to severe levels of burden (Brooks et al., 1986). During the first year after the injury, approximately one third of relatives reported high levels of anxiety, and one fifth to one fourth were considered depressed (Livingston et al., 1985a). The Glasgow researchers additionally noted that the ability of family members to function in familial roles declined during the first year, particularly within their marital relationship (Livingston et al., 1985a). Oddy and his colleagues in Britain found that 39% of family members were significantly depressed 1 month after the injury (Oddy et al., 1978a). Consistent with research findings from Scotland, about one fourth of relatives in the British studies were considered depressed at 6 and 12 months postinjury (Oddy et al., 1978a).

Prevalence rates reported by researchers reflect the proportion of family members experiencing significant distress at a given point in time. Consequently, the number of relatives who are highly distressed at some point during the first year or so postinjury may be much greater than the figures reported above. In addition, individuals who do not report clinically significant levels of depression or anxiety may nevertheless experience strong feelings of sadness, loss, and tension. For example, Lezak (1978) described the lasting emotional burden of caregivers as a "chronic pall on their lives" (p. 594).

Because a substantial proportion of relatives report high levels of distress and burden, clinicians and researchers have been interested in identifying the major correlates and sources of strain. Readily apparent stressors include injury severity and the injured person's residual deficits. In most studies, indices of injury severity, such as the length of coma or post-traumatic amnesia, have not been strongly associated with relatives' distress (e.g., Oddy et al., 1978a). The lack of a strong association between injury severity and relatives' distress is not surprising, as the former is only a gross predictor of subsequent disability. The absence of significant correlations may also reflect the homogeneity of research samples on the dimension of injury severity. Researchers who directly compared families of persons with severe injury to those of persons with mild injury found significant differences in the extent to which relatives reported anxiety, burden, and impaired psychosocial role functioning (e.g., Livingston et al., 1985b). Finally, the relationship between injury severity and family distress may not be linear. For example, Brooks et al. concluded that although relatives of the most severely injured individuals consistently reported high burden, relatives of less severely injured persons varied on burden ratings.

However, the injured person's residual physical and cognitive problems are stressful to family members. Clinical observations have suggested that family members are generally more disturbed by cognitive, emotional, and behavioral changes than by residual physical and language difficulties (e.g., Lezak, 1978; Thomsen, 1974). Systematic investigations have corroborated clinical impressions by documenting that personality, emotional, and behavioral problems are correlated with high burden and emotional distress (e.g., Brooks & McKinlay, 1983; McKinlay et al., 1981; Oddy et al., 1978a; Rosenbaum & Najenson, 1976). In addition, Rosenbaum and Najenson demonstrated that the cognitive, emotional, and behavioral problems resulting from head injury were more stressful for caregivers than were the primarily physical problems resulting from spinal cord injury.

The increased responsibilities and altered roles of family members after head injury also predict relatives' distress. Research conducted by Kozloff (1987) and Jacobs (1988) documented that family members often assume additional roles and responsibilities to compensate for the increased dependence of the injured person and decreased contact and support from those outside the family. These researchers did not evaluate the relationship between increased responsibilities and emotional status. However, Rosenbaum and Najenson (1976) found that depression levels among wives were strongly associated with altered familial roles and increased responsibility for household tasks and activities.

The relative's relationship to the injured person may predict subsequent distress and burden. Several writers (e.g., Panting & Merry, 1972; Thomsen, 1974) have commented that marital relationships are more readily strained following a head injury than are parental relationships. This may be explained by the more dramatic role changes that occur when a spouse is disabled, and the greater number of responsibilities typically assumed by spouses in comparison to parents. Despite these suggestions, researchers have not documented a significant difference in burden, distress, or impaired psychosocial functioning between spouses and parents. The only exception to this is the Mauss-Clum and Ryan (1981) survey, which found that wives more often reported negative emotional reactions than mothers. It may be that the type of relationship (i.e., parental versus marital) is significantly associated with outcome variables not yet explored (e.g., durability of the relationship, relationship satisfaction, or family functioning).

Research has not yet systematically explored possible moderator variables of relatives' distress and burden, such as their personal resources (e.g., coping skills), and the services or support available to them. Preliminary evidence suggests these factors may prove to be important predictors of family reactions. For example, Livingston (1987) found that the psychiatric and medical status of relatives prior to the injury was highly predictive of their emotional status and psychosocial functioning following the injury. Brooks et al. (1987) reported that the relative's sense of burden was related to believing that help was available if needed.

In summary, a substantial proportion of family members report feelings of burden, emotional distress, and an impaired ability to function normally in their psychosocial roles. Available research also points to the nature and extent of the person's disability following head injury as an important contributor to these adverse reactions. Other factors that have yet to be fully explored include the extent to which family members assume increased responsibilities, personal/psychological resources of family members, and the availability of extrafamilial support and services.

Limitations of Research on Family Reactions

Although researchers have begun to address the repercussions of head injury on family members, several factors limit the utility of this information as a basis for education and development of programs and interventions. The vast majority of this research was conducted on British and Scottish populations. However, coordinated services for head-injured individuals are virtually nonexistent in the United Kingdom (McKinlay & Pentland, 1987). Differences in the cultures and rehabilitation service delivery systems between the United States and other countries call into question the extent to which research findings may be applicable to American populations. In addition, available research in this area is characterized by insufficient empirical support of ideas, reliance on self-report of information, failure to employ well-validated measures, and a lack of precision in describing and/or selecting samples. These limitations need to be addressed in order to advance our understanding of the ways in which head injury affects the family.

Empirical findings have not always supported observations derived from clinical experience with families of head-injured persons. For example, Lezak (1978, 1986, 1988) has argued that negative emotional reactions are common and expected in response to significant characterological alterations. However, even studies that evaluated relatives of persons with severe injury found variability in distress levels reported by relatives (Livingston et al., 1985a). Discrepancies between observations and empirically derived data underscore the importance of evaluating clinical impressions through systematic investigation. Research that explores subject and moderator variables will help clarify under what conditions, or in what families, significant distress or impaired family functioning can be expected.

A major methodological limitation within this area of research has been the reliance on self-reported information, which is typically collected from the relatives of persons with head injury. Self-reported information may be biased for a variety of reasons. For example, responses may be affected by family members' emotional distress, animosities toward the head-injured person, or tendencies to exaggerate or minimize complaints. Consequently, self-reported information should be supplemented by data from other sources. However, researchers and clinicians should consider potential biases from each source of data. For example, many persons with head injury are often unaware of serious problems that affect family functioning. Staff members typically view the head-injured individual in a structured institutional setting or may have limited contact with him or her. Assessments of the person with head injury also occur in a structured setting and may not reveal many of the problems that become apparent in real-life settings. Furthermore, many skills, including initiative, organizational skills, and planning ability, are difficult to assess quantitatively. Nevertheless, independent sources of information should be considered in order to fully understand relationships between the head-injured person's functioning and family reactions.

The utility of information obtained from relatives has been limited by a failure to employ well-validated or standardized measures. For example, the British researchers (e.g., Weddell et al., 1980), who investigated friction within the family, based their conclusions on semistructured interviews. The actual methodology used was not specifically described, which makes it difficult for other researchers to replicate their findings. Rosenbaum and Najenson (1976) incorporated items tapping some aspects of family functioning into their questionnaire, but little information was provided about the development and properties of this instrument. Unfortunately, for certain variables of interest (e.g., residual deficits), measures with established reliability and validity do not yet exist. However, existing measures of psychological distress and family functioning with demonstrated validity and reliability should be employed in future research. The use of well-established measures facilitates replication of research findings and comparisons across studies.

Another methodological problem concerns the selection of relatives who are evaluated. Some studies have examined any relative, while others have limited their focus to primary caregivers or female relatives/caregivers. Little research has addressed the influence of family member characteristics, such as age, sex, relationship to the head-injured person, and amount of time spent with the head-injured individual on family outcome. These subject variables could best be explored via large, multisite studies or surveys. Researchers who do not select subjects in order to control potentially important variables must carefully describe their samples. In addition, correlations between subject variables and dependent measures should be reported when possible.

A broad spectrum of head-injured individuals should be included to evaluate targeted subject variables. For example, including individuals who vary on injury severity or extent of disability will clarify relationships between the head-injured person's status and family reactions. Similarly, other factors, such as time since injury or time since discharge, could be investigated by examining individuals who vary on these dimensions.

Research addressing the prevalence and nature of distress and impaired functioning among families of head-injured persons in the United States is lacking. Information available from abroad may be of limited utility considering differences between European and American populations. In addition, researchers must employ validated assessment instruments, carefully describe their samples, and incorporate multiple sources of information in order to adequately characterize family reactions. Attention to these limitations will improve our understanding of family responses to head injury.

Implications for Future Research on Family Reactions

Explanations of family outcome following head injury will be inherently complex. Many factors contribute to the health and well-being of individual family members, and to the functioning of the family unit. Individual research projects can address selected aspects of family reactions, contributing piecemeal to an overall conceptualization of family outcome. Numerous areas require further investigation and elaboration. In particular, information is needed regarding the changes in family reactions over time, the influence of moderator variables on distress levels or impaired family functioning, and the impact of head injury on the family as a unit.

A major goal of future studies should be to characterize family outcome over time. Time postinjury is important because of the implied relationship to various processes, including the head-injured person's recovery, his or her resumption of responsibilities, and the family's adjustment process. Most research investigating emotional distress has addressed only the first year postinjury. Ideally, studies should focus on reactions within the same families over time, and follow families for several years. Investigators have typically reported on family reactions at certain time intervals, such as 3, 6, and 12 months postinjury. Researchers interested in assessing the impact of recovery and adjustment processes should also consider tying evaluations to markers in the head-injured person's rehabilitation (e.g., evaluating emotional distress at discharge). Delineating stressors associated with different phases of rehabilitation, and evaluating the relationship between stressors and distress or family functioning are of particular importance. Even the retrospective questioning of family members about stressors would help identify targets for assessment and intervention, given the dearth of existing data.

Researchers have primarily evaluated the impact of stressors (e.g., residual of the head-injured person problems) on family members' emotional status. There has been little empirical inquiry into the importance of potential moderator variables, such as intrafamilial and extrafamilial resources, in buffering the adverse effect of stressors. For example, it may be that relatives who employ effective personal coping skills nevertheless experience high distress at certain times postinjury. Perhaps only families that receive ongoing external support (e.g., respite services, social support) in addition to internal resources and coping skills can continue to function well despite the significant disability of a family member. These and other questions of primary importance have not been addressed thus far. Within a general framework of exploring family outcome over time, researchers should focus on identifying important moderator variables in addition to the previous emphasis on stressors.

Investigators have typically focused on reactions of a particular family informant. Studies of families after head injury should incorporate assessment of the family unit as well. Fortunately, family researchers have developed instruments that provide quantitative information on family functioning. For example, Epstein, Baldwin, and Bishop (1983) have developed the Family Assessment Device (FAD) based on the McMaster Model of Family Functioning (Epstein, Bishop, & Levin, 1978). This 53-item self-report questionnaire contains a General Functioning subscale and six specific subscales labeled: Problem Solving, Communication, Roles, Affective Responsiveness, Affective Involvement, and Behavior Control. The FAD characterizes the relative health or dysfunction of the family unit on each dimension. This scale is easily administered and cut-off scores based on normative data are available. In addition, although the FAD has not been applied to head-injured populations, it has proven useful in research with persons who have had a stroke and their families (e.g., Evans et al., 1987). Furthermore, clinician impressions of family functioning can be quantified by using a parallel rating scale (Epstein, Baldwin, & Bishop, 1982).

A second self-report instrument likely to contribute to a better understanding of family outcome is the Family Adaptability and Cohesion Evaluation Scales (FACES II; Olson, Sprenkle, & Russell, 1979; FACES III; Olson, Portner, & Lavee, 1985). This 20-item questionnaire focuses on two major dimensions of family functioning. Family Adaptability is defined as the extent to which the family system is flexible and subject to change; items in this subscale measure family leadership, discipline, child control, and roles. Family Cohesion refers to the emotional bonding among family members; items in this subscale reflect mutual support, family boundaries, shared time, and shared activities. Scores place families at one of four levels on each dimension, which results in 16 possible family subtypes. Extreme ratings on either dimension are not necessarily considered pathological. Administration procedures call for family informants to provide both actual and ideal family ratings. Consequently, the questionnaire has the advantage of providing an index of family members' satisfaction with their family.

Researchers interested in incorporating self-report measures of family functioning are referred to Bishop and Miller (1988) and Zarski, DePompei, and Zook (1988) for a more complete review. Those interested in clinician ratings of family functioning are referred to Carlson and Grotevant (1987) for a comparative review of family rating scales. Employing measures derived from theoretical models will help identify key elements that relate to a family's ability to promote the health of individual members. Clinically derived inventories and structured interviews will highlight areas of particular importance to families faced with issues specific to head injury. Clinical and theoretical assessment approaches will provide complementary information.

Knowledge regarding family reactions to head injury remains incomplete. Researchers have provided evidence that head injury can result in a severe burden on the family. Additional investigation is needed to better understand the specific circumstances that contribute to family distress. Future research should focus on characterizing family reactions over time and the importance of resources both within and outside the family unit. Finally, increased attention to the functioning of the family as a unit is recommended.

FAMILY NEEDS RESEARCH

In addition to the focus on emotional reactions and changes in family relationships, researchers have recently begun to explore family needs. Interest in this area stems from the assumption that attention to family needs will bolster the family's coping resources, resulting in reduced emotional stress and better quality care for persons with head injury. Existing research has primarily focused on the personal needs of relatives during the initial hospitalization of critically ill patients. Investigators have also begun to address the long-term rehabilitation needs of head-injured individuals and their families.

Mauss-Clum and Ryan (1981) investigated needs for professional help at the time of injury for a sample of wives and mothers of adults with central nervous system dysfunction. They administered a needs questionnaire developed by Molter (1979) for use with families of critically ill patients. Relatives of neurologically impaired patients reported that during the initial hospitalization the following needs were the most important: 1) the need for a clear and kind explanation of the patient's condition and treatment, 2) discussion of realistic expectations, and 3) emotional support. During the acute care phase, needs for financial and resource counseling were rated as least important. Family members also indicated whether their needs were met. Approximately half of the sample was satisfied with the degree of emotional support and patient status information that was provided. However, less than one fourth indicated that they were allowed an opportunity to discuss realistic expectations about the patient's recovery. Finally, respondents identified persons who provided emotional support at the time of the injury. Half of the wives and mothers reported that friends and family were important sources of emotional support. Forty-three percent indicated that a physician met this need. Approximately one fifth of the sample identified nurses, social workers, and

clergy as important sources of emotional support.

Mathis (1984) used Molter's (1979) questionnaire to compare needs reported by families of patients with acute brain injuries to families of critically ill patients without central nervous system involvement. There was considerable overlap in the top 10 needs reported by each group. Both groups indicated that needs for information pertaining to the patient's status and reassurance about the quality of medical care were among the most important. In addition, needs to feel hope and to have questions answered honestly were considered very important by both groups. Overall, relatives of patients with brain injury rated needs as more important compared to families of critically ill patients without brain injury.

Very few studies have addressed long-term rehabilitation needs of head-injured persons and their families. McCaffrey, Pollock, and Burns (1987) presented results of a telephone survey conducted by the New York State Head Injury Association in 1984. About half of the sample was made up of family members. The remainder included primarily head injury survivors, although friends and professionals were included as well. Time postinjury, injury severity, and the age of injured persons varied widely. The most frequently reported needs were for family support (62%), special social opportunities (47%), counseling opportunities (47%), and special therapies (43%; e.g., cognitive rehabilitation). Results underscored the lack of resources that might otherwise bolster the head-injured person's family and social support system. Importantly, family needs were frequently reported despite the fact that nearly half the sample comprised individuals who suffered no loss of consciousness.

Ostby, Sakata, and Leung (1988) focused on patient and family needs for rehabilitation services. They administered a Needs Assessment Questionnaire to a sample of 58 head-injured persons or relatives of injured persons who had received acute care hospital and/or rehabilitation services. Respondents were divided into four groups based on the rehabilitation services they had received. Groups also varied on the severity of initial injuries. Results pertaining to needs expressed across groups are of most interest to the present review. The only need that was frequently reported by respondents in all groups was the need for training the family how to deal with the head-injured family member. Services needed by the majority of respondents in three of the four groups included family education, job training and work programs, social and recreational services, and financial assistance. In two of the four groups, most people indicated a need for more educational materials, counseling, and help in the head-injured person's transition from home to work. Ostby and his colleagues suggested that the variation among needs reported by the four rehabilitation groups implied that services received and injury severity influence perceived needs. However, many needs were common to individuals with head injury and their families regardless of group differences. Ostby et al. therefore concluded that despite the provision of "coherent" rehabilitation services, persons with head injury and their families experienced persisting problems and long-term needs for rehabilitation services.

Summary of Family Needs Research

In summary, during the initial hospitalization of patients, family members have emphasized needs for information about the patient's medical status, reassurance about the quality of medical care, discussion of realistic expectations about the patient's prognosis, and emotional support. As expected, the need for services relevant to long-term issues, such as financial and resource counseling, were considered least important during the early phase of rehabilitation. Later on in the rehabilitation process, head injury survivors and family members continued to report the need for information/education and emotional support (e.g., counseling, family support). In addition, needs for a variety of services relevant to community reintegration came to the fore. Ostby et al. (1988) found that families often requested ongoing assistance in learning to deal effectively with their head-injured family member. Other long-term needs of primary importance included

services focused on returning the injured person to vocational and social roles.

Unfortunately, only limited information is available on family needs following head injury. Mauss-Clum and Ryan (1981) and Mathis (1984) addressed needs only during the acute medical crisis and their studies included a heterogeneous patient population. Although McCaffrey et al. (1987) and Ostby et al. (1988) investigated needs for long-term rehabilitation services, these researchers combined information from head injury survivors, family members, and others, obscuring possible differences in the perceptions of needs. Generally, researchers have not evaluated the relationship between reported needs and potentially important head-injured person and family characteristics.

Implications for Future Family Needs Research

Family needs are apt to change as a function of time postinjury, the injured person's deficits, and the phase of rehabilitation. Studies have not provided longitudinal data and consequently it is not known how needs change over time. Other variables describing persons with head injury and their families, such as preinjury functioning and family composition, will likely be associated with needs as well. Further research is required to evaluate the relationship between head-injured person and family characteristics and family needs. Families of persons with traumatic brain injury are a heterogeneous group. Ideal rehabilitation programs will provide for these diverse needs by matching family and head-injured person characteristics to available services and interventions.

Researchers interested in family needs lack established assessment instruments. Progress in evaluating family needs requires the development of reliable and valid instruments designed specifically for persons with traumatic brain injury. Kreutzer, Camplair, and Waaland (1988) have developed the self-report Family Needs Questionnaire (reproduced in Appendix B, Chapter 16, this volume) designed to assess both the importance of family needs and the extent to which needs have been met. Items were selected to cover the range of family needs throughout the rehabilitation process. This will allow researchers to evaluate changes in the relevance and importance of needs over time. Assessment of the extent to which needs have been met is likely to provide an important gauge for evaluating the successfulness of family intervention programs. Preliminary data based on 60 family members of brain-injured outpatients have provided support for the representativeness of questionnaire items and clinical utility of the instrument (Camplair & Kreutzer, 1989). Further analyses will focus on the questionnaire's usefulness with inpatient populations.

In some instances, researchers who addressed family needs combined perceptions of head-injured persons and family members. Priorities may very well differ between these two groups, and family members will likely report a greater range of needs. Consequently, the head-injured person's and the family member's perceptions should be evaluated separately. Development of a needs questionnaire for persons with traumatic brain injury that parallels the format of questionnaires intended for family members is suggested. Information collected separately from injured persons and their families will allow investigation of interactions between the injured person's outcome, family outcome, head-injured person's needs, and family needs.

Researchers have investigated family and head-injured person's report of needs to the exclusion of input from rehabilitation professionals. Certainly, families' opinions should be weighted heavily due to their role as primary caregivers, and as consumers of rehabilitation services. However, research by Romano (1974) and Gardner (1973) suggests that family perceptions are colored by powerful emotional reactions, such as denial and anger. Consequently, researchers should also incorporate data obtained from experienced clinicians. Comparisons between different sources of family needs data can serve as a basis for dialogue between providers and beneficiaries of rehabilitation and support services.

In conclusion, family needs following head injury have received only cursory attention. One barrier to systematic investigations of this important topic is the unavailability of a standardized methodology. Further development of assessment instruments is needed before significant progress can be made. Researchers should develop instruments to reflect perceptions of head-injured persons and professionals in addition to those of family members. Future research should evaluate changes in family needs over time. Relationships between needs and head-injured person's or family's characteristics should also be examined. Of particular interest will be the correlation between family needs and services or interventions rendered. Family perceptions of needs in this case can be considered an index of their satisfaction with support from rehabilitation professionals.

CONCLUSIONS

Fortunately, researchers and clinicians have helped draw attention to the burden so often reported by family members following head injury. Their burden is reflected in the high prevalence of emotional distress and alterations in family relationships. Existing research has underscored the strain produced by significant changes in the injured person's emotional and behavioral functioning. However, family members of severely injured persons are not universally distressed. Positive influences, including familial, community, and professional resources, evidently help preserve and maintain adaptive family functioning. Unfortunately, methodologically sound research is relatively scarce and additional work is clearly needed. For example, the relative contribution of factors other than the head-injured person's residual deficits has not been adequately evaluated to date. Further identification of factors related to distress and burden will alert rehabilitation professionals to risk factors that contribute to impaired family functioning, helping to minimize family distress.

Investigations of family needs during the hospitalization and rehabilitation of persons with head-injury have indicated that families often require long-term emotional and social support as well as education regarding rehabilitation services and the effects of injury. Families involved in the process of community integration report a relatively greater range of needs than families involved in acute rehabilitation. Limited outpatient rehabilitation services, prolonged social isolation, and slowing of the recovery process likely affect the needs of family members. Longitudinal research addressing family needs is required in order to fully appreciate changing priorities. Additional research delineating family needs and their relationship to familial and head-injured person characteristics will facilitate program development and help to empirically establish service priorities.

Identification of mechanisms by which families cope following head injury and facilitate or hinder injured persons' reentry into the community will be furthered by research that describes the relationship between family reactions and family needs. The extent to which families report that needs are being met will likely be predictive of distress levels and the adequacy of coping skills. For the present, it can be assumed that the provision of ongoing support to families will help maintain the health of the entire family system.

Researchers and clinicians must fully appreciate the family's abilities and limitations in providing support to head-injured persons. Families not only suffer due to the strains imposed by head injury, but they often serve as the primary vehicle for returning head injury survivors to vocational, avocational, and social roles. A thorough understanding of family outcome is a prerequisite for the development of effective family treatment strategies aimed at ameliorating family distress and facilitating the head-injured person's community reintegration. Fortunately, research on family reactions and needs following traumatic brain injury has progressed since the early 1970s. Ongoing collaboration between researchers and clinicians will continue to advance knowledge about family outcome.

REFERENCES

Beck, A.T. (1972). *Depression: Causes and treatment*. Philadelphia: University of Pennsylvania Press.

Bishop, D.S., & Miller, I.W. (1988). Traumatic brain injury: Empirical family assessment techniques. *The Journal of Head Trauma Rehabilitation, 3,* 16–30.

Brooks, N., & McKinlay, W. (1983). Personality and behavioral changes after severe blunt head injury: A relative's view. *Journal of Neurology, Neurosurgery, and Psychiatry, 46,* 336–344.

Brooks, N., Campsie, L., Symington, C., Beattie, A., & McKinlay, W. (1986). The five year outcome of severe blunt head injury: A relative's view. *Journal of Neurology, Neurosurgery, and Psychiatry, 49,* 764–770.

Brooks, N., Campsie, L., Symington, C., Beattie, A., & McKinlay, W. (1987). The effects of severe head injury on patient and relative within seven years of injury. *Journal of Head Trauma Rehabilitation, 2*(3), 1–13.

Camplair, P.S., & Kreutzer, J.S. (1989, June). *Psychosocial needs of families of adult head injury survivors: Development of the Family Needs Questionnaire.* Paper presented at the 13th Annual Postgraduate Course on Rehabilitation of the Brain-Injured Adult and Child, Williamsburg, VA.

Carlson, C.I., & Grotevant, H.D. (1987). A comparative review of family ratings scales: Guidelines for clinicians and researchers. *Journal of Family Psychology, 1*(1), 23–47.

Epstein, N.B., Baldwin, L.M., & Bishop, D.S. (1982). *McMaster Clinical Rating Scale.* Unpublished manuscript, Brown/Butler Family Research Program, Providence, RI.

Epstein, N.B., Baldwin, L.M., & Bishop, D.S. (1983). The McMaster Family Assessment Device. *Journal of Marital and Family Therapy, 9*(2), 171–180.

Epstein, N.B., Bishop, D.S., & Levin, S. (1978). The McMaster Model of Family Functioning. *Journal of Marriage and Family Counseling, 4,* 19–31.

Evans, R.L., Bishop, D.S., Matlock, A., Stranahan, S., Smith, G.G., & Halar, E.M. (1987). Family interaction and treatment adherence after stroke. *Archives of Physical Medicine and Rehabilitation, 68,* 513–517.

Gardner, R.A. (1973). *The family book about minimal brain dysfunction.* New York: Jason Aronson.

Goldberg, D. (1978). *Manual of the General Health Questionnaire.* Windsor, Berkshire: NFER Publication Co.

Grad, J., & Sainsbury, P. (1963). Evaluating a community care service. In H. Freeman & W.L. Farndale (Eds.), *Trends in the mental health services* (pp. 303–317). London: Pergamon Press.

Hoenig, J., & Hamilton, M.W. (1967). *The desegre-*

gation of the mentally ill. London: Routledge & Kegan Paul.

Hurwitz, N. (1960). The measurement of marital strain. *American Journal of Sociology, 10,* 610–615.

Jacobs, H.E. (1988). The Los Angeles Head Injury Survey: Procedures and initial findings. *Archives of Physical Medicine and Rehabilitation, 69,* 425–431.

Katz, M.M., & Lyerly, S.B. (1963). Methods for measuring adjustment and social behavior in the community. I. Rationale, description, discriminative validity and scale development. *Psychological Reports, 13,* 503–535.

Kozloff, R. (1987). Networks of social support and the outcome from severe head injury. *Journal of Head Trauma Rehabilitation, 2*(3), 14–23.

Kreutzer, J., Camplair, P., & Waaland, P. (1988). *Family Needs Questionnaire.* Richmond, VA: Medical College of Virginia, Rehabilitation Research and Training Center on Severe Traumatic Brain Injury.

Lezak, M.D. (1978). Living with the characterologically altered brain injured patient. *Journal of Clinical Psychiatry, 39,* 592–598.

Lezak, M.D. (1986). Psychological implications of traumatic brain damage for the patient's family. *Rehabilitation Psychology, 31*(4), 241–250.

Lezak, M.D. (1988). Brain damage is a family affair. *Journal of Clinical and Experimental Neuropsychology, 10*(1), 111–123.

Livingston, M.G. (1987). Head injury: The relative's response. *Brain Injury, 1*(1), 33–39.

Livingston, M.G., Brooks, D.N., & Bond, M.R. (1985a). Patient outcome in the year following severe head injury and relatives' psychiatric and social functioning. *Journal of Neurology, Neurosurgery, and Psychiatry, 48,* 876–881.

Livingston, M.G., Brooks, D.N., & Bond, M.R. (1985b). Three months after severe head injury: Psychiatric and social impact on relatives. *Journal of Neurology, Neurosurgery, and Psychiatry, 48,* 870–875.

Mathis, M. (1984). Personal needs of family members of critically ill patients with and without acute brain injury. *The American Association of Neuroscience Nurses, 16,* 36–44.

Mauss-Clum, N., & Ryan, M. (1981). Brain injury and the family. *Journal of Neurosurgical Nursing, 13*(4), 165–169.

McCaffrey, R.J., Pollock, J., & Burns, P.G. (1987). An archival analysis of the needs of head injured survivors in New York State: Preliminary findings. *Archival Analysis, 4,* 174–177.

McKinlay, W.W., Brooks, D.N., Bond, M.R., Martinage, D.P., & Marshall, M.M. (1981). The short-term outcome of severe blunt head injury as reported by relatives of the injured persons. *Journal of Neurology, Neurosurgery, and Psychiatry, 44,* 527–533.

McKinlay, W.W., & Pentland, B. (1987). Developing rehabilitation services for the head injured: A UK perspective [Editorial]. *Brain Injury, 1*(1), 3–4.

Molter, N.C. (1979). Needs of relatives of critically ill patients: A descriptive study. *Heart & Lung, 8,* 332–337.

Oddy, M., Coughlan, T., Tyerman, A., & Jenkins, D. (1985). Social adjustment after closed head injury: A further follow-up seven years after injury. *Journal of Neurology, Neurosurgery, and Psychiatry, 48,* 564–568.

Oddy, M., & Humphrey, M. (1980). Social recovery during the year following severe head injury. *Journal of Neurology, Neurosurgery, and Psychiatry, 43,* 798–802.

Oddy, M., Humphrey, M., & Uttley, D. (1978a). Stresses upon the relatives of head-injured patients. *British Journal of Psychiatry, 133,* 507–513.

Oddy, M., Humphrey, M., & Uttley, D. (1978b). Subjective impairment and social recovery after closed head injury. *Journal of Neurology, Neurosurgery, and Psychiatry, 41,* 611–616.

Olson, D.H., Portner, J., & Lavee, Y. (1985). *FACES-III: Family Adaptability and Cohesion Evaluation Scales.* St. Paul: University of Minnesota, Family Social Science.

Olson, D.H., Sprenkle, D., & Russell, C. (1979). Circumplex model of marital and family systems: I. Cohesion and adaptability dimensions, family types and clinical applications. *Family Process, 18,* 3–28.

Ostby, S., Sakata, R., & Leung, P. (1988, June). *Head injury rehabilitation: Persistence of problems and perceived needs within two years post-treatment.* Paper presented at the 12th Annual Postgraduate Course on Rehabilitation of the Brain-Injured Adult and Child, Williamsburg, VA.

Panting, A., & Merry, P.H. (1972). The long-term rehabilitation of severe head injuries with particular reference to the need for social and medical support for the patient's family. *Rehabilitation, 38,* 33–37.

Romano, M.D. (1974). Family response to traumatic brain injury. *Scandinavian Journal of Rehabilitation Medicine, 6,* 1–4.

Rosenbaum, M., & Najenson, T. (1976). Changes in life patterns and symptoms of low mood as reported by wives of severely brain injured soldiers. *Journal of Consulting and Clinical Psychology, 44*(6) 881–888.

Snaith, R.P., Ahmed, S.N., Mehta, S., & Hamilton, M. (1971). Assessment of the severity of primary depressive illness. *Psychological Medicine, 1,* 143–149.

Snaith, R.P., Bridge, G.W.K., & Hamilton, M. (1976). The Leeds Scales for the self-assessment of anxiety and depression. *British Journal of Psychiatry, 128,* 156–165.

Teasdale, G., & Jennett, B. (1974). Assessment of coma and impaired consciousness: A practical scale. *Lancet, 2,* 81–84.

Thomsen, I.V. (1974). The patient with severe head injury and his family. *Scandinavian Journal of Rehabilitation Medicine, 6,* 180–183.

Thomsen, I.V. (1984). Late outcome of very severe blunt head trauma: A 10–15 year second follow-up. *Journal of Neurology, Neurosurgery, and Psychiatry, 47,* 260–268.

Weddell, R., Oddy, M., & Jenkins, D. (1980). Social adjustment after rehabilitation: A two year follow-up of patients with severe head injury. *Psychological Medicine, 10,* 257–263.

Weissman, M.M., & Bothwell, S. (1976). Assessment of social adjustment by patient's self-report. *Archives of General Psychiatry, 33,* 1111–1115.

Zarski, J.J., DePompei, R., & Zook, A. (1988). Traumatic head injury: Dimensions of family responsivity. *The Journal of Head Trauma Rehabilitation, 3,* 31–41.

CHAPTER 15

Family Response to Childhood Traumatic Brain Injury

Pamela Kaye Waaland

Traumatic brain injury is the primary cause of death and disability among youth in the United States today (Frankoski, 1985; Rivera & Mueller, 1986). Epidemiological studies (Levin, Benton, & Grossman, 1982) suggest that 41% of pediatric deaths and 35% of injuries are caused by brain trauma, which far exceeds all other causes of mortality and morbidity in youth. Youth (individuals from birth through adolescence) also are at higher risk for brain injury relative to the adult population. Incidence studies (Annegers, 1983; Kalsbeek et al., 1980) indicate that one sixth of all injuries occur before age 14. This figure jumps to nearly one half of all injuries when including the age range of 15 to 25, which constitutes the group at highest risk for injury.

Children also are more likely to survive traumatic brain injury relative to adults (Jennett & Teasdale, 1981). This undoubtedly reflects age trends in the causes of injury (Goldstein & Levin, 1987). Falls and parental abuse are primary causes in preschool years (Annegers, 1983); children from ages 5 through 14 are more often injured in sports-related, pedestrian, and bicycle accidents. Children over 14, as are adults, are most frequently injured in moving vehicle accidents (Klauber, Barrett-Connor, Marshall, & Bowers, 1981). As in all age groups, boys incur head injuries more frequently than girls (Field, 1976). Boys are also two to four times more likely to sustain head injury and four to six times more likely to die from head injury (Annegers et al., 1980).

Higher incidence and survival rates among youth implicate higher rates of family survivors. Family survivors, as do persons with head trauma, often experience significant frustration, helplessness, and despair (Lezak, 1978). Family members must without preparation adjust to a "new" person. This person may have extensive impairment and immense, immediate needs that must be met by family members. Behavioral and intellectual consequences of the child's injury alter roles and responsibilities, relationships with friends and family, and life priorities for all family members. Daily activities, family vacations, and finances typically are curtailed in these families. Finally, severe limitations in community resources further tax family members' coping abilities.

This chapter addresses three major aspects of family adjustment to pediatric head injury. As summarized in Table 15.1, any attempt to understand family functioning and needs must address the complex interface among the child with head injury, family members, and their biopsychosocial system. To assist clinicians and researchers in better meeting the needs of child and family survivors, the chapter begins with a summary of current research knowledge. This discussion addresses four major areas affecting family adjustment: 1) head-injured child characteristics, 2) family characteristics, 3) social environment, and 4) community resources. To date, our understanding of family adjustment to pediatric head injury has been based primarily on informal observations and generalizations from adult popu-

The research on which this chapter is based was partly supported by Grant #133AH70049 from the National Institute on Disability and Rehabilitation Research, United States Department of Education.

Table 15.1.   Factors related to family adjustment

Characteristics of child with head injury

Cognitive, sensorimotor, and socioemotional se-
   quelae
Developmental stage
Preinjury adjustment

Characteristics of family

Parental psychiatric status, attitudes, skills, so-
   cioeconomic status, and marital relationship
Sibling coping strategies, psychiatric status, gen-
   der, birth order, age, and preinjury adjustment
Family structure, cohesion, and adaptability
Family/child developmental stage

Social environment

Family socioeconomic status
Stressful life events
Social support network

Community resources

Family educational programs
Academic and vocational programs
Respite care, recreational, and other extracurricu-
   lar programs
Medical and therapeutic services

Cultural factors

Cultural/subcultural norms regarding disabilities
Public policy

lations. The latter generalizations can be very
misleading due to the overriding importance of
developmental issues. Consequently, investigations of family adjustment to other disabling
childhood conditions are incorporated into the
discussion. In addition, assessment issues and
instruments useful in evaluating family adjustment and needs are reviewed, and intervention
issues unique to families coping with pediatric
head injury are discussed. The chapter concludes
with a summary of the current research and treatment status as well directions for future research.

CHARACTERISTICS OF
THE CHILD WITH HEAD INJURY

"What can we expect for our child in the future?" is one of the most frequent questions
asked by family members. Because of common
misconceptions regarding cognitive sequelae,
families often receive contradictory information
from professionals and develop unrealistic expectations. In particular, many clinicians and researchers create expectations for greater resi-

lience and more complete recovery in childhood
versus adulthood. These expectations in turn
may contribute to the maladaptive family coping
patterns discussed in this chapter. Consequently,
factors guiding cognitive, emotional, and vocational outcome are briefly reviewed.

Cognitive and Sensorimotor Sequelae

Head-injured persons' ability to process information and learn from experience will influence
not only their adjustment, but also the adjustment of family members. Unfortunately, families typically cannot be provided clear guidelines
or prognostic information. Researchers have de-
bated the nature or even existence of a common
pattern of cognitive sequelae following mild to
moderate injury in childhood. Probably the
greatest debate concerns when a child is considered at risk. Depending upon the investigation,
one can expect transient or limited sequelae for
children unconscious from less than 1 day (Levin
& Eisenberg, 1979) to children unconscious 2 or
more weeks (Chadwick, Rutter, Brown, Shaffer,
& Traub, 1981, Chadwick, Rutter, Shaffer, &
Shrout, 1981). In general, however, strong and
direct relationships have been obtained between
injury severity (based on duration of coma or
post-traumatic amnesia) and assessed cognitive
ability for coma duration of 24 hours or greater
(Levin & Eisenberg, 1979).

Recovery trends are somewhat similar for
adults and children. Substantial recovery has
been noted to occur during the first 4 months,
followed by slower gains for several years
postinjury (Ewing-Cobbs & Fletcher, 1987; Rutter, Chadwick, & Shaffer, 1983). Children often
are impaired in their ability to express themselves, process visuospatial relations, think conceptually or sequentially, and produce efficient
motor output (Ewing-Cobbs & Fletcher, 1987).
Persistent attention and memory impairments
are particularly problematic for children, as
these deficits create significant parenting and
learning problems.

Sensorimotor disorders in childhood often
are transient relative to more persistent cognitive
disorders. Most investigators have documented
impressive resolution of focal motor impairments, sensory deficits, and daily living skills

(Boll, 1983). For example, Bruce et al. (1979) report that 90% of children with severe head injury showed good recovery or only moderate disability despite pervasive neurological deficit. As a consequence of resolved sensorimotor impairments, clinicians and family members often overestimate the child's capabilities. Nevertheless, cognitive sequelae present the greatest obstacle to social and vocational success (Levin et al., 1982).

Clearly, age at the time of injury can be expected to affect the child's learning abilities and the family's adaptation. Early research led clinicians to expect greater recovery from traumatic brain injury during childhood. However, the concept of greater neuroplasticity in childhood has not been consistently supported. First, this assumption was based primarily on sequelae to nontraumatic focal brain injury (Dennis & Kohn, 1975). Recent investigations (Rasmussen & Milner, 1977) suggest that increased plasticity occurs only for interhemispheric (and, more specifically, linguistic based) rather than for intrahemispheric transfer of functions. Second, greater "plasticity" appears restricted to primarily the first 2 years of life and is at the expense of a general decline in intellectual potential (Rasmussen & Milner, 1977).

Third, recent studies comparing outcome of head injury in children versus adolescents clearly do not support the view that recovery is enhanced in children (Wider, Schlesner, Grumme, & Kubicki, 1979; Levin et al., 1982). Indeed, there is increasing consensus among researchers that head injury typically produces different and more severe cognitive sequelae during childhood than comparable trauma in adolescence or adulthood (Ewing-Cobbs & Fletcher, 1987; Ewing-Cobbs, Fletcher, & Levin, 1986). Expressive language and motor functions are particularly vulnerable for children under 6 (Ewing-Cobbs, Fletcher, & Levin, 1986). Increased vulnerability undoubtedly reflects immature neuroanatomy and the lack of empirically based treatment strategies for the developing child.

Finally, the extent of cognitive impairment may not manifest itself fully during early childhood or preadolescence. Black and colleagues' (1971) longitudinal follow-up in adolescence suggests that many children with head injury may "grow into" deficits with developmental demands for verbal encoding, fluent language, and higher level reasoning. This finding highlights the need for long-term clinical follow-up. Clinical experience suggests that many family members fail to make the connection between early traumatic brain injury and later academic or social failure. This leads to misattributions and unnecessary frustration for both family and child.

Unfortunately, most available knowledge of pediatric cognitive sequelae is based on formal test findings rather than day-to-day behavior. As Ben-Yishay and Diller (1983) have pointed out, many children with traumatic brain injury pass the standardized tests, yet fail at life. Because of the highly structured test situation, children often can compensate for impairments in judgment, problem solving, and organization (Telzrow, 1987). Again, this often leads professionals and family members alike to develop unrealistic hopes and expectations for the youth.

Socioemotional Characteristics

Socioemotional and personality changes following head injury are often the most distinctive symptoms and the most problematic for caregivers. Flach and Malmros (1972) found over one fourth of their sample to be "socially maladjusted" nearly a decade after their injury; they and other researchers have reported equally high rates of psychiatric or behavioral sequelae (Brink et al., 1970; Flach & Malmros, 1972; Klonoff & Paris, 1974). These sequelae undoubtedly produce the greatest stress and anxiety among family members coping with home-management problems (Lezak, 1978; Telzrow, 1987).

Relative to childhood populations, psychiatric sequelae to head injury in adults have been well documented (McLean, Temkin, Dikmen, & Wyler, 1983; Prigatano, 1987). Symptomatology includes: disinhibition; depression; irritability; anxiety; impaired social awareness; and unrealistic self-appraisal, paranoia, and aggression (McLean et al., 1983; Prigatano, 1987). Unfortunately, there does not appear to be a unitary syndrome or predictable behavior pattern in childhood, with the exception of increased "inappropriate" behavior. Published reports of childhood behavioral sequelae range from increased hyperactivity and distractibility to lethargy and withdrawal (Black et al., 1971; Brink et al., 1970). One study suggests that approximately half of youth with traumatic brain injury suffer from underarousal or lethargy, and half suffer from overarousal and hyperactivity (Filley, Cranberg, Alexander, & Hart, 1987).

There is some indication that emotional and behavioral differences among youth with traumatic brain injury may be age related. That is, younger children tend to display heightened activity, distractibility, and aggression whereas older children evidence increased affective disturbance, impulsivity, and decreased initiative (Brink et al., 1970). Somatic complaints, including headaches, eating problems, and sleep disturbance, tend to occur among all age groups (Black et al., 1971; Klonoff & Paris, 1974). Age-related differences have obvious implications for family intervention approaches, which are discussed later in this chapter. Further, parents and clinicians alike often have difficulty distinguishing between behavior problems caused by neurological impairment versus those secondary to parent and child reaction to the emotional trauma surrounding brain injury. These types of diagnostic issues further cloud effective parenting and family intervention.

Notably, recovery trends are strikingly different for cognitive sequelae relative to psychiatric sequelae. In contrast to declines in cognitive deficits, psychiatric and behavior sequelae show surprising upward trends following head injury. Indeed, Chadwick, Rutter, Brown, et al. (1981) and Chadwick, Rutter, Shaffer, and Shrout (1981) found both the incidence and severity of psychiatric disorder to increase steadily over a 2-year follow-up of their sample. These findings highlight the need to isolate factors placing children at higher risk for psychiatric sequelae and to focus on early family intervention among this group of children.

Preinjury Characteristics

Recent investigations report a strong relationship among preinjury behavior, the occurrence of head injury, and postinjury adjustment (Rutter et al., 1983; Brown, Chadwick, Shaffer, Rutter, & Traub, 1981). That is, children who incur a head injury often display preexisting problems with impulsivity, inattention, and aggression; these behaviors tend to be exacerbated by head injury.

Brown et al. (1981) systematically addressed psychiatric sequelae in their prospective study. The mild to moderate head injury group and orthopedic control group did not differ in rates of *new* disorder at any of the follow-up assessments based on clinical interview or questionnaire data. The child's physical disbility, age, or sex was not reliably related to psychiatric disorder. However, *preinjury* behavior disturbance was related to postinjury disorder among this group, and appeared exacerbated by head injury. Further, youth with preexisting problems were more often engaged in inappropriate, prohibited activities at the time of their injury. Similarly, Black et al. (1971) reported preinjury behavior problems in one third of their clients.

These findings suggest that what professionals interpret as "family denial" may at times reflect family complacency to preexisting behavior problems. Consequently, successful interventions may be more difficult to implement due to deeply entrenched family interaction and child behavior patterns.

CHARACTERISTICS OF THE FAMILY OF THE CHILD WITH HEAD INJURY

Parent Characteristics

Parents coping with pediatric head injury, as do their children, differ from their counterparts in a number of respects. These parents tend to show higher rates of marital instability and divorce (Klonoff, 1971; Rune, 1970). Further, they are more likely to have a history of mental disorder (Rune, 1970). Finally, this group of parents tends to have more limited income, social status, and social advantages when compared with parents of noninjured children (Rutter, Chadwick, Shaffer, & Brown, 1980; Brown et al., 1981).

Findings of Brown and colleagues (1981) implicate family adjustment as a primary determinant of psychiatric outcome for youth with mild to moderate head injury. That is, children with high levels of psychosocial adversity (as assessed by family stability, parent psychiatric history, and socioeconomic status) were more likely to develop psychiatric disorder. Indeed, psychosocial adversity was better able to predict psychiatric outcome than any other variable, including injury severity. Not surprisingly, a high percentage of these children were engaged in prohibited or unsupervised activities at the time of their injury. These findings are consistent with other published reports in implicating poor parental supervision and practices as contributing to childhood head trauma. Incidence studies (Annegers, 1983) also suggest these children are two to three times as likely to incur a second injury, further accentuating their high-risk status.

Unrealistic parent expectations and practices undoubtedly contribute to postinjury adjustment differences noted among Brown et al.'s (1981) sample. Although family characteristics have not been systematically assessed among head-injured populations, follow-ups of children with severely handicapping conditions highlight the importance of family characteristics on child adjustment (Mink, Nihira, & Meyers, 1981; Nihira, Mink, & Meyers, 1981). Good parenting (as judged by observations and interviews addressing child-rearing practices, attitudes, and quality of the home environment) bore a strong, direct relationship to child adaptive behavior, home manageability, and school adjustment. Parenting skills also were predictive of long-term gains made by this group of children.

Thus, while more socially advantaged parents may experience greater problems accepting their child's limitations, their increased resources, family stability, and education appear to reduce the risk of head injury and enhance outcome. Collectively, the above investigations are in concordance with Mednick's developmental study of schizophrenia in emphasizing the concept of "at-riskness" for disorder or sequelae. Unfortunately, preliminary research data suggest that families in the most adverse, high-risk, conditions are the least likely to receive or follow through with needed services.

Sibling Characteristics and Adjustment

To date, no studies have addressed preinjury characteristics of siblings. Based on preinjury

differences in persons with head injury, their parents, and family socioeconomic advantages, one would postulate siblings to be at increased risk for a multitude of adjustment problems as well. Irrespective of their preinjury status, siblings clearly are adversely affected by their sibling's injury. Parents' time and emotional resources typically are drained by caregiving demands and concerns for the injured child. Parents may have little or no time for attending to the adjustment problems of their other children, let alone transporting them to extracurricular activities, assisting in homework, or providing for their developmental needs.

Clinicians may be equally lax in assessing the needs of siblings if clinical focus parallels research interest. Although literature related to family adjustment is burgeoning, there are no systematic investigations of sibling adjustment to head injury. Consequently, the adjustment of children to siblings with other types of disabilities may provide guidelines.

Farber's (1959) seminal research indicated that the greater the impairment and dependence of a handicapped family member, the poorer the adjustment of his or her nonhandicapped siblings. More recent work, however, suggests that this relationship may be applicable only for children from less socially advantaged families (Grossman, 1972). In particular, children from families with fewer financial resources typically are burdened with greater responsibility for their handicapped sibling and household tasks. Not surprisingly, these children are at higher risk for behavior and emotional problems.

Birth order, gender, and family size also are predictive of objective burden and socioemotional adjustment of nonhandicapped siblings. In particular, older female siblings appear at greatest risk for behavioral and emotional problems (Cleveland & Miller, 1977; Grossman, 1972). Again, those at greatest risk—youth who are the oldest, female or from a small family—are also those who bear the greatest responsibility for caring for the handicapped child. Not surprisingly, Sullivan (1979) has found that siblings of developmentally disabled children experience greater stresses and mature earlier than their peers. Other investigators (Trevino, 1979) have corroborated increased risk for a wide variety of emotional problems among siblings of handicapped and chronically ill children. These children must learn to nurture, rather than be nurtured, and often give up play time, social activities, and other integral developmental experiences.

Not surprisingly, parental attitude toward the disabled child is strongly predictive of sibling adjustment (Graliker, Fisher, & Koch, 1962; McHale, Simeonsson, & Sloan, 1984). Children of parents who share a healthy attitude toward their child's disability tend to display fewer behavioral problems in both home and school. Under these conditions, children having handicapped siblings may actually experience beneficial effects. These positive effects included higher levels of empathy, tolerance, and self-esteem. Hopefully, future research will elucidate the contributory roles of parent attitude, family role flexibility and cohesion, and sibling preinjury adjustment on outcome.

Family Reactions following Traumatic Brain Injury

As suggested, coping reactions of individual family members undoubtedly are influenced by the family unit's ability to readjust roles and adapt to the changed family member. Although the incidence of pediatric head trauma is relatively high, there are virtually no published investigations of family longitudinal adjustment or reactions to the childhood head injury. However, systematic investigations of reactions to congenital handicaps (Turnbull & Blacher-Dixon, 1980), developmental disabilities (Gardner, 1973), and adult head injury (Lezak, 1986) suggest that there are fairly predictable responses in reaction to these traumatic experiences. These findings suggest individuals often progress through a series of stages in moving toward family readjustment or, alternatively, dysfunction.

The pioneering work of Kubler-Ross (1969) and Lezak (1986) suggest commonalities between family reactions to terminal illness and brain injury of a family member. Polinko, Barin, Leger, and Bachmen's (1985) clinical description of family reactions to childhood head trauma is strikingly similar to Lezak's (1986) model derived from head injury in adulthood. Both link stages of perceptions of the injured persons, future expectations, and coping mechanisms to stages of recovery of the head-injured individual. Generally, the family's initial elation that the head-injured person will live moves from expectations for complete recovery to depression and mourning when it becomes apparent that deficits are relatively permanent. A summary of Polinko et al.'s (1985) model and clinical prescriptions paralleling each stage appear in Table 15.2.

According to this model, family members initially experience shock and denial. During

Table 15.2. Common family reactions and clinical prescriptions during different postinjury stages

Stage	Reaction	Clinical role
1. Injury to stabilization	Shock, denial, and panic	Simplified, consistent information Support Reassure about the quality of care
2. Return to consciousness	Relief; massive denial	Stabilize family resources and roles; orient slowly to possible realities Attend to siblings' needs
3. Rehabilitation phase	Variability: continued denial; anxiety and guilt; anger/depression	Normalize feelings and needs Focus on family communication Address physical, social, and supportive needs of family members
4. Return to community	Depression, anger, and grief	Promote nondefensive attitude Normalize family dyads Facilitate transition Work toward acceptance and action

Adapted from Polinko, Barin, Leger, and Bachman (1985).

this first phase, the parents' major concern is that the child survive. At the same time, family members are bombarded with technical language, medical technology, and, at times, contradictory reports. In order to cope with overwhelming circumstances, family members often "shut out" negative information. In the second stage, after the child regains consciousness, the family experiences relief, elation, and often massive denial. Family members tend to focus on similarities between present and past behavior and on minor improvements in order to justify often unrealistic beliefs about recovery.

During the third stage, typically coinciding with rehabilitation, family members may maintain a hopeful attitude. However, they begin to become discouraged and concerned by the head-injured child's slowed progress. At this point, family members may begin to express anxiety, guilt, anger, depression, or some combination of these feelings. These feelings may be indirectly expressed as discontentment with the child's rehabilitation program, anger toward professionals and other family members, resentment toward parents of noninjured children, or a "why me?" attitude. The fourth stage often is precipitated by the child's return to the community. In particular, changes in the child's curriculum, social life, and learning abilities often increase parents' awareness of the relative permanence of impairments and elicit grief. Optimally, this stage will lead to increased acceptance and healthier family adjustment.

These stages have been empirically validated in a study of parents of severely handicapped children (Eden, cited in Blacher, 1984). However, the final stage of "acceptance" does not appear to represent a uniform outcome. The author cautioned that "acceptance" should be viewed as a fluid state that family members may reach on differing time lines, or perhaps not at all. Similarly, Jacobs's (in press) review suggests family acceptance of the adult with head injury often is influenced by preinjury family typology, resources, coping history, and the role of the head-injured individual. These factors as well as preinjury family attitudes may account for the wide variability in family members' response to the head injury survivor.

Furthermore, Romano's (1974) early work suggests that adjustment to the "changed" head-injured person may represent an obstacle to acceptance not apparent with death or developmental disabilities. Romano found family members of adults with head trauma evidenced persistent, protracted denial of disabilities often resistant to counseling. Common forms of denial reported by Romano include: 1) fantasies about recovery, 2) verbal denials ("He always had a bad temper"; "He never talked much"), and 3) inappropriate reactions to the head-injured person's behavior (resulting from denial of disabilities or unrealistic expectations). Family denial may be intensified among pediatric populations. Because of the child's dependent, immature status, the family can more easily minimize inappropriate behaviors or attribute them to preinjury status. Family members also can easily maintain hopes that the child will "outgrow problems" despite research suggesting the contrary. Denial may be magnified among parents of children with preinjury adjustment problems due to similarities between preinjury and postinjury maladjustment.

Siblings undoubtedly go through similar stages in adjusting to the child's disability. However, their feelings often are expressed indirectly due to their emotional immaturity and tendency to be "sheltered" from information during their sibling's hospitalization.

To date, sibling reactions to head injury have not been assessed. However, Powell and Ogle (1985) provide expectations in their review of common reactions experienced by siblings of handicapped children. Typical reactions include resentment, anger, and jealousy; frustration, fear, and embarrassment; and reactive guilt, isolation, and depression. These feelings are often manifested in aggression, crying, or irritability among young children and antisocial behavior or depression among older children. A subset of children seem to adopt the "perfect" child or caregiving role in response to guilt and parental demands. Declining school performance also is common. Although commonalities among family members' reactions have not been investigated, one would expect sibling reactions to parallel parent coping reactions.

Family as a System

Strong family denial of head injury sequelae may create unhealthy interactions among family members and the child with head injury. According to systems theory (Minuchin, 1984), maladaptive coping strategies of any family member will affect the behavior patterns and coping strategies of all family members as well as their relationship with systems outside of the family.

Consistent with this theory, dysfunctional family and community interaction patterns are more frequently noted among families of children with autism (Helm & Kozloff, 1986). In particular, these families often evolve into a "closed" system by isolating themselves from "outsiders" and focusing exclusively on the autistic child's needs. Rogers and Kreutzer (1984) note that isolation also is a common pattern among families of adults with head injury. These families find it easier to remain at home due to difficulties obtaining respite care, adapting to the head-injured adult's limited physical capacity, or coping with the embarrassment of inappropriate community behavior.

Harris (cited in Morgan, 1988) describes four patterns observed among families of children with autism (see Table 15.3). Family studies (Wright, Granger, & Sameroff, 1984) of children with other types of disabilities and chronic illness support Harris's topology. Similarly, Farber (1959) found higher rates of marital discord, parental inconsistency and overprotectiveness, and maladjustment of the disabled child among families displaying persistent, unhealthy coping strategies.

Harris's subtypes (cited in Morgan, 1988) although oversimplified, bear a striking resemblance to our clinical "typology" of dysfunctional family patterns among children with head injury. For example, fathers in traditional or "breadwinner" roles often have more limited contact during the children's hospitalization and provide less direct support upon their return home. As a consequence, fathers are more likely to downplay their children's limitations. In contrast, mothers or primary caregivers more often experience intense guilt, depression, and fear that may translate into overindulgent or overprotective parenting practices.

Family theory (Minuchin, 1984) also emphasizes the bidirectionality that exists among parent-child behavior. In particular, postinjury child behavior changes undoubtedly alter parental behavior, which in turn intensifies child behavioral sequelae. The circularity of parent-child

Table 15.3.   Family interactional patterns in response to childhood disability

Subtype	Family members	Behavior
"Poor sick child"	Parent–Injured child	Overindulgence and failure to set limits Belief the child is "sick" and not responsible for behavior Exclusion of other parent and other siblings
"It's just the three of us"	Parent–Injured child	Both parents overinvolved with injured child Lack of discipline or full-time commitment to remediation Exclusion of other siblings
"This child has come between us"	Parent–Injured child	One parent's overinvolvement creates overt marital conflict and disengagement Enclusion of marital dyad
"Mother's little helper"	Parent-Sibling	Mother joins forces with an older child to care for the injured child Father is excluded from these interactions and involvement with the injured child Dyads between the father and other children or outside systems (e.g., work relations)

Adapted from Morgan (cited in Powell & Ogle, 1985).

behavior and its contribution to symptomatic behavior of family members have not been directly investigated. However, in their follow-up of 231 children 2 years postinjury, Konoff and Paris (1974) noted an increased incidence of disturbed parent-child relations, parent anxiety related to residual impairments, and overprotectiveness. This published report is unique in its focus on changes in parent behavior. Nevertheless, the researchers did not address the relationship between parent behavior and child adjustment.

Clearly, practitioners are well advised to sequentially assess family interaction patterns in order to promote healthy marital, parent-child, and family-community relations.

SOCIAL ENVIRONMENT OF THE FAMILY

As noted previously, family financial, educational, and social status predict not only how the family will adjust, but whether a youth will sustain head injury. However, research with families of children with developmental disabilities suggests it may not be these family factors per se that put families at greater risk (e.g., Bristol, 1984; McKinney & Petersen, 1987). Rather, families with greater adversity also may have more limited support to help them cope with emotional, caregiving, and financial burdens. In particular, the availability of quality support appears to be an important determinant of marital satisfaction, family adjustment, and prognosis for the child with head injury (McKinney & Petersen, 1987; Powell, 1979; Weintraub, Brooks, & Lewis, 1977.)

McKinney and Petersen (1987) reported that perceived support and control over life events were more powerful predictors of high-risk children's outcome than more objective socioeconomic stressors. Social support and perceived control accounted for over one-half of the variance in behavior problems and two-thirds of the variance in school problems; socioeconomic status accounted for only one-tenth of the variance in either behavioral or school adjustment. Social support appeared to be a particularly potent predictor of outcome for children reared in high stress conditions.

Similarly, Bristol (1984) found adaptation in families of children with autism to be more strongly influenced by the quality of social support than by social status or child characteristics such as severity of impairment. The most potent predictor of family adaptation was the amount of perceived support the mother received from her husband. Mothers who reported greater marital support experienced lower levels of depression and greater acceptance of the child. Greater support from extended family members correlated with quality parenting practices and marital satisfaction. Bristol (cited in Bristol & Schopler, 1984) also found support to correlate with parents' perception of burden or stress. Mothers in the low versus high stress group differed in perceived support received from their spouse, extended family, and friends.

In later comparing these families with a control group, Bristol (cited in Morgan, 1988) found similarities on a number of family interactional and adjustment measures, including family relationships and personal growth. However, families of autistic children showed a stronger belief in God and adherence to moral standards. Bristol suggests that strong faith and church support serves as a sustaining force for many families of disabled children.

Although some similarities exist, many of Bristol's (1984; Bristol, cited in Morgan, 1988) findings are discordant with those of Brooks et al.'s (1987) longitudinal investigation of family adjustment to severe head injury in adulthood. In both investigations, perceived burden was not related to severity of client deficits. However, Brooks and colleagues did not obtain the expected relationship between subjective burden and social support evident among Bristol's sample. Unfortunately, methodological differences obscure the contribution made by stage of development, type of disability, and assessment techniques, among other factors. Clearly, direct comparison between adult and child populations is needed to clarify differing family needs. In particular, clarification of the *type* of support (e.g., family members versus others; social versus service oriented) needed as a function of family and injured child characteristics could greatly enhance clinical efforts.

COMMUNITY CHARACTERISTICS

Subsequent to their child's head injury, parents experience understandable feelings of confusion, anxiety, and helplessness. These feelings often are greatly intensified by inadequate understanding of the child's injury, prognosis, and needs. The family's reported need for appropriate *information and education* in adult populations has been well established (Molter, 1979; Norris & Grove, 1986). Similarly, few families of children with head injury are adequately prepared to accommodate the children's behavioral changes and multiple needs.

Several research findings (Blacher, 1984; Granger, 1983) suggest that the availability of appropriate parent education programs may greatly enhance outcome for children with disabilities. Granger (1983) systematically assessed the adjustment of mothers of handicapped children who were enrolled in intervention programs promoting either high or low levels of parent involvement. The highest level of anxiety was experienced by mothers with little external support and in low-involvement intervention programs. Conversely, the least anxiety was reported by mothers with high support in high-involvement intervention programs. Although not directly assessed, both enhanced parenting skills and subjective feelings of competency likely contribute to the improved outcome. Similarly, Blacher (1984) found family adjustment and outcome for the injured child to be enhanced for parents with greater feelings of competency and knowledge of their child's disabilities. Unfortunately, outpatient intervention programs are seldom available for families of children with head injury.

Although education may facilitate family adjustment, it will not compensate for parent strain created by inadequate *community resources*. Parents often are faced with the demands of transporting their child to doctor and therapist appointments, managing inappropriate behavior, and addressing school-related prob-

lems. High rates of depression, isolation, and dissatisfaction among family members (Lezak, 1988) are not surprising when considering the hardships they face in attempting to reintegrate the head-injured child into the community.

The availability of appropriate community resources clearly can reduce the incidence of parent "burnout" (Bristol & Schopler, 1984). Marcus (1984) cited lack of available respite care as a primary cause of burnout among parents coping with childhood disabilities. Other stressors cited included lack of suitable therapeutic or supportive services and associated parental neglect of personal needs. DeMyer and Goldberg (1983) investigated family service needs at varying developmental stages for children with autism. Notably, respite care, financial assistance, and appropriate educational services were among the top four, and the only needs cited consistently at every developmental stage.

To date, needs among families of children with head injury have not been systematically assessed. However, informal clinical assessment suggests the need for appropriate educational services ranks high. Problems in obtaining appropriate educational placement and curricula for children with head injury are well documented (Savage, 1987; Telzrow, 1987). In contrast to the multitude of specialized adult rehabilitative programs, educators seldom receive specialized training in head injury. A survey of special educators in Vermont (Savage, 1987) indicated that only 5%–8% had received any information about head injury in their graduate or undergraduate programs. Parents surveyed by Rosen and Gerring (1986) cited the following obstacles to successful academic reentry: lack of teacher understanding, uncooperative and insensitive mainstream teachers, loss of friends and social isolation of their child, parental isolation, inappropriate classroom placement, and parental strain from helping their child with homework.

ASSESSMENT OF FAMILY ADJUSTMENT

The preceding discussion highlights the complex interplay of factors affecting family adjustment following pediatric head injury. Ideally, a thorough assessment of these factors will help the clinician to develop intervention strategies tailored to specific family needs. The reader is referred to Bishop and Miller (1988) for a complete review of the psychometric properties of major assessment techniques useful in assessing family adjustment to head injury. The present discussion focuses on assessment tools the clinician may find useful in assessing family response to traumatic brain injury in childhood.

Clinical Interview

Although less "scientific" than formal assessment devices, a thorough clinical interview is essential to establish rapport, observe customs and interaction patterns, and formulate treatment plans for family members. The clinical interview should culminate in a comprehensive understanding of the family. This includes the family's background, cultural values, religious beliefs, and educational levels; history of psychiatric, learning, and medical problems, including any hospitalizations and arrests among family members; specific family roles and structure; and parenting skills and practices. As indicated in the preceding sections, family and client preinjury history play an important role in outcome and, ideally, in the type of intervention strategies selected by the sophisticated clinician.

In many cases, the family has been transitioned from a number of settings in the past (i.e., from acute care to rehabilitation to outpatient services). In these situations, clinician communication with other professionals and review of records prior to the interview is essential. Families often have difficulty adjusting to new settings and health care providers. These difficulties are heightened when clinicians are ignorant of the family background and treatment history.

By the end of the first or second meeting with the family, the clinician should be able to answer the following questions from the family's perspective:

Whose "fault" is the injury (e.g., parents, family, professionals)?

How are individual family members coping with the problem (e.g., denying, withdrawing, fighting, blaming, pitying, crying, work-

ing, turning to religion, escaping through drugs or alcohol)?

Has the family received appropriate education regarding the child's sequelae, needs, and prognosis?

Have other professionals been seen in the past?

What professionals are currently involved (e.g., physicians, therapists, school personnel, attorneys)?

What was the child's family role (e.g., "achiever", "black sheep") preinjury?

What beliefs do family members hold regarding the child's status?

How realistic are their current and future expectations?

How "far" are they looking ahead?

How have family interaction patterns and roles changed since the child's injury (e.g., family outings or childcare responsibilities)?

How has the child's injury affected family contacts with support systems? intimate and sexual relations? personal time?

What services and support systems are currently available to the family and child?

How satisfied are parents with services (e.g., school, community programs, respite care, specialized therapies)?

How effectively do family members use available services?

What unusual demands does the child place on family members (e.g., behavior outbursts; sleep, eating, or sexual disturbance; dependence on others to care for hygiene or transportation needs)?

How open are family members to outside interventions?

Shapiro (1983) has proposed a series of interview questions to illuminate sibling understanding of and response to the head-injured child's disabilities. These questions, presented below, have been adapted for siblings of children with head injury:

How did you find out about your sibling's injury?

What is your understanding of your sibling's disabilities?

What are your feelings toward your sibling at different times?

What special responsibilities have you had to take on since your sibling's injury?

Do you volunteer to help your sibling or do your parents "make you"?

How have your parents' relationships with each other and with you changed since the injury?

Does your family spend more or less time together since the injury?

Are you nervous you may need to take responsibility for your sibling some day?

Do people at school, church, or in other places act differently toward you when they find out about your sibling?

Has your sibling's injury affected your social life, relationships, or dating?

Has your sibling's injury affected your future goals and plans?

During the initial interview, it is particularly important to determine why the family seeks assistance and what it hopes to gain from professional services. Responses may vary from "fixing" the head-injured child to following the family attorney's advice to strengthen the child's legal case. Interventions then can be "reframed" to address the family's particular agenda and ultimately to increase its commitment to treatment. The clinician also should determine if the family has sought prior services in the past; and, if so, why services were terminated. The clinician subsequently can coordinate services with other involved professionals, avoid repeating unsuccessful interventions, and identify individuals expecting a "quick fix" to likely chronic problems.

Although the clinician may wish to initially interview the parents and the child with head injury individually, siblings and extended family members should be incorporated into sessions as soon as feasible. These family members provide critical sources of information. Furthermore, the clinician focusing on individual treatment often obtains an unrealistic portrayal of family life that can only be clarified through observation of family interactions and problem-solving strategies. The clinician can detect family organization patterns, including individual family roles, disengagement or overinvolvement of particular

members, and unhealthy attitudes toward the client. Finally, important family- or client-related issues candidly discussed by parents may be inappropriately avoided or minimized in the presence of their children. Children in turn may develop behavior problems to divert attention away from central problems or to obtain attention. Again, these types of observations can guide treatment planning. The interested reader is referred to Minuchin (1984) for comprehensive guidelines to isolate family interactional patterns and roles.

For the clinician or researcher who desires a more objective interview, Bishop and Miller (1988) review available semistructured interview instruments. The Camberwell Family Interview assesses specific strategies the family uses to cope with psychiatric illness of a member. The McMaster Structured Interview for Families and the Standardized Clinical Family Interview address more global issues such as family structure, communication patterns, and problem-solving skills.

Standardized or Quantifiable Assessment Techniques

Standardized assessment techniques provide a more objective method of categorizing family strengths and weaknesses; these tools also enable the clinician to assess the effectiveness of intervention strategies at various points during treatment. As Bishop and Miller (1988) have pointed out, it is difficult but necessary to differentiate between *family functioning* and *objective family burden*. Family functioning refers to family organization, structure, and patterns of interaction. In contrast, "burden" encompasses objective problems the family faces in caring for the child with traumatic brain injury (e.g., financial expenses, transportation problems) or their subjective perception of burden (Livingston & Brooks, 1988).

The two most popular and up-to-date self-report measures of family functioning include the Family Adaptability and Cohesion Evaluation Scales (FACES-III; Olson, Portner, & Lavee, 1985) and the McMaster Family Assessment Device (FAD; Epstein, Baldwin, & Bishop, 1983). (See Bishop & Miller, 1988, for a review of these and other measures.) FACES-III is theoretically grounded in the circumplex model of family and marital systems (Olson, Russell & Sprenkle, 1983) and assesses family adaptability and cohesion. The clinician may also opt to use a second version of this 20-item scale, which assesses the respondent's "ideal" versus perceived view of the family. The discrepancy is used to measure the respondent's level of family satisfaction. FACES-III is reported to have good reliability and discriminative validity, although its construct and concurrent validity have been questioned (Bishop & Miller, 1988). The Family Assessment Device appears be more psychometrically sound and provides information on seven different dimensions ranging from problem solving and communication to affective responsiveness and degree of closeness of family members.

Although quantifiable data are not available, Rosenthal and Young (1988) have proposed the use of their Family Diagnostic Assessment technique in assessing family functioning. Family members are observed carrying out assigned tasks (which may range from a list of family problems or assisting the client in carrying out self-help tasks) to assess family interactional patterns. The author has found this technique to be quite useful in detecting parental overprotection, unrealistic expectations for the client, or punitive parenting approaches.

Clinical assessment of family burden or stress often helps the clinician better understand the adaptive value of seemingly dysfunctional family behavior. Due to the multiple stresses posed by the child with head injury, a thorough evaluation should include measures of family social support (O'Grady & Metz, 1987; Procidano & Heller, 1983); and objective or perceived stresses (Abidin, 1983; McCubbin, Patterson, & Wilson, 1981). The Children's Social Support Questionnaire (O'Grady & Metz, 1987) is unique in its focus on the quality of social support available to children and their caregivers. This 19-item Likert-type scale assesses: 1) support directly available to the child; 2) support available to the primary caregiver; and 3) the general level of support provided in the family environment. Although internal consistency and

test-retest reliability coefficients are high, normative data are not available.

The Parenting Stress Index (Abidin, 1983) was specifically developed to diagnose the relative magnitude of stress in the parent-child system and addresses three major source domains of stressors: 1) child characteristics, 2) caregiver characteristics, and 3) situational/demographic life stressors. Stressors identified range from objective life events such as the death of a family member, the caregiver's judgment of child behavior, and subjective feelings of burden regarding parenting responsibilities. The reliability and validity of this 120-item scale have been well established.

Probably one of the most important, but most seldom assessed areas affecting family adjustment is satisfaction of salient needs. Although norms are not available, Molter (1979) has developed a Family Needs Scale based on 45 frequently expressed needs of family members of adults with traumatic brain injury. Respondents indicate the extent to which various needs are met and the type of professional who has addressed each need. This scale has recently been modified (Kreutzer, Waaland, & Camplair, 1988) to address the specific needs of families of pediatric clients. (See Appendix B, Chapter 16, this volume.) This 40-item scale addresses the relative importance of various needs, ranging from information and services to social support, and family members' perceptions of the extent to which these needs are met.

When inappropriate parental attitudes or behaviors are suspected, the Adult-Adolescent Parenting Inventory (Bavolek, 1984) can provide helpful diagnostic information and intervention guidelines. This 32-item scale assesses parental expectations of children, level of empathy toward child needs, value of physical punishment, and appropriateness of parent-child roles. Bavolek has linked patterns of dysfunction in these various areas to particular intervention needs and strategies.

Finally, the Child Behavior Checklist (Achenbach, 1981) provides a measure of parents' perceptions of behavior problems and competencies of their children (ages 2–16). The scale assesses a variety of behavior problems ranging from depression, withdrawal, and anxiety to aggression, somatization, and hyperactivity. The author routinely asks teachers to fill out a corresponding version to determine the extent to which parents' perceptions are consistent with those of significant others. With all self-report measures, both parents (and other family members as appropriate) should complete forms independently to determine their level of agreement on particular issues. A self-report version is also available for teenagers, which provides a comparison between the child's and parent's perception of problem areas. Discrepancies in ratings can provide a starting point for interventions and for techniques to facilitate more open discussion among family members.

FAMILY INTERVENTION ISSUES

The preceding sections highlight the multitude of demands placed on family members following traumatic brain injury. To address family and patient needs, most major hospitals have developed treatment teams. Unfortunately, the quality of family services often is dependent upon family geographic location, financial status or insurance benefits, the experience or cooperative efforts of team members, and the family's willingness to accept services. As summarized elsewhere (Rosenthal & Young, 1988; Waaland & Kreutzer, 1988), comprehensive family interventions ideally should incorporate a full range of services: family education, support groups, networking, and advocacy, as well as family, marital, parent, or individual therapy services. Long-term planning and intervention also are essential to address the unique needs of the family and the child with head injury.

Family Education

Upon the head-injured child's return home, the primary burden of care falls on family members. Children typically are returned home as soon as possible due to the lack of appropriate rehabilitation facilities and mandate of public education to provide for their specialized needs. However, families of children with head injuries typically are ill prepared to cope with the multitude of home-management problems and coordination of community needs. Unfortunately, poor preparation may culminate in poor outcome. Numerous investigators (see Jacobs, in press, for a comprehensive review) have noted that educating family members to provide positive support favorably influences outcome, while inappropriate family understanding and behavior can greatly retard the head-injured child's progress. Consequently, it is essential to provide family members with a thorough understanding of the head-injured child's disabilities, prognosis, and needs.

During the youth's hospitalization, family education can include active participation in therapies and family conferences with team members (Rosenthal & Young, 1988; Waaland & Kreutzer, 1988). The family conference helps family members understand the nature and extent of the child's limitations and provides a forum to address their concerns or questions. When family members are included as active "therapists," they can often channel maladaptive feelings of helplessness and anger into productive involvement in the head-injured child's recovery (Jacobs, in press). For each interventions to be effective, team members must provide nontechnical explanations and patiently model intervention strategies adjusted to the family's educational level and needs. Parents can be asked to chart management problems during trial home visits. Problems noted then can be addressed in family sessions. Home intervention specialists may be utilized to assure generalization of strategies into the home and provide services on an out-patient basis.

Family education groups also provide an effective method for imparting information to family members. In one of the author's ongoing programs, families attend a six-session series with speakers from a variety of disciplines (i.e., physiatry, neurology, social work, psychology, education, and nursing). This provides a comprehensive understanding of clients needs, a forum for discussing problems, and an opportunity to network with other parents. Parents also are provided with lists of available community services, educational literature, and audio or videotapes.

Parent and Individual Therapy

Subsequent to the child's head injury, parents typically feel confused, inadequate, and helpless. They often receive contradictory advice and information from well-meaning friends and relatives, which further compromises their parenting self-confidence. These feelings are particularly pronounced for first-time parents. Although emotional support is important, parents also rely on the clinician to provide practical guidelines and home intervention strategies. Family concerns include management of anger outbursts, noncompliance, and overdependence as well as the development of appropriate social and daily living skills. Deaton (1987) provides an excellent discussion of behavioral strategies and environmental modifications tailored for children with head injury.

Family members, as well as the child with head injury, likely will require periodic counseling to address their individual needs and concerns. The level of intervention may vary from consultation to address normal adjustment problems to more intensive psychological or psychiatric involvement when family members present symptoms of severe depression, psychosomatic disorder, or other clinical syndromes. As noted earlier in this chapter, the high incidence of premorbid psychiatric and adjustment problems necessitates careful monitoring of individual family members. Due to the clinician's need to shift roles and alliances within the family system, it is advisable to make appropriate referrals for family members showing evidence of or more intensive individual needs.

Family Therapy

Through early and appropriate family intervention, long-term maladaptive family coping patterns often can be avoided. Particularly since many families coping with head injury evidence preexisting family adversities, the most helpful approach for family members is a competency-based model. This model focuses on family strengths and remediation or bypassing family weaknesses rather than viewing behavior as dysfunction. Based on this model, reports or feedback should emphasize strengths, gains, and positive intervention strategies. As a general rule, the clinician should provide the family members with a should for every "should not" and a "can" for every "cannot." Paradoxical interventions (Weeks & L'Abate, 1982) and other types of brief, strategic family therapy approaches will not effectively address the multiple needs of families coping with head injury.

Changing Family Needs

From the onset of a child's head injury, the need for *continuity of family care* from setting to setting is imperative. Parents frequently articulate feeling "dumped" from one system to another and ill prepared for the child's reentry into the home. Such feelings may contribute to the "therapeutic resistance" noted to characterize many families of persons with head injury (Romano, 1974). Consequently, it is important to establish a network of continuous care, beginning with intensive care in the hospital setting and ending with successful family, academic, and community integration.

In the event follow-up services will not be provided by hospital-based personnel, it is essential to involve outpatient health care professionals during late rehabilitation phases. Their involvement ideally should include attendance of client staffings and family and treatment team meetings, and education regarding intervention programs.

Family needs and therapeutic interventions will vary not only as a function of family differences, but also as to the postinjury stage. As noted in Table 15.1, families initially will respond with shock and panic to the trauma of the threatened loss of a loved one and to the rapid readjustments required of all family members. During the crisis phase, explanations and educational efforts should be simplified and consistent. This type of consistency requires good communication and teamwork among interdisciplinary team members. Inclusion of family members in interdisciplinary team conferences provides an excellent medium for facilitating family education and consistency of explanations given by staff members.

Although family members require orientation to potential long-term changes in their loved one, family resistance to harsh realities should be addressed with a patient attitude. The inexperienced therapist who insists the family "accept" the child's long-term disabilities often only serves to intensify family isolation and a "we-them" attitude toward professionals.

During later stages of rehabilitation, normalization of feelings of anger, guilt, or depression in combination with actively addressing the family's practical and emotional needs often can help to minimize family resistance. Parents often require "permission" or even direct prescriptions to spend time nurturing siblings, their marital relationship, and particularly their own needs. Because of overriding guilt, the individual's need for personal time often must be restated as "in the client's best interest" to facilitate therapeutic compliance. This includes emphasizing the head-injured child's need for autonomy and family members' need to model appropriate family and community behavior.

The child's reentry into the community often precipitates crisis in the family. At this stage, marital conflict, inappropriate family alliances, and unhealthy coping strategies tend to be heightened. The establishment of a network and appropriate services prior to the head-injured child's return home can alleviate many of these problems. However, more intensive therapeutic intervention likely will be required at this juncture to address family problems.

During this stage, parents often develop intense feelings of anxiety or guilt that interfere with their ability to modify inappropriate parenting practices. Many parents are aware of the inappropriateness of their practices, but require assistance in developing alternative behaviors. For example, one parent in the author's practice experienced intense guilt and blamed herself for her child's bicycle accident. She subsequently prohibited all her children (ages 5, 9, and 13) from riding bicycles and participating in other healthy activities. As an alternative, she was advised to have her children wear bicycle helmets and participate in an area safety program. Because of her inability to "do nothing," she was asked to unobtrusively monitor their adherence to rules and develop a "bicycling exam" to demonstrate her children's newly developed competency. Through similar interventions, she gradu-

ally was able to develop a healthier, more relaxed attitude toward parenting. As a consequence, overdependency displayed by younger children and rebellion by her teenage child also were significantly reduced over a 2-month period.

Parent conflict regarding the head-injured child's needs represents a second typical family problem. One parent (typically the mother) may be overly concerned by the child's poor progress and overinvolved with caring for his or her needs. In contrast, the other parent may fail to acknowledge or may minimize the child's deficits, and avoids contact with both spouse and child. In this situation, the goal is to increase contact between the uninvolved parent and the child. The uninvolved parent is charged with many of the more difficult child-care tasks typically provided by the primary caregiver. The primary caregiver in turn is charged with spending quality time with other children or taking care of neglected personal needs. Both parents are required to spend individual time together (with no discussion of family-related issues) toward the goal of promoting the head-injured child's "sense of mastery." These interventions can help both parents develop a more balanced perspective and reduce resentment regarding the burden of care and neglected marital needs.

Due to changing *developmental needs* of clients, the clinician working in pediatric head injury should have a thorough knowledge of developmental stages and needs. Thus, family interventions and child management programs of necessity should be tailored to the head-injured child's specific developmental level.

Based on Erickson's theory, disruption at various developmental levels will have a differing impact on the child's adjustment. For example, parent-child bonding is often disturbed as a consequence of head injury in infancy. Consequently, the parent may require involvement in an infant stimulation program. The goal of such programs is to increase parental sensitivity to child cues and facilitate infant responsiveness through appropriate positioning, exercises, and controlled rate of stimulation.

Parents of preschool children will require help in providing a "safe" environment for the child to explore through "babyproofing" and other environmental strategies. Because of the child's limited understanding of consequences and "peak" behavior management problems, preschool children with disabilities are vulnerable targets for parent abuse. Thus, parents require structured behavior management strategies that decrease physical punishment and negative parenting behaviors. Unless bonding has been disrupted by long-term hospital stays, children at this age also profit from involvement in a structured, center-based remedial program or nursery school program as appropriate. Respite care also may prevent caregiver "burn-out," common among parents of preschoolers with head injury, and neglect of other family members' needs.

For the child functioning at the latency-age level, the focus of intervention gradually shifts from home and family to school and peers. Cognitive intervention strategies (e.g., self-monitoring and reward, social skills training, and problem-solving approaches) and logical consequences begin to replace structured behavioral approaches in the home. It is particularly important for parents and teachers to learn to break down tasks and modify expectations at this stage to promote successful mastery. Areas of nonacademic strength such as music, competitive or noncompetitive sports, art, or crafts should be developed to foster social skills and self-identity. These types of interventions also help the child avoid overidentification with the "sick role." Children who fail to develop such strengths often use symptomatic behavior as a source of attention and identity.

Adolescence often precipitates significant adjustment problems for the head-injured child as well as for family members. The adolescent experiences increased growth spurts, hormonal changes, social stressors, and academic demands. These stresses often intensify home-management problems and unhealthy parent-child interactions. Depression is common due to the adolescent's increased awareness of differences from others and the resulting self-perception as "damaged." Driver's rights, heralding a rite of passage to adulthood, often are restricted secondary to sensorimotor or cognitive impairments. Many adolescents, particularly males, engage in inappropriate risk taking, experimentation with drugs and alcohol, and other acting-out behaviors in an attempt to fit in socially. Due to poor inhibition and emerging sexual needs, sexual promiscuity is particularly problematic for adolescents with head injury.

Typical adolescent management problems often precipitate family crises. During adolescence, it is particularly important to reduce parental overprotection and anxiety while at the same time helping the client to accept personal limitations. The behavior management strategies effective with the latency-age child often precipitate rebellion as the same child reaches adolescence. Hospitalization may be necessary to reduce parent-adolescent conflict and to protect the acting-out adolescent. At this stage, vocational and independent living skills become primary. For the clients ultimately unable to function autonomously or in a supervised group home setting, the family will need assistance in formulating long-range plans.

Finally, the potential for the client to "grow into" later problems (Black et al., 1971) highlights the need for *long-term follow-up*. Such long-term follow-up might be accomplished through yearly checks at a head injury clinic, well checks, case management calls to monitor family needs, or alternative services. At each follow-up visit, the clinician should obtain information from school personnel, family members, and the client. Service needs, ranging from adaptive aids to school programming to therapy needs of family members, should be updated. The findings of Brooks and colleagues (1987) suggest that family adjustment problems may intensify over time. Consequently, the needs of not only the client, but also the parents and siblings require careful monitoring.

Social Support and Networking

Particularly during the early postinjury stages families should be encouraged to utilize support systems in order to avoid maladaptive patterns of family isolation. Rogers and Kreutzer (1984) outline a "network intervention strategy" designed to identify family needs, anticipate potential problems, and provide resources to address these issues. Interventions might include extended family, friends, school or community service representatives, and clergy. As friends and others may avoid the family due to feelings of helplessness, positive prescriptions undoubtedly decrease the likelihood of family isolation.

Effective use of available support systems is particularly important for families returning to geographically isolated areas. Service providers in more rural areas are unlikely to be educated in the specialized needs of the child with head injury. Clients may return from the sophisticated medical center to rural areas with few services available. Informal support systems become much more critical in these types of situations. Irrespective of locality, friends and extended family are critical members of the "treatment team." Indeed, family members typically report friends and family rather than professional staff to be most important in meeting their needs (Mauss-Clum & Ryan, 1981).

In addition to preexisting social networks, other families who have experienced pediatric head injury provide an important source of support and guidance. Networking with other family survivors helps to reduce feelings of isolation, self-pity, and the perception that "no one else could understand." Family members often find it easier to disclose their fears, anger, and "unacceptable thoughts" to others who have experienced similar circumstances. Such family contacts typically are available through the local chapter of the National Head Injury Foundation or parent-to-parent programs. When local programs are not established, the clinician is well advised to establish an informal network among families. Based on Alcoholics Anonymous and other successful self-help programs, families should be put in contact with "veteran" members who have more extensive experience and are realistic about family needs.

Support groups also provide an excellent opportunity to establish family-to-family support networks. Although support groups and other informal networks are often available, programs typically focus on parent or client needs and exclude siblings. This is unfortunate, since sibling needs are the least likely to be met through other resources. In their model program, Conder and Conder (1988) demonstrated improved sibling adjustment (as assessed by the Child Behavior Checklist [Achenbach, 1981]) subsequent to participation in a group for sib-

lings of head-injured children. Children in their group were given a brief orientation to effects of brain injury and encouraged to share their concerns or emotional reactions. Coping solutions and ways of helping the head-injured child were exchanged. Parents observed group interactions from an outer circle toward improving parental understanding of sibling concerns. Although the latter group consisted of children from ages 4 to 14, the author has noted youth to profit from groups tailored to their specific developmental level and needs. Similar to parent groups, youth often form special bonds and mutually help one another overcome feelings of isolation and anger.

Community Resources and Advocacy

In addition to their personal and social needs, families of children with head injury face immense practical needs. In order to serve as an effective advocate, the clinician must be conversant with available community resources. These resources may range from financial assistance and medical facilities to respite care and educational and vocational programs. Fortunately, the National Head Injury Foundation and its state chapters provide an important source for information, support, and referral. In addition to providing support and educational programs for families, the National Head Injury Foundation is directly involved in influencing public policy and attitudes, coordinating needed services and programs, and making referrals for appropriate services.

Adult rehabilitation facilities and supportive programs specializing in head injury have grown exponentially in the past decade. In contrast, children typically are discharged into the community with the assumption that parents and schools will bear the burden of care. Unfortunately, needed training and support are typically unavailable to enable these individuals to function as "therapists." As noted previously, few educators have knowledge of the specialized needs of the child with head injury. Furthermore, although children with handicapping conditions are lawfully required to receive appropriate services, traumatic brain injury is not recognized as a unique handicapping condition. These children do not fit into preexisting categories and often "fall through the cracks" without appropriate professional advocacy.

Consequently, clinicians working with children with head injury should be conversant with available educational programs and assist family members in effectively advocating for their child. (Many of these issues are outlined in Chapter 18, this volume.) Families, often overwhelmed by home-management problems upon the child's return home, often are further stressed by delayed or inappropriate educational placement. Ideally, referral for special educational services should be made during the child's hospitalization to assure a smooth transition into the family and community. Because family members often hold unrealistic expectations for the child upon initial hospital discharge, they should be prepared for changes in the child's placement and curriculum.

A member of the treatment team well versed in educational issues should accompany parents to the child's eligibility meeting and advocate for needed services. Due to the variety of neuropsychological and medical sequelae, the child with head injury often can receive the most flexible programming through the category of "other health impaired." However, placement may vary from regular classroom placement with resource assistance or adjunctive (physical, occupational, or speech) therapies to a self-contained classroom or temporary homebound program. The family's advocate also should participate in developing goals and objectives outlined in the child's individualized education program (IEP).

Poor educational planning frequently results in unnecessary family stress and anxiety. As noted by Rosen and Gerring (1986), parents often cited teacher insensitivity, child social isolation, and personal strain from assisting their child with homework as obstacles to family adjustment. Again, many problems can be anticipated and prevented through scheduling modifications and appropriate programming. For example, the child may not initially be able to tolerate full-day services, classroom changes, or public transportation. Consequently, the clinician can recommend scheduling modifications. The child also may require extended (12-month) services when learning regressions are likely.

Helping professionals also can assist the family through educating and providing ongoing consultation to school personnel. Teachers can be asked to contact the clinician directly concerning major behavioral problems. Teachers often ask parents to "fix" or provide a solution to inappropriate school behavior, which can intensify family stress and anxiety. As social problems can be equally distressing for family members, establishing a social support system for the child also can facilitate successful academic reentry. This might include developing a "buddy" system or having a session with classmates prior to the child's reentry to dispel peer misunderstanding and fears. In order to avoid parent-child "power struggles" centering on homework, parents might be advised to obtain an after-school tutor; also, teachers should be advised to reduce homework assignments. As school adjustment represents a measure of child progress and success to many parents, family adjustment undoubtedly can be enhanced by appropriate educational planning and services.

SUMMARY AND FUTURE DIRECTIONS

In conclusion, the rapid onset and traumatic aftereffects associated with pediatric head injury place a tremendous burden on family members. Although children are more likely to survive traumatic head injury, they are at greater risk for long-term sequelae. Expressive language functions and capacity for future learning often are seriously compromised. Furthermore, children also are at risk to "grow into" cognitive deficits and psychiatric sequelae. In contrast to cognitive deficits, the incidence of psychiatric disorder appears more related to preinjury adjustment, age, and family characteristics. Unfortunately, there is no knowledge base to accurately predict outcome. The younger the child, the less information is known about long-term child and family adjustment. This is particularly problematic for family members who seek guidance in planning for the child's future and often are presented with contradictory professional opinions.

Families least equipped to handle a pediatric head injury are most likely to be victimized. These families have higher rates of psychosocial adversity ranging from poor education, low income, and crowded living conditions to parental pathology, marital discord, and divorce. Based on family response to other types of childhood disabilities and chronic diseases, the availability of social support and parental attitude toward the disability are potent predictors of family adjustment and should be addressed by the clinician. Siblings of the head-injured child—particularly the eldest or female—also are at risk for a variety of socioemotional problems. Unfortunately, the needs of siblings are seldom addressed by researchers or clinicians.

To work effectively with family members, clinicians should be sensitive to "stages" of adjustment, which parallel stages of adjustment to death. With respect to adults with head injury, the family typically experiences massive denial and shock, followed by periods of anger, guilt, and depression. Acceptance—an ultimate goal—may never be reached, depending upon family coping strategies.

As with any crisis, family members are at risk to develop maladaptive coping strategies and interactional patterns without appropriate clinical intervention and support. The clinician ultimately must function as educator, advocate, therapist, friend, and community networker (Waaland & Kreutzer, 1988). Families need assistance in avoiding patterns of isolation, client overprotection, unhealthy guilt, mutual blaming, and a "defeatist attitude" that often develop subsequent to head injury. Families are in particular need of education, practical services such as respite care and financial assistance, and community networking. Among other needs, support from extended family and community rank high. As the school represents the major rehabilitation facility for children, prompt, appropriate, and flexible educational programming also ranks high among family needs. Finally, the family requires continuity of services to include

prepared transition at every level of rehabilitation, long-term follow-up, and a full range of services. Needed services may range from home intervention specialists to specialized case managers trained to coordinate doctor visits, community services, referrals, and advocacy needs.

Unfortunately, much of our knowledge regarding pediatric head injury is based on generalizations from adult populations and clinician speculation rather than a research base. A number of areas clearly should be addressed in future investigations. These issues include the relationship between family adjustment and client outcome to: 1) preinjury risk factors, 2) developmental stage, 3) availability and type of support systems, and 4) family needs and how these needs change as a function of family and child developmental stage. It also is important to determine what cognitive, emotional, and behavioral problems are most problematic for family members. Lezak (1988) has eloquently summarized the impact of adult sequelae to head injury on family adjustment. However, clinicians do not have similar information to guide their interventions in childhood populations. In particular, problematic behaviors and family needs likely change developmentally and with time postinjury.

The ideal design for many of these questions is longitudinal. By following families over time, we can better understand the dynamic interplay among child and family life cycles with characteristics of the family preinjury and the injury itself. It is also critical to use research designs that account for the bidirectional relationship among family members; that is, not only how the head-injured child's behavior affects family functioning but also how the family affects the adjustment of the head-injured child and his or her siblings. It is hoped that future efforts will help us better serve families facing the trauma of pediatric head injury.

REFERENCES

Abidin, R.R. (1983). *Parenting Stress Index.* Charlottesville: University of Virginia.

Achenbach, T.M. (1981). *The Child Behavior Check-*

list. Burlington: University of Vermont, University Associates in Psychiatry.

Annegers, J.F. (1983). The epidemiology of head

trauma in children. In K. Shapiro (Ed.), *Pediatric head trauma* (pp. 1–10). New York: Futura Press.

Annegers, J.F., Grabow, J.D., Kurland, L.T., & Laws, E.R. (1980). The incidence, causes, and secular trends of brain injury in Olmsted County, Minnesota, 1935–1974. *Neurology, 30,* 912–919.

Bavolek, S. (1984). *Adult-Adolescent Parenting Inventory.* Schaumburg, IL: Family Development Associates.

Ben-Yishay, Y., & Diller, L. (1983). Cognitive remediation. In M. Rosenthal, E. Griffith, M. Bond, & D. Miller (Eds.), *Rehabilitation of the head injured adult* (pp. 367–380). Philadelphia: F.A. Davis.

Bishop, D.S., & Miller, I.W. (1988). Traumatic brain injury: Empirical family assessment techniques. *The Journal of Head Trauma Rehabilitation, 3,* 16–30.

Blacher, J. (1984). A dynamic perspective on the impact of a severely handicapped child on the family. In J. Blacher (Ed.), *Severely handicapped young children and their families: Research in review* (pp. 3–50). Orlando, FL: Academic Press.

Black, P., Blumer, D., Wellner, A.M., & Walker, A.E. (1971). The head injured child: Time course of recovery, with implications for rehabilitation. In *Proceedings of an International Symposium on Head Injuries.* Edinburgh, Scotland: Churchill Livingstone.

Boll, T.J. (1983). Minor head injury in children—Out of sight but not out of mind. *Journal of Clinical and Child Psychology, 12,* 74–80.

Brink, J.D., Garret, A.L., Hale, W.R., Woo-Sam, J., & Nickel, V.C. (1970). Recovery of motor and intellectual function in children sustaining severe head injuries. *Developmental Medicine Child Neurology, 12,* 565–571.

Bristol, M.M. (1984). Family resources and successful adaptation to autistic children. In E. Schopler & G.B. Meisbov (Eds.), *Issues in autism: Vol. III. The effects of autism on the family* (pp. 289–310). New York: Plenum.

Bristol, M.M., & Schopler, E. (1984). A developmental perspective on stress and coping in families of autistic children. In J. Blacher (Ed.), *Severely handicapped young children and their families: Research in review.* Orlando, FL: Academic Press.

Brooks, D.N., Campsie, L., Symington, C., et al. (1987). The effects of severe head injury upon patient and relative within seven years of injury. *Journal of Head Trauma Rehabilitation, 2,* 1–13.

Brown, G., Chadwick, O., Shaffer, D., Rutter, M., & Traub, M. (1981). A prospective study of children with head injuries: III. Psychiatric sequelae. *Psychological Medicine, 11,* 63–78.

Bruce, D.A., Raphaely, R.C., Goldberg, A.E., Zimmerman, R.A., Bilaniuk, L.T., Schult, L., & Kuhl, D.E. (1979). Pathophysiology: Treatment and outcome following severe head injury in children. *Child's Brain, 5,* 174–191.

Chadwick, O., Rutter, M., Brown, G., Shaffer, D., & Traub, M. (1981). A prospective study of children with head injuries: II. Cognitive sequelae. *Psychological Medicine, 11,* 49–61.

Chadwick, O., Rutter, M., Shaffer, D., & Shrout, P. (1981). A prospective study of children with head injuries: IV. Specific cognitive deficits. *Journal of Clinical Neuropsychology, 3,* 101–120.

Cleveland, D., & Miller, N. (1977). Attitudes and life commitments of older siblings of mentally retarded adults: An exploratory study. *Mental Retardation, 15,* 38–41.

Conder, & Conder (1988). *Paper presented at the 12th annual conference of the Postgraduate Course on Rehabilitation of the Brain Injured Adult and Child,* Williamsburg, VA.

Deaton, A.V. (1987). Behavioral change strategies for children and adolescents with severe brain injury. *Journal of Learning Disabilities, 20,* 581–589.

DeMyer, M.K., & Goldberg, P. (1983). Family needs of the autistic adolescent. In E. Schopler & G.B. Mesibov (Eds.), *Autism in adolescents and adults* (pp. 225–250). New York: Plenum.

Dennis, M., & Kohn, B. (1975). Comprehension of syntax in infantile hemiplegics after cerebral hemidecortication: Left hemisphere superiority. *Brain and Language, 2,* 472–482.

Epstein, N.B., Baldwin, L.M., & Bishop, D.S. (1983). The McMaster Family Assessment Device. *Journal of Marital and Family Therapy, 9*(2), 171–180.

Ewing-Cobbs, L., & Fletcher, J.M. (1987). Neuropsychological assessment of head injury in children. *Journal of Learning Disabilities, 20,* 526–535.

Ewing-Cobbs, L., Fletcher, J.M., & Levin, H.S. (1985). Neuropsychological sequelae following pediatric head injury. In M. Ylvisaker (Eds.), *Head injury rehabilitation: Children and adolescents* (pp. 71–90). San Diego, CA: College-Hill Press.

Ewing-Cobbs, L., Fletcher, J.M., & Levin, H.S. (1986, February). *Neuropsychologic functions following closed-head injury in infants and preschoolers.* Paper presented at the meeting of the International Neuropsychological Society, Denver, CO.

Farber, B. (1959). Effects of a severely mentally retarded child on family integration. *Monographs of the Society for Research in Child Development, 21.*

Field, J.H. (1976). *Epidemiology of head injury in England and Wales.* London: Her Majesty's Stationery Office.

Filley, C.M., Cranberg, M.D., Alexander, M.P., & Hart, E.J. (1987). Neurobehavioral outcome after closed head injury in childhood and adolescence. *Archives of Neurology, 44,* 194–198.

Flach, J., & Malmros, R. (1972). A long-term follow-up study of children with severe head injury. *Scandinavian Journal of Rehabilitation Medicine, 4,* 9–15.

Frankoski, R.F., Annegers, J.F., & Whitman, S.C. (1985). Epidemiological and descriptive studies: Part I. In D. Becker & J.J. Povlishock (Eds.), *Central nervous system trauma: Status report* (pp. 33–45). Bethesda, MD: National Institutes of Health, National Institute of Neurological and Communicative Disorder and Stroke.

Gardner, R.A. (1973). *The family book about minimal brain dysfunction.* New York: Jason Aronson.

Goldstein, F.C., & Levin, H.S. (1987). Epidemiology of pediatric closed head injury: Incidence, clinical characteristics, and risk factors. *Journal of Learning Disabilities, 20,* 518–525.

Graliker, B.V., Fishler, K., & Koch, R. (1962). Teenage reaction to a mentally retarded sibling. *American Journal of Mental Deficiency, 66,* 838–843.

Granger, R.D. (1983). A study of the effect of concepts of development, social support, and involvement in community interaction programs upon the stress experienced by mothers of handicapped children. Unpublished master's thesis. University of Illinois at Chicago.

Grossman, F.K. (1972). *Brothers and sisters of retarded children.* New York: Syracuse University Press.

Helm, D.T., & Kozloff, J.A. (1986). Research on parent training: Shortcomings and remedies. *Journal of Autism and Developmental Disorders, 16,* 1–22.

Jacobs, H.E. (in press). A rationale for family involvement in long-term traumatic head injury rehabilitation. In D.E. Tupper & K.D. Cicerone (Eds.), *The neuropsychology of everyday life.* Boston: Klewer Academic Publishing.

Jennett, B., & Teasdale, G. (1981). *Management of head injuries.* Philadelphia: F.A. Davis.

Kalsbeek, W.D., McLaurin, R.L., Harris, B.S., & Miller, J.D. (1980). The national head injury and spinal cord injury survey: Major findings. *Journal of Neurosurgery, 53,* S19–S31.

Klauber, M.R., Barrett-Connor, E., Marshall, L.F., & Bowers, S.A. (1981). The epidemiology of head injury: A prospective study of an entire community—San Diego County 1978. *American Journal of Epidemiology, 113,* 500–509.

Klonoff, H. (1971). Head injuries in children: Predisposing factors, accident conditions, and sequelae. *American Journal of Public Health, 61,* 2405–2417.

Klonoff, H., & Paris, R. (1974). Immediate, short-term, and residual effects of acute head injuries in children: Neuropsychological and neurological correlates. In R.M. Reitan & C.A. Davidson (Eds.), *Clinical neuropsychology: Current status and applications* (pp. 179–210). New York: Halstead Press.

Kreutzer, J.K., Waaland, P.K., & Camplair, P. (1988). *Family Needs Questionnaire.* Richmond: Medical College of Virginia, Rehabilitation Research and Training Center on Severe Traumatic Brain Injury.

Kubler-Ross, E. (1969). *On death and dying.* New York: Macmillan.

Lange-Cosack, H., Wider, B., Schlesner, H., Grumme, T., & Kubicki, S. (1979). Prognosis of brain injuries in young children (one until five years of age). *Neuropaediatrie, 10,* 105–127.

Levin, H.S., Benton, A.L., & Grossman, R.G. (1982). *Neurobehavioral consequences of closed head injury.* New York: Oxford University Press.

Levin, H.S., & Eisenberg, H.M. (1979). Neuropsychological outcome of closed head injury in children and adolescents. *Child's Brain, 5,* 281–292.

Lezak, M.D. (1978). Living with the characteriologically altered brain injured patient. *Journal of Clinical Psychiatry, 39,* 592–598.

Lezak, M.D. (1986). Psychological implications of traumatic brain damage for the patient's family. *Rehabilitation Psychology, 31,* 241–250.

Lezak, M.D. (1988). Brain damage is a family affair. *Journal of Clinical and Experimental Neuropsychology, 10,* 111–123.

Livingston, M.G., & Brooks, D.N. (1988). The burden on families of the brain injured: A review. *The Journal of Head Trauma Rehabilitation, 3,* 6–15.

Marcus, L.M. (1984). Coping with burnout. In E. Schopler & G.B. Mesbov (Eds.), *The effects of autism on the family* (pp. 311–326). New York: Plenum.

Mauss-Clum, N., & Ryan, M. (1981). Brain injury and the family. *Journal of Neurosurgical Nursing, 13,* 165–169.

McCubbin, H., Patterson, J., & Wilson, L. (1981). Family inventory of life events and changes. In H. McCubbin & J. Patterson (Eds.), *Family stress, resources, and coping: Tools for research, education, and clinical intervention.* St. Paul: University of Minnesota Press.

McHale, S.M., Simeonsson, R.J., & Sloan, J.L. (1984). Children with handicapped brothers and sisters. In E. Schopler & G. Mesibov (Eds.), *The effects of autism on the family.* New York: Plenum.

McKinney, B., & Petersen, R.A. (1987). Predictors of stress in parents of developmentally disabled children. *Journal of Pediatric Psychology, 12,* 133–150.

McLean, A., Temkin, N.R., Dikmen, S., & Wyler, A.R. (1983). The behavioral sequelae of head injury. *Journal of Clinical Neuropsychology, 5,* 361–376.

Mink, I.T., Nihira, K., & Meyers, C.E. (1981, August). *Stressful life events in families with retarded children.* Paper presented at the meeting of the American Psychological Association, Los Angeles.

Minuchin, S. (1984). *Families and family therapy.* Cambridge, MA: Harvard University Press.

Molter, N.C. (1979). Needs of relatives of critically ill patients: A descriptive study. *Heart & Lung, 8,* 332–337.

Morgan, S.B. (1988). The autistic child and family functioning: A developmental–family systems perspective. *Journal of Autism and Developmental Disorders, 2,* 263–280.

Nihira, K., Mink, I.T., & Meyers, C.E. (1981). Relationship between home environment and school adjustment of TMR children. *American Journal of Mental Deficiency, 86,* 8–15.

Norris, L.O.,& Grove, S.K. (1986). Investigation of selected psychosocial needs of family members of critically ill adult patients. *Heart & Lung, 15,* 194–199.

O'Grady, D., & Metz, J.R. (1987). Resilience in children at high risk for psychological disorder. *Journal of Pediatric Psychology, 12,* 3–23.

Olson, D.H., Portner, J., & Lavee, Y. (1985). *FACES-III: Family Adaptability and Cohesion Evaluation Scales.* St. Paul: University of Minnesota, Family Social Science.

Olson, D.H., Russell, C.S., & Sprenkle, D.H. (1983). Circumplex model of marital and family systems: Theoretical update. *Family Process, 22,* 69–83.

Polinko, P.R., Barin, J.J., Leger, D., & Bachman, K.M. (1985). Working with the family. In M. Ylvisaker (Ed.), *Head injury rehabilitation* (pp. 91–116). San Diego: College-Hill Press.

Powell, D. (1979). Family-environment relations and early child rearing: The role of social networks and neighborhoods. *Journal of Research in Development and Education, 13,* 1–11.

Powell, T.H., & Ogle, P.A. (1985). *Brothers & sisters-A special part of exceptional families.* Baltimore: Paul H. Brookes Publishing Co.

Prigatano, G.P. (1987). Psychiatric aspects of head injury: Problem areas and suggested guidelines for research. *BNI Quarterly, 3,* 2–8.

Procidano, M.E., & Heller, K. (1983). Measures of perceived social support from friends and from family: Three validation studies. *American Journal of Community Psychology, 11,* 1–24.

Rasmussen, T., & Milner, B. (1977). The role of early left-brain injury in determining lateralization of cerebral functions. *Annals of the New York Academy of Sciences, 29,* 355–369.

Rivera, F.P., & Mueller, B.A. (1986). The epidemiology and prevention of pediatric head injury. *Journal of Head Trauma Rehabilitation, 1,* 7–15.

Rogers, P.M., & Kreutzer, J.S. (1984). Family crises following head injury: A network intervention strategy. *Journal of Neurosurgical Nursing, 16,* 343–346.

Romano, M. (1974). Family response to traumatic head injury. *Scandinavian Journal of Rehabilitation Medicine, 6,* 1–4.

Rosen, C.D., & Gerring, J.P. (1986). *Head trauma: Educational reintegration.* San Diego: College-Hill Press.

Rosenthal, M., & Young, T. (1988). Effective family intervention after traumatic brain injury: Theory and practice. *The Journal of Head Trauma Rehabilitation, 3,* 42–50.

Rune, V. (1970). Acute head injuries in children. *Acta Paediatrica Scandinavica,* (Suppl. 209).

Rutter, M., Chadwick, O., & Shaffer, D. (1983). Head injury. In M. Rutter (Ed.), *Developmental neuropsychiatry* (pp. 83–111). New York: Guilford Press.

Rutter, M., Chadwick, O., Shaffer, D., & Brown, G. (1980). A prospective study of children with head injuries: I. Design and methods. *Psychological Medicine, 10,* 633–645.

Savage, R.C. (1987). Educational issues for the head-injured adolescent and young adult. *Journal of Head Trauma Rehabilitation, 2,* 1–10.

Shapiro, B. (1983). Informational interviews. *Sibling Information Network Newsletter, 2,* 5.

Sullivan, R.C. (1979). Siblings of autistic children. *Journal of Autism and Developmental Disorders, 9,* 287–298.

Telzrow, C.F. (1987). Management of academic and educational problems in head injury. *Journal of Learning Disabilities, 20,* 536–545.

Trevino, F. (1979). Siblings of handicapped children: Identifying those at risk. *Social Casework, 60,* 488–493.

Turnbull, A.P., & Blacher-Dixon, J. (1980). Preschool mainstreaming: Impact on parents. In J.J. Gallagher (Ed.), *New directions for exceptional children* (Vol. 1.). San Francisco: Jossey-Bass.

Waaland, P.K., & Kreutzer, J.S. (1988). Family response to childhood traumatic brain injury. *Journal of Head Trauma Rehabilitation, 3,* 51–63.

Weeks, G.R., & L'Abate, L. (1982). *Paradoxical psychotherapy: Theory and practice with individuals, couples, and families.* New York: Brunner/Mazel.

Weintraub, M., Brooks, J., & Lewis, M. (1977). The social network: A reconsideration of the concept of attachment. *Human Development, 20,* 31–47.

Wright, J.S., Granger, R.D., & Sameroff, A.J. (1984). Parental acceptance and developmental handicap. In J. Blacher (Ed.), *Severely handicapped young children and their families: Research in review.* Orlando, FL: Academic Press.

CHAPTER 16

A Practical Guide to Family Intervention following Adult Traumatic Brain Injury

Jeffrey S. Kreutzer, Nathan D. Zasler,
Patricia Stiles Camplair, and Bruce E. Leininger

The purpose of this chapter is to provide clinicians with an overview of interventions intended to enhance family adaptation to adult traumatic brain injury. Family interventions can assume many forms and can be implemented by a variety of persons in different roles. Despite variation in treatment strategies the goals for most families are similar. The goals of family intervention strategies following adult traumatic brain injury are to improve the emotional well-being of individual family members and the functioning of the family unit. Educated and emotionally stable families provide the injured individual with appropriate support and participate fully as members of the rehabilitation team.

Community integration presents a new series of formidable challenges to families and persons with traumatic brain injury. One must consider that discharge from an acute rehabilitation facility often follows a plateau in progress that may lead to increased pessimism over prospects for complete recovery. Lezak (1986) has suggested that a period of depression often follows periods of minimal improvement. Following stabilization and discharge, the family may first begin to appreciate that the head-injured person's problems are likely to be long term, if not permanent. Simultaneously, support provided

by the acute care rehabilitation team is withdrawn—which leads to apprehension. Many communities lack transitional living, outpatient rehabilitation, day rehabilitation, and vocational rehabilitation services. Family members who are able to maintain work, family, and household responsibilities while the person with traumatic brain injury was provided full-time care during acute rehabilitation must now provide for the individual's needs.

Following discharge, insurance coverage for rehabilitation may be exhausted or may not include outpatient services. Families may have to devote considerable time to seeking, visiting, and evaluating treatment facilities. In some cases, services may be too far away or simply unavailable within a day's traveling distance. In other cases, lengthy daily travel may be required to allow the person with traumatic brain injury to participate in outpatient rehabilitation services on a regular basis. Family members providing transportation may need to give up their jobs or reduce work hours, which exacerbates financial stresses.

The Jacobs (1988) investigation of the long-term impact of severe head injury helped clarify the sources and nature of stresses on families. One hundred forty-two family members of per-

This work was partly supported by Grants #H133B80029 and #G0087C0219 from the National Institute on Disability and Rehabilitation Research, United States Department of Education.

sons with severe head injury who were more than 1 year postinjury were interviewed. In more than one third of all cases, the injured person required constant supervision. One family member's income was typically sacrificed, yielding an average annual family income loss of $28,000. In nearly one third of the cases, family members reported that most or all of their financial resources were exhausted by medical bill payments.

The work of epidemiological and family researchers (e.g., Frankowski, Annegers, & Whitman, 1985; Kurtzke, 1982) and clinical experience has helped in characterizing the head injury population and their caregivers. Most persons with traumatic brain injury are males in their 20s. A typical case may involve an individual who moved away from his family's residence prior to injury. The individual probably held a job or attended school. He may have married and fathered children who were likely to be less than 5 or 6 years old at the time of his injury. Following the injury, the individual was discharged from the acute rehabilitation setting to live with his parents or spouse. Caregivers, usually spouses and parents, typically bear the burden of providing financial support and transportation to and from therapies, work, and appointments with physicians. The family unit living in the same household may consist of an adult with head injury, his mother and father, and occasionally other siblings. In other cases, a household may consist of the person with brain injury, his spouse, and their children. Otherwise, the injured person may live with unrelated persons who assume caregiving responsibilities (e.g., girlfriend, friends).

For purposes of providing an organizational framework the authors of this chapter have chosen to describe seven approaches to community intervention intended to benefit families of persons with traumatic brain injury. Discussion focuses on family education, support groups, networking, advocacy, family therapy, marital therapy, and sexual counseling. Many families will require several different types of intervention simultaneously. Furthermore, family intervention is undoubtedly a dynamic process that ideally conforms to the needs of the person with traumatic brain injury and his or her family.

Changes in family conflicts and coping skills often become apparent when new rehabilitation services are initiated, treatments are completed, and third-party coverage changes. In addition, the authors acknowledge there is some overlap between family intervention strategies. However, overlap is beneficial and inevitable given that family, professional, and community support teams ideally share the responsibility of attaining optimal outcome.

STRUCTURED APPROACHES TO FAMILY INTERVENTION

Family Education

Family education focuses on providing selected family members with information about traumatic brain injury and specific information about the injured individual. Information concerning brain injury includes material about personality, intellectual, psychomotor, perceptual, and neurological changes following injury. Families should also be educated about available types of rehabilitation therapies, support and advocacy groups, and the costs of available treatments. Research by Leske (1986), Norris and Grove (1986), and Molter (1979) has established that the need for information pertaining to the effects of injury or illness ranks among the highest needs of family members. Education provides reassurance to family members who may be confused and overwhelmed. Systematic educational efforts also permit families to develop reasonable expectations about rehabilitation and improvement, and allow them to become more effective members of the rehabilitation team.

There are various means of presenting information to families. Eisner and Kreutzer (1988) have suggested that clinicians develop a library of resource materials. Potential resources include articles from professional journals in addition to booklets written by professionals especially for family members and laypersons. Materials pertaining to traumatic brain injury should be carefully selected and made available based on the family's specific needs. Care should be taken to eliminate materials that require a formal medical education. In appropriate cases, family members may be encouraged to attend professional meetings and conferences that focus on traumatic brain injury. Unfortunately, many families do not have a sufficient educational background to benefit from these meetings, and may find the information presented confusing or overwhelming. Clinicians are also encouraged to network with local head injury support groups including those affiliated with the National Head Injury Foundation. Local support groups often have libraries of information selected for family members, and sponsor educational meetings and conferences targeted to family audiences.

The National Head Injury Foundation has established a library of educational materials and has developed a catalog (National Head Injury Foundation, 1988). Family members should be encouraged to review the catalog and purchase relevant materials. Prices for written information typically range from $1.50 to $7.50, which covers the cost of printing, mailing, and handling. Videotape and audiotape materials, which in many cases were produced for family members, are also available. Furthermore, the four Rehabilitation Research and Training Centers on Traumatic Brain Injury supported by the National Institute on Disability and Rehabilitation Research each have a mission to provide training as well as to establish national clearinghouses of information on traumatic brain injury (Thomas, 1988). The research and training centers are in the development phase, having been funded for 5-year periods beginning in early 1988. These centers will provide educational information to both family members and professionals.

Over the course of acute rehabilitation, information on the head-injured person's status, prognosis, and treatment is often conveyed to family members during rehabilitation team meetings. Ideally, family members are encouraged to participate and ask questions. Responses to questions should be provided in understandable terms. Outside team meetings, family members may also receive information from specific team members either designated by the staff or selected by the family.

Caution is urged over the assumption that family members retain relevant facts beyond the time of discharge. In many cases, stresses on the family interfere with information storage. Addi-

tionally, because of denial or preoccupation with immediate therapeutic issues, family members may not be willing or able to fully retain information relevant to long-term disability. In fact, effective family education often requires relatively greater effort following discharge from acute rehabilitation. For example, communication with the family is typically more difficult unless the person with traumatic brain injury is a participant in an organized rehabilitation program housed under one roof. Physical distance and the lack of outpatient programs, especially in rural communities, disrupt the process of regularly providing information in an integrated format.

Lack of coordinated service delivery following discharge from acute rehabilitation can be especially traumatic to the family and the head-injured individual, and can result in at least partial loss of gains realized during inpatient hospitalization. Additionally, the absence of a coordinated team effort to educate families about the course of therapy and the head-injured person's prognosis contributes to anxiety among family members. For example, therapists in different outpatient settings may offer differing opinions about the client's prognosis and appropriate treatment options. A case management approach is therefore recommended to reduce family anxieties yielding overall benefits in rehabilitation progress. If designated case managers are unavailable, one of the professionals providing outpatient services should agree to assume a case management role. This professional should facilitate communication among other professionals providing services as well as communication between professionals and family members. The case manager is also encouraged to organize outpatient team meetings where feasible. Team meetings can especially help professionals in different settings communicate efficiently, develop an integrated treatment plan, and present a unified impression of the client's needs, goals, and prognosis.

In addition to team meetings, individual professionals are also encouraged to schedule regular meetings that include family members to provide feedback regarding progress. In every case, jargon should be avoided and information should be presented in lay terms. The use of professional jargon contributes to family members' feelings of being overwhelmed, and can also create feelings of distrust, confusion, and lack of confidence in professionals.

Family Support Groups

Family support groups provide opportunities for emotional support, education, and social networking. Groups are typically composed of family members of persons with brain injury; however, participants often include extended and immediate family. Occasionally, persons with brain injury also participate. Rehabilitation professionals are often involved in starting support groups because of their knowledge of group dynamics and head injury. The formal role of professionals often diminishes over time as family members develop a sense of kinship and the group process gains inertia and proceeds in an orderly fashion.

There are several unique characteristics of family support groups. First, experienced family members have benefited from extensive trial-and-error problem solving, professional guidance, and information gathering. The knowledge they can share with less experienced family members is invaluable, and there is no substitute for actual experience. Families readily learn from storytelling and sharing experiences. Second, group problem-solving processes may elicit less defensiveness than family or individual psychotherapy sessions directed by professionals. Individuals often respond more positively to confrontation directed by other families rather than by professionals. Family members are often responsive to advice from others who "really know what it feels like." Third, the group can accommodate many different personal styles. The anxious, talkative individual who exercises some restraint can often find a patient audience. Those who choose to say little can learn a great deal by listening to others. Finally, family support groups offer an important beginning for social relationships, which evolve naturally through the expression of similar concerns and interests. Support groups help compensate for the loss of social contact that commonly follows traumatic brain injury.

Professionals have a unique and valuable role as educators and facilitators in family support groups. Professionals have clinical and academic knowledge that can be imparted to family members. Questions about the effects of injury, medications, and rehabilitation therapies often arise and can be readily addressed. Special training in group processes and dynamics helps professionals assume roles as facilitators. For example, an individual who dominates group discussion may need assertive feedback. Soliciting opinions from less active group members helps remedy domination. In some cases, family members need to be told that each situation is unique. Caution about expecting too little or too much based on another individual's experience may need to be expressed. A timid family member with pressing problems may benefit from encouragement to speak up. Group meetings during which professionals can comfortably relax while families appropriately address issues of mutual concern often yield the most benefits.

There are differing opinions over whether persons with brain injury should participate in the same group as family members. Those who believe in separating the two groups emphasize that persons with brain injury and family members confront very different issues. Some clinicians argue that frequently recurring conflicts create an undesirable atmosphere of group tension. Persons with brain injury may complain about overprotectiveness and insensitivity. Family members may complain about rebelliousness, uncooperativeness, poor self-awareness, and aggressiveness. Joint groups may affect participants' willingness to be open and honest, which reduces the benefits of group problem solving.

Others argue that groups that combine persons with head injury and family members provide a unique opportunity to deal actively with conflicts in a supportive and constructive environment that allows simulation of conflicts that occur at home. The person with head injury and family each present their side. Comments offered by other injured persons and family members contribute to presentation of a balanced set of opinions. Families with good problem-solving skills can serve as appropriate models. Effective problem solvers often convey feelings of hope that ultimately serve to reduce feelings of helplessness among group members.

Family support groups have many distinct advantages over other clinical techniques. Group members often leave feeling that they have given as much as they have received. Helping others is clearly a positive experience. Those who apologize for having focused too much on themselves are most often responded to with reassurance and an invitation to help others at a later date. Additionally, financially stressed families often express concern over the cost of professional services. There is usually no charge for participating in family support groups. One might argue that the weekly or biweekly format of support groups does not permit timely assistance in crisis situations. However, support group members frequently contact each other outside formal meetings. Often, an external social and emotional support network evolves that may be available 24 hours a day, 7 days a week.

Family Networking

Family networking is a process of developing the extended family and social system to share the burden of care for clients and provide mutual support. Research by Jacobs (1988), Mauss-Clum and Ryan (1981), and Kozloff (1987) has strongly underscored the need to actively solicit support from extended social systems for persons with traumatic brain injury and their families. Kozloff reported that following head injury social network density increases and the size of social networks diminishes. In other words, persons with head injury have to depend on fewer people for greater social support relative to preinjury. The number and quality of friends may be reduced, which leaves the burden of support primarily on the immediate family. Lezak (1978) has also commented that families often become socially isolated. She reported frequent conflicts between immediate and extended family members over how to best care for the individual with head injury. Disagreements pertaining to the head-injured person's care and guilt about overburdening relatives increase the family's reluctance to solicit help from others.

More than a decade ago, Speck and Attneave (1973) and Rueveni (1979) began developing social network interventions for families of persons with mental illness including schizophrenia and severe depression. The primary purpose of intervention was to create an effective system that could be mobilized to help the immediate family avoid crises, and to intervene collectively when unavoidable crises occurred. Immediate and extended family, friends, co-workers, and acquaintances were invited to a series of meetings focused on identifying current and potential problems, possible solutions, and means of implementing effective strategies. The role of professional facilitators diminished over time during these meetings and the group functioned with increasing autonomy. Speck and Atteneave described the development of a "network effect." The group problem-solving process helped establish a sense of cohesion, kinship, and willingness to share responsibility.

Rogers and Kreutzer (1984) described and illustrated the application of social network strategies for persons with traumatic brain injury and their families. Social network groups were adapted to include rehabilitation professionals and family members of other injured persons as well as immediate family, extended family, coworkers, and acquaintances. Social networking entails a series of group meetings that usually begin with introductions, descriptions of relationships, and education into the effects of the injury. In addition to problem solving over potential problems, the primary tasks include development and maintenance of an extended support system. Furthermore, a grieving process may occur during which members describe their memories of the person prior to his or her injury in contrast to the present character.

Immediate family members are encouraged to discuss their guilt about placing an unreasonable burden on others. Network members are encouraged to support the immediate family and to be assertive in responding to requests for support. Soliciting agreement that such feelings will be discussed openly and assertively provides relief from guilt for the immediate family. Respite care can sometimes be equitably shared among several families in the network. Inevitably, coordinating and sharing group resources provides a more powerful support structure than several individuals working independently.

Two to three meetings may be required to establish the "network effect." After the initial meetings a group meeting every 3–6 months helps maintain the community system. As old problems are solved, new problems arise. Problems often can be anticipated and addressed proactively. More frequent meetings and subgroup gatherings may be necessary during crises. The difficulties of arranging meetings are nominal given the value of extended networks in providing respite and preserving the often vulnerable emotional health of primary caregivers.

Family Advocacy

Family advocacy entails working with families to help them take full advantage of existing community resources, to modify existing resources to better meet the needs of persons with head injury, and to develop needed services. The National Head Injury foundation and local support groups have become increasingly active in advocacy efforts. Advocacy is also provided by rehabilitation professionals including social workers, psychologists, and case managers.

Advocacy for new services typically proceeds in a series of steps. First, a high priority service need is identified. Second, the advocate attempts to locate an existing service delivery system that, if modified, could meet the identified need. The advocate may provide assistance in the planning and implementation of appropriate modifications. If development of a new service delivery system is required, the advocate would help plan the system to best meet the needs of the persons with head injury. Following system development, an assessment process takes place to establish that the plan was properly implemented and to assess whether additional changes for optimal effectiveness are required. Additionally, advocates work to demonstrate cost-effectiveness in attempts to secure funding by third-party payers and in the development and modification of service delivery systems.

More recently, family advocacy has focused on developing therapies to enhance community integration following discharge from acute rehabilitation. For example, many communities do not offer a complete spectrum of outpatient rehabilitation services. If appropriate services cannot be found, family members spend considerable time supervising the head-injured individual at home (Jacobs, 1988). Otherwise,

family members may devote their time to transporting the individual with brain injury to and from distant rehabilitation facilities and waiting on site during therapy. Improved cost-effectiveness could be established by having experienced head injury consultants educate therapists serving other disabilities. Teaching other professionals about the special needs of persons with head injury allows for the appropriate adaptation of services that might not be otherwise available.

Even when appropriate services exist in the community, their availability may be limited by the unwillingness of insurance companies or government agencies to provide coverage for necessary services. Rehabilitation professionals may convince third-party payers to cover services through the use of logic and carefully prepared arguments. The most convincing arguments usually are based on the fact that providing services will likely reduce long-term costs related to the illness. (See Chapter 9, this volume, for a discussion of how to obtain funding for day rehabilitation.)

The supported employment model of vocational rehabilitation has illustrated the benefits of family advocacy to help persons with head injury return to the work force (Wehman et al., 1988; Wehman et al., 1989). Supported employment is a comprehensive, cost-effective service delivery model that places primary emphasis on helping persons with traumatic brain injury find and maintain competitive employment. Little time is devoted to preplacement activities, whereas considerable emphasis is placed on worksite intervention and long-term monitoring. Wehman and colleagues have found that success can be enhanced substantially by helping families obtain outpatient rehabilitation services. Recreational, substance abuse, and social programs were developed in the community and within the vocational program to supplement employment services. Family therapy, marital therapy, and family support groups services were also provided. Initial program benefits have included reducing family stresses, providing respite, and allowing family members to work outside the home instead of serving as full-time caregivers.

Professionals are encouraged to be knowledgeable about rehabilitation services available within and outside their communities. Many family members have questions about the availability and suitability of rehabilitation resources. Horror stories or unmitigated praise from other families contribute to confusion and anxiety. Family intervention reasonably includes helping families obtain additional information about resources and helping them make informed decisions about treatment choices. Additionally, families may need reassurance about their decisions given the variability in treatment approaches within the same community and even within the same discipline. Finding additional resources helps provide respite, and reduces feelings of helplessness and being overwhelmed. Identifying social and recreational activities may be at least as important as finding resources for traditional rehabilitation services during community integration.

Although advocacy is essential for all families and persons with head injury in the process of community integration, it may be most crucial for children with traumatic brain injury (Waaland & Kreutzer, 1988). Although school systems are required by law to provide an appropriate education, academic resources are often limited. Furthermore, many school systems have limited experience and are ignorant of the special needs of children with head injury. Professionals and support groups can be helpful in several ways. First, receptive school systems may agree to or request a series of in-service programs or other educational presentations for teachers about head injury. Second, families who are having problems with school systems can benefit from networking with other families who have successfully negotiated educational services. Third, knowledgeable and experienced rehabilitation professionals can help in the development of appropriate individualized education programs (IEPs). Their participation is often reassuring to families who have concerns about the adequacy of offered academic services. Relative to school personnel, families are more likely to view head injury professionals as fair and objective. Fourth, the combined efforts of rehabilitation professionals and support groups may be necessary to pressure reluctant school personnel to provide appropriate services. However, cau-

tion should be exercised in criticizing the school administration. Their intentions are usually good despite their apparent aim to limit requested services.

Family Therapy

Family therapy focuses on the entire family unit, which includes the person with traumatic brain injury and his or her immediate family. Extended family members may be involved in therapeutic efforts depending on the strength of their relationship with the head-injured individual and frequency of contact. A primary assumption underlying family therapy is that the family is an interactive system (Satir, 1972; Terkelsen, 1980). Accordingly, changes in one element of the system necessarily result in changes in other members within the system. A second assumption is that families develop particular behavior patterns. The therapist initially works to identify adaptive and maladaptive behavior patterns. The ultimate goal is to increase the frequency of adaptive behaviors and minimize or eliminate maladaptive behaviors. This section discusses the application of family therapy techniques to families of persons with traumatic brain injury to facilitate community integration.

Therapy is appropriate for nearly all families of persons with traumatic brain injury and helps reduce feelings of grief, loss, and helplessness. Therapeutic goals may also include ongoing education, and improved affect, problem solving, communication, and cohesiveness. Family roles and responsibilities are necessarily shifted as the head-injured person's abilities and psychological status change. Therapists can help negotiate and equitably reassign responsibilities previously assumed by the injured family member. Injury-related stresses also contribute to anxiety and conflict among family members. Consequently, stress reduction and rebuilding the family into an effective team are critical goals. Therapy services are available through psychologists, social workers, and rehabilitation counselors.

During the therapeutic process, family members express grief, which stems from the realization that the injured person has suffered

permanent changes. Personality changes following brain injury are common and often the most
distressing (Lezak, 1978). In many cases, families struggle with ignorance regarding the long-
term effects of injury, with hopes that the injured
person will return to normal, with unfounded
beliefs that the effects of injury are only temporary, and with fears that disabilities will be permanent or perhaps even progressive and fatal.

Unfortunately, feelings of grief, fear, and
exhaustion are complicated by frustrations arising from the lack of community services. The
development of rehabilitation programs for community integration has seriously lagged behind
the development of acute rehabilitation and neurosurgical intervention. Frustrations occasionally are inappropriately directed at service providers, particularly when providers are unable to
offer long-term solutions to chronic problems.
Fortunately, family therapy provides a forum for
constructive discussion of frustrations. Initially,
therapists can encourage family members to reflect on the source of their negative and conflicting feelings. Concurrently, clinicians should
take an active problem-solving approach aimed
at the family's greatest needs.

Family members may assume personal responsibility for their inability to find or pay for
services, or for the head-injured person's lack of
progress. Clinicians should help family members acknowledge their inherently human limitations in meeting the brain-injured individual's
needs. Active approaches include seeking additional sources of funding and service providers
inside or outside the home community. Therapists and family members may offer to work with
community agencies serving other disabilities to
adapt services to accommodate the special needs
of those with head injury. If active approaches
fail, families should be encouraged to temporarily suspend their search for services or support. In the meantime, patience, acceptance, and
reassurance that they have done all that is hu-
manly possible may remain as the only constructive alternative. Sensitive therapists should be
especially generous in praising family members
for their diligent efforts even though their attempts at problem solving may fail.

Clinicians with prior experience in a mental
health clinic or in outpatient psychiatric settings
will find the process of working with families of
persons with head injury to be different in at least
four major ways. First, many families in mental
health settings are self-referred. In the case of
traumatic brain injury, families are often recommended for therapy or occasionally pressured
into therapy by rehabilitation professionals. Referrals for families of persons with brain injury
are often made routinely with the concepts of
proactive intervention and prevention in mind.
Consequently, the family's initial confusion
about the need for referral and resistance to participate in therapy may be relatively great. Second, in nearly every case, family problems arise
partly from loss and grieving. Third, relative to
mental health problems, head injury is a recent
phenomenon. Within the last 10–15 years, improved medical care has contributed to significantly higher survival rates from severe injuries.
Consequently, the brain injury field has many
more unexplored avenues, unproven therapies,
and unanswered questions than the mental health
field. Fourth, repeated confrontation of immediate family members is rarely appropriate. Families who are unwilling to accept recommendations or evaluation results should be responded
to with patience, reassurance, and education.
Confrontation simply increases stress levels and
distrust for professionals, and further diminishes
the likelihood of a desirable outcome.

Despite difficulties in scheduling sessions
convenient to all parties, family intervention has
a number of distinct advantages over marital or
individual therapy. In regard to assessment,
bringing the family together allows for the process of enactment (Minuchin, 1974). Enactment
refers to the fact that family conflicts and maladaptive interactions are often simulated in the
therapeutic setting. The therapist is afforded the
unique opportunity to observe actions and reactions among family members that likely parallel
processes in the home environment. Family intervention provides an opportunity for all family
members to present their perspective on the
causes and solutions to problems. Furthermore,
objectivity is increased by soliciting views from

each family member. Participation of the whole family enables the clinician to help the family develop a sense of mutual ownership for problems. Efforts to cast blame and scapegoat can be identified and actively discouraged.

Ideally, family therapy should initially include all family members who live with the head-injured person and extended family members who are actively involved in caregiving. Children often perceive that their needs have been neglected following injury to another family member. The family session provides children with an opportunity to be reassured that their needs are important and they are still loved. Children should be actively encouraged to ask questions and their level of understanding should be assessed. In most cases, they have difficulty understanding and accepting the brain-injured person's characteriological changes. Unusual shifts in family roles and responsibilities contribute to children's confusion. Unfortunately, they are prone to blame themselves for negatively perceived changes. For example, aggressive or inappropriate behavior directed by the person with head injury toward children may contribute to development of poor self-esteem and diminished self-worth. Dislike and avoidance may replace love and affection if the injured family member displays negative personality attributes, especially irritability, aggressiveness, and frequent temper outbursts. Therapy provides a unique opportunity for children to be educated about the effects of injury and to express their negative feelings in a safe environment.

Family therapy may be most necessary in families of divorce, especially in cases of childhood injury. Divorce frequently follows a lengthy period of marital conflict. The conflict stresses children and other members of the extended family. Parents and other family members often have difficulty giving up negative feelings toward one another even years after the final decree is signed. Establishment of new relationships for former spouses frequently adds to jealousy and conflict. Unfortunately, the head-injured child is often the victim of postdivorce animosities. Anger may surface in the form of arguments over appropriate rehabilitation and

caregiving. Parents may disagree about the child's ability to resume responsibility. For example, one parent may allow the child to drive against a professional's advice. The child may view that parent more positively than the parent who enforces the professional's recommendations. In cases where the injured child is harmed by conflicts between divorced parents the therapist may require both parents and their new partners to negotiate and develop consistent child-rearing approaches. The skilled clinician can help divorced couples recognize their animosities toward one another and enable them to become more sensitive to the harm their animosities may be causing. Parents ultimately state that their intentions are to do what is best for their child. The therapist must use these stated intentions to bring about agreement between feuding parties.

Clinicians should keep in mind that disputes over child-rearing practices may also exist in families with intact marriages. Stresses on marital systems may increase antagonism between spouses, and, again, the child with head injury may ultimately be the victim. Intervention strategies in this situation are nearly identical to the situation involving divorced family members. It is hoped that proactive intervention will help families remain intact and thus avoid problems arising from divorce and dissolution.

Furthermore, family members should be encouraged to keep in mind that conflicts are not entirely avoidable. They are a natural part of all relationships and provide a valuable opportunity to develop communication and negotiation skills. Belief on the part of family members that all conflicts are avoidable and destructive will only contribute to stresses and paradoxically increase the likelihood of additional conflicts. Therefore, a primarily role of clinicians is to help families develop constructive conflict resolution strategies.

Family support and communication systems inevitably are compromised by the many long-term stresses, changes, and frustrations following traumatic brain injury. Gordon (1975) has described the "no-lose" method of resolving family conflict that involves a six-step process.

First, conflicts should be identified and defined. Second, the family participates in generating potential alternatives for problem resolution. Third, the pros and cons of each solution are discussed. Fourth, the best solution is chosen. Fifth, specific strategies for implementing the solution are applied. Finally, the family evaluates whether the solution was effective. If the solution is not entirely effective, a return to earlier steps is indicated. Such structured problem-solving techniques have been proven effective in a variety of situations and have been used extensively by practitioners of behavior therapy (Goldfried & Davison, 1976).

Marital Therapy

Marital therapy focuses on the marital dyad. Many of the problems and techniques applicable for treatment of family problems are relevant to marital therapy. In circumstances where scheduling problems, severe family conflict, or problems of marital intimacy exist, the therapist may choose to work with the couple rather than the family unit. Additionally, marital therapy techniques are relevant to unmarried couples living together or intimate couples living apart. Services are typically provided by licensed professionals such as psychologists, psychiatrists, and social workers.

Jackson (1972) has provided a useful framework for analysis of marital problems. Marriage has four characteristics, in addition to sexual aspects, that may be affected by the occurrence of traumatic brain injury. First, although individuals may be driven to marriage partly by the need to conform, marriage is a voluntary relationship. Second, marriage is intended to be lifelong, as denoted by the vow "Till death do us part." Third, marriage is primarily an exclusive relationship in which both partners primarily depend on one another and are relatively independent of others. Couples usually work to develop a marital unit that in many ways is independent from their families of origin. Fourth, marriage is goal oriented, characterized by assignment and sharing of tasks that vary depending on family composition. Furthermore, Jackson has stated that regardless of selected roles, marriage

evolves as a negotiated relationship between two interactive individuals.

The reader is asked to consider the situation in which the person with the head injury is the husband. The wife of a head-injured husband is often denied the comfort and resources of a previously supportive partner. Wives often report that their injured husband has emotionally regressed and acts more childlike than their children. Mauss-Clum and Ryan (1981) reported that many wives feel they are married to a stranger, or married but feel they have no husband. At 1–6 years postinjury, Thomsen (1974) noted that 80% of family members reported personality changes including childishness, irritability, restlessness, and emotional instability. Most distressing were acts of verbal or physical aggression directed at spouses by their head-injured husbands. Mauss-Clum and Ryan found that nearly one fourth of wives surveyed had been verbally abused or threatened with physical violence.

Although marriage is initially entered into voluntarily, many wives of men with traumatic brain injury feel trapped. Divorce is considered less often during the early stages of recovery; thoughts of divorce are more frequent during the process of attempted community integration as wives first begin to consider that their marital relationship has been permanently changed for the worse. Lezak (1978) has commented that social pressures and guilt very likely sustain many unsatisfactory postinjury relationships. Understandably, people would have a difficult time living with their conscience believing they "deserted" a marital partner because they could not bear the consequences of their disability. Presently, there is no research to suggest that the divorce rate among couples with head injury is any higher than the normal population. To maintain personal satisfaction and the marriage, the uninjured spouse must eventually learn to accept the permanent changes following head injury.

The self-sufficiency Jackson (1972) described tends to be exacerbated following head injury. Except for the needs for financial and rehabilitation support, research suggests that families become less reliant on others and more socially isolated following injury (Kozloff,

1987; Lezak, 1978). Lezak (1978) has described the situation as pathological and an almost inevitable consequence of the brain-injured person's characterological aberrations. Fortunately, many families can be encouraged to reach out to community support groups such as religious and head injury support organizations. Emotional and physical distance from extended family often arises as a consequence of guilt about overburdening others in a relationship that is not mutually beneficial. Conflicts among spouses and the head-injured person's parents over appropriate caregiving behaviors also contribute to distance among family members.

The ability of spouses to carry out and effectively share former roles is seriously compromised by head injury. Healthy family members are required to assume former roles of the brain-injured person. At least temporarily, the spouse of a person with traumatic brain injury must often completely assume the role of two adults. For example, the victim of injury is often male and the primary breadwinner. His traditional roles may include home and automobile maintenance, and managing family finances. Wives may be unprepared to assume these traditionally male roles. Furthermore, the wife must assume the role of mother and father to the children. The wife may need to find a job or increase work hours to meet financial obligations. Seeking rehabilitation services, assuming complete responsibility for parenting, and simultaneously maintaining employment results in high stress.

To provide effective treatment, clinicians must first consider the demands of the healthy spouse's postinjury responsibilities in comparison to those held preinjury. Stresses related to increased responsibility are dynamic, multidimensional, and occasionally hidden behind an attitude of stoicism. Children's reactions, the presence of extended family, and financial stresses must also be considered by the clinician. Frustrations often arise during the process of seeking rehabilitation services in the community that are often either unavailable or unaffordable. Many researchers (e.g., Ben-Yishay, Silver, Piasetsky, & Rottok, 1987; Fawber & Wachter, 1987) have commented on the failure or lack of vocational rehabilitation programs. The evolu-

tion of successful vocational rehabilitation programs would contribute immensely toward the reduction of fiscal and emotional stressors on family systems.

Especially if the head-injured spouse has severe cognitive and behavioral problems, therapy sessions held independently with the uninjured spouse may necessarily precede sessions including both parties. Initial goals may include stress management, education, and development of behavior intervention programs. Sessions involving both partners allow a unique opportunity for airing individual frustrations. Husbands with head injury may argue that they have been treated like children, have no voice in family decisions, and have had numerous privileges taken away. Conversely, the wife may argue that the husband behaves like a child, is not trustworthy, acts aggressively, and is insensitive. Ideally, marital therapy will result in increased empathy between spouses. Often, partners make negative assumptions regarding one another's intentions. Wives may benefit from knowing their husband's behavior is partly a consequence of physiological changes. Husbands may benefit from knowing their wives are frustrated and overburdened, yet attempt to act in their best interests. In summary, the therapist acts as a mediator and facilitator, conveying an impression of neutrality, and allowing each spouse to speak their opinions without interruption or criticism.

Both spouses may require help in resolving their grief if they have not yet learned to accept the relatively permanent changes of injury. Grieving requires a discussion of the origins of the marital relationship. Partners are encouraged to describe the initial feelings, interests, and attraction to one another that characterized the beginning of the relationship. Questions about why each person committed to marriage helps renew positive feelings. Discussion should include perceived changes relative to preinjury in marital roles, communication patterns, feelings, and stresses. The therapist should inquire as to how family career, retirement, and child-rearing goals also have been changed. Finally, both spouses should be encouraged to state their postinjury personal goals and the goals for their relationship. Each person should be asked to share responsibility for problem resolution and indicate how they intend to improve the marriage by changing their personal behavior.

In every case, the therapist should inform couples that change is a lengthy process that requires patience and effort from both parties. Establishment of reasonable expectations for change helps reduce frustrations and disappointments. Marital partners should be informed that additional difficulties are likely and unavoidable. However, the ultimate goal is long-term satisfaction, which necessarily involves learning from both mistakes and successes.

Sexual Counseling

Sexual counseling usually is initiated in the context of marital relationships. However, counseling may be undertaken with injured persons without partners and those engaged in intimate relationships. Educational efforts should include family members and caregivers whenever possible.

Sexual concerns become increasingly prominent during community integration. It is critical to realize that sexuality issues will potentially change over time as neurological and functional recovery occur. Early in the course of recovery, head-injured persons and therapy staff are preoccupied with improvements in activities of daily living, ambulation, cognition, and communication skills. As substantial progress is made in each of these areas, concerns regarding sexual, vocational, and social functioning become more prominent. Jackson (1972) has indicated that a mutually satisfying sexual relationship is one of several fundamental characteristics underlying satisfying marriages. Sexual satisfaction is also interrelated with self-esteem, affect, and social skills.

Satisfying sexual relationships have physical, emotional, and psychological components. The physical aspects of disability often interfere with normal sexual functioning, which adds to depression, diminished self-esteem, and frustrations for both sexual partners (Neistadt & Freda, 1987). Intimacy partly reflects interpersonal sensitivity and is a critical element of a mutually satisfying sexual relationship. Self-centeredness, childishness, irritability, and other charac-

terological alterations arising from traumatic brain injury interfere with the development and maintenance of intimate relationships. Consequently, clinicians should consider that successful marital or family counseling may be a prerequisite or concomitant of sexual counseling.

Clinical experience and research suggest that disturbances in sexuality are commonplace after traumatic brain injury (Kreutzer & Zasler, 1989; Lezak, 1978). Unfortunately, sexuality is a topic that is infrequently discussed after traumatic brain injury with either the head-injured person, his or her spouse, or parents. The authors recommend that the subject be addressed in every intake interview to determine the need for additional assessment, counseling, and other forms of intervention. Sexuality may not be an issue for everyone, but rehabilitationists must address all areas of function to be truly holistic in their approach. Sexuality is simply another means by which one communicates with others in one's environment, whether they be strangers or intimate sexual partners.

There are major psychological and physiological obstacles that the person with a traumatic brain injury faces in attempting to meet their sexual needs and appropriately express their sexuality. Obstacles include social isolation, physical barriers, communication disorders, decreased self-esteem, and distorted body image. Negative spousal and societal attitudes toward sexuality and disability, misinformation, and ignorance also complicate the picture. Libido is generally decreased, although there are rare instances where hypersexuality occurs (Kreutzer & Zasler, 1989).

Males report a variety of sexual problems including inability to attain and/or maintain an erection, or to ejaculate in a timely fashion. Physiological changes arising from traumatic brain injury may occur at the genital level and elsewhere in the nervous system. As a general rule for both sexes, sexual dysfunction and diminished frequency of intercourse are more common among persons with more significant injuries. From a treatment perspective, it is imperative that clinicians differentiate between true libidinal changes and inappropriate or disinhibited behaviors that are sexual in nature. Furthermore, appropriate treatment may also be hindered by difficulties in determining the extent to which dysfunction is organically versus functionally based.

Professionals who address sexual concerns must feel comfortable with their own sexuality before they can appropriately respond to clients' concerns. They also must possess adequate knowledge of sexual neurophysiology, anatomy, and development. Counselors must also obtain an understanding of the compensatory techniques and treatments that are available for sexual problems and the common personal and societal attitudes toward such solutions. Conversely, professionals should be well aware of limitations in their knowledge about physiological and psychological aspects and intervention techniques. Education and counseling about sexuality issues is often most effective if rehabilitation professionals representing several disciplines, each with respective areas of expertise, share in the responsibility of intervention.

Proper assessment in terms of an adequate sexual history and physical exam is critical in the neuromedical work-up of sexual dysfunction after traumatic brain injury. Some key points when eliciting sexual information are to provide a private atmosphere, allow adequate time, be frank yet empathetic, use terminology that the client understands, do not assume sexual preference, and remain aware of one's own sexuality. Furthermore, therepeutic success can be enhanced by varying intervention strategies to accommodate individual differences among clients representing different cultures and having different religious beliefs.

Information about prior sexual experience should be elicited from every client who enters into a rehabilitation program. Data pertaining to sexual experience help clinicians to better define the clients' needs and those of their sexual partner. The client and his or her partner should be questioned about current and past sexual functioning and practices, partner and client satisfaction with sex life, relationship history, and past medical history, including sexually transmitted diseases. A complete review of past and present medications is essential. Information should be obtained about illicit and prescription drug use to fully assess the potential contribution of these agents to concomitant sexual dysfunction.

Sexual history taking needs to be thorough and specific if any clues to the problem are to be gained. If someone was not sexually active prior to the injury, the obstacles faced are much different from those of the individual who was very sexually active. Female clients who are having orgasmic dysfunction need to be questioned about the techniques they find most effective to achieve orgasm. Inquiries about the amount and adequacy of vaginal lubrication should also be made. Males with erectile dysfunction should be questioned about the quality of erections with intercourse, oral sex, and manual manipulation (partner/self), and whether they ever experience penile tumescence upon awakening.

Clients and their partners should be questioned about their personal sexual preferences and "priorities." For many couples, effective intervention may be as simple as suggesting alternative positions or prescribing assistive devices such as dildos or vibrators. In some cases, relationships may have deteriorated because intimacy at a very basic level has been disrupted (e.g., the spouse cannot caress, hold, or kiss his partner in the same manner as before his brain injury). At times, grief counseling may be required because the uninjured partner may no longer find the client physically attractive or capable of meeting his or her emotional needs because of characteriological changes. In other cases, the healthy spouse may be too exhausted or overwhelmed by stresses related to the illness. Ingenuity and creativity must often be relied upon to help find respite for overburdened spouses.

The physical exam for persons with sexual dysfunction begins when the client first enters the exam room. Observation of mobility status can provide clues regarding "sexual mobility" skills. Skills in activities of daily living (e.g., undressing) should also be observed to give the examiner a sense of manual dexterity, upper extremity strength and coordination, and so forth. Spasticity, particularly in the hip abductors, should be assessed. General hygiene, including bladder and bowel management, should always be checked. A standard physical exam should include examination of the skin, head and neck, pulmonary and cardiovascular systems, abdomen, recto-genital structures, and musculoskeletal system (Ducharme, Gill, Biener-Bergman, & Feritta, 1988). A complete neurological examination should be performed including evaluation of the neuro-urological system. The neurological examination provides the examiner with information regarding the intactness of motor, sensory, and autonomic nerves involved with sexual function.

Rehabilitative management of sexual dysfunction after traumatic brain injury may be multifaceted depending upon the problems at hand. Compensations for sensorimotor deficits, cognitive remediation, behavior management, proper bowel/bladder/ostomy management, increasing joint range of motion and/or stability, controlling spasticity, and managing genital sexual dysfunction are all potential interventions that can be offered. Relative increases or decreases in libido can be addressed pharmacologically and behaviorally. Erectile dysfunction can be treated with oral medications, penile implants, external devices, and alternate sexual techniques (e.g., "stuffing," or placing the semierect or flaccid penis into the vagina). Theoretically, ejaculatory dysfunction can be treated pharmacologically. Premature ejaculation generally can be managed utilizing the "squeeze technique." Problems related to inadequate vaginal lubrication can be remedied through a combination of strategies, which include use of lubricants (e.g., K-Y Lubricating Jelly), dildos, and vibrators.

Sexuality is a controversial topic for persons with traumatic brain injury. Issues concerning sexual expression for clients who do not have sexual partners must often be addressed. The authors believe that an acceptable outlet for sexual release must be provided to those clients who have chronically ungratified sexual needs. Masturbation should be encouraged as a form of sexual release as long as it is done in the appropriate environment. If necessary, the brain-injured person can be provided with erotic reading material, pictures, or videotapes. Some health care professionals have advocated the use of "sexual surro-gates" for persons with disabilities. Due to the litigious nature of our society at present and Judeo-Christian moral and ethical beliefs, the authors believe that such solutions, although sound in principle, may be perceived as too radical by most clients, families, and society.

Effective intervention often requires referral to other specialists. For example, counselors should consider appropriate referral to psychologists, urologists, physiatrists, obstetricians, or endocrinologists for further work-up. Other issues that need to be addressed with brain-injured persons are topics of birth control, sexually transmitted disease, and sexual abuse. Decisions over who should or should not be sexually active are often difficult to make. Generally, clients who have been deemed competent and have the capability to understand and remember the ramifications of their actions are *probably* capable of being sexually active in a responsible manner.

All attempts must be made to teach clients and partners healthy sexual attitudes. The counselor should: 1) debunk the myth that sexual intercourse culminating in orgasm is essential for sexual satisfaction; 2) provide education regarding the relative contribution of psychological and physiological factors to sexual behavior; 3) explain how sexual disorders can result from the brain injury itself; 4) approach sexual problems with a mature, professional attitude to help clients and partners feel comfortable; and 5) acknowledge that clients and partners may initially feel uncomfortable about discussing problems. Counselors should discuss and help brain-injured persons and their partners determine what changes can be made, work toward effecting those changes, and accept problems that cannot be changed. Many persons with traumatic brain injury simply require permission to acknowledge their sexuality.

In conclusion, sexual satisfaction is an important part of the human experience. Rehabilitation professionals are encouraged to address sexuality issues throughout the continuum of care. Interventions directed at optimizing sexuality and relationships should be considered as critical as efforts directed at optimizing physical, cognitive, avocational, and vocational outcomes.

INTERVENTION STRATEGIES FOR SELECTED PROBLEMS

Clinicians' and researchers' descriptions of family reactions to brain injury generally are very similar. The similarity of perceptions among professionals very likely reflect the fact that families' long-term reactions are usually normal responses to an unexpected event that has long-term negative consequences. General descriptions and suggestions to alleviate some family problems were provided in previous sections of this chapter. Following is a more complete description of several relatively dangerous problems that occur in the context of community integration and a series of specific suggestions for intervention. The discussion focuses on denial, anger, guilt, blame, overprotectiveness, and aggressive behavior.

Denial

Denial is an unwillingness or inability to acknowledge the negative effects of traumatic brain injury on the family or the client. Individual rehabilitation professionals and the rehabilitation team are specially trained to evaluate persons with traumatic brain injury. Their evaluation enables them to provide a relatively accurate description of the head-injured person's abilities, suggestions for additional treatment, and a set of prognostic statements. Families and rehabilitation teams ideally should share similar views. However, psychological factors and differences in opinions among professionals may contribute to overly optimistic family views about the impact of injury and prognosis. Professionals must assume responsibility for educating family members to eliminate naiveté and ignorance that are distinct from denial.

Denial unfortunately may lead to distrust of and anger toward professionals, and pursuit of unreasonable goals for the person with brain injury. This can result in wasted time and effort, guilt, and frustration, which further add to existing distress. Denial may occur either overtly or covertly. Family members may simply state that the results of an evaluation, prognostic statement, or recommendation for therapy are inaccurate or inappropriate. For example, a client's mother might suggest that the clinician "really doesn't know" the client. In some instances, clinicians' professional qualifications may be questioned.

In extreme cases, the family might decide that the previously valued rehabilitation team is unqualified to help the head-injured person and may initiate "doctor shopping." The family then brings the client to a series of rehabilitation professionals until one is found who agrees with the family's perspective. "Doctor shopping" is distinct from the process of reasonable decision making that involves information gathering. Inappropriate anger and mistrust toward previously valued professionals along with unwillingness to accept the validity of similar opinions provided by different professionals helps distinguish pathological from reasonable searches for services.

Clinicians are encouraged to view denial as an indication of a family member's stress and coping ability. Denial sometimes may be a healthy way of maintaining hope or coping with an otherwise overwhelming situation. Denial is most pathological when clients are not permitted to participate in prescribed rehabilitation programs. Fortunately, over time, denial often yields in the face of patience and ongoing family support. Families are better able to assimilate bad news a little at a time than all at once. Some reassurance can be gained from the fact that families learn from experience, although experience can sometimes be a cruel teacher. After failures resulting from denial, the family may return to rehabilitation professionals for help. The family is more likely to return if the clinician has been gentle and supportive in the past, rather than harsh and confrontational. Unfortunately, clinicians sometimes wrongly view denial as their own personal failure either to be "strong enough" or appropriately educate the family.

Several techniques can be used to reduce the likelihood and potential adverse effects of denial. The results of regular evaluations should be conveyed with minimal use of jargon— providing information in layperson's terminology demonstrates a sensitivity to the family. The head-injured person's strengths and potential should be emphasized in the context of reasonable expectations. Following presentation of results, family members should be actively encouraged to ask questions. Clinicians should be sensitive to the fact that some family members do not ask questions simply because they fear that professionals will perceive them as ignorant. Therefore, family members should be encouraged to paraphrase and summarize information to demonstrate their understanding. Written copies or summaries of reports should be provided. The team meeting is likely to be stressful and families can only remember part of what they have heard. Providing the name and phone number of a contact person who can reiterate and provide additional information at a later time will also prove helpful. Furthermore, family members will benefit from a follow-up phone call to inquire about additional questions. Although no questions may arise during the call, families will be reassured that they are important and that professionals are concerned about their needs.

Inconsistent views among team members can also contribute to denial. Consider the situation in which a family member attends a team meeting to discuss the client's employment potential. One team member says the client will never work. Another states that the client might be able to work after 2 years of prevocational training. A third team member states that the client could work within a week if provided with a vocational counselor. The family is likely to be quite confused by the different opinions provided. Family members may end up disliking those who provide more pessimistic views, even though these views may be more accurate. To avoid such difficulties, professionals are encouraged to integrate the results of their reports, negotiate among themselves prior to communicating with the family, and provide consistent information to family members. Struggles over who is right and wrong on the part of professionals will only lead to confusion, distrust, and ultimately a worse outcome for the client and his or her family.

Anger, Guilt, and Blame

One hundred percent of the mothers and 84% of the wives of adults with brain injury surveyed by Mauss-Clum and Ryan (1981) reported they were frustrated. The percentages of wives and mothers reporting feelings of anger were 63% and 45%, respectively. Nearly half of all wives and one fifth of mothers reported feelings of guilt. Gardner (1973) has also reported that family members react similarly to having children with brain dysfunction.

Anger, which often arises from frustration, as well as guilt and blame are clinically interrelated phenomena. The presence of each emotion and the resulting behavior affects the quality and intensity of the others. For example, anger on the part of family members may be a consequence of the head-injured person's aggressive behavior. The family may respond by punishing the client or withdrawing affection. The client who perceives that he or she is being punished may become more frustrated and therefore behave more aggressively. Unfortunately, anger is a more likely response to an aggressive client than is empathy. Frustrations arising from lack of services and financial stressors may be directed toward service providers, the person with brain injury, or other family members.

Family members often attempt to recognize the source of their anger and cast blame. In the case of unavailable services, community and rehabilitation professionals may be blamed. Members of the insurance industry and politicians also may be held responsible. However, blame is most destructive when inappropriately directed at family members. Parents may criticize each other because of the head-injured child's lack of progress. The husband might accuse the wife of failing to follow the child's rehabilitation program. The wife might accuse the husband of being responsible for the client's problems because he works too much and has too little time to spend with the injured child. Blame is often inappropriately directed toward the client due to the confusing psychological and physiological consequences of traumatic brain injury. For example, the family might declare the client unworthy of help because "he is unwilling to help himself." Apparent unwillingness may actually reflect depression and motivation arising from physiological changes. Unfortunately, blame directed by the parents toward the person with head injury is likely to make the situation worse. In fact, family members sometimes blame themselves for the client's apparent lack of motivation.

Guilt results when anger is directed toward oneself. In some situations, family members blame themselves for the client's injury or lack of progress. Frequent statements beginning with "I should have" or "I could have" suggest the presence of guilt. Unfortunately, guilt contributes to family members' depression. Depression is nearly universal and begins during the grieving process as family members begin to realize that the injured person will never be the same. In some circumstances, guilt is a consequence of family members feeling overly responsible for the client's behavior. For example, a mother might state, "My son wouldn't have hit his boss and lost his job if only I would have spent more time teaching him how to behave."

Family members first must be helped to appropriately recognize and label their feelings. They respond better when they themselves provide labels for their feelings rather than a professional who uses jargon. Questioning by the skilled clinician can effectively elicit clients' descriptions of feelings. Clients must often be assured that anger, guilt, and blame are normal reactions to their situation. Sometimes family members feel embarrassment because of feelings that they are abnormal or crazy. Family members are comforted by hearing that they are normal people reacting normally to a very abnormal situation.

Anger is energizing and the clinician can help the family use their anger constructively. Frustrations about lack of services can be directed toward seeking information and services, such as working to develop new services and improving existing services. Family members can be encouraged to network with other families and prepare reports or petitions for community agencies, politicians, or insurance carriers.

Exercise and recreational activities also can serve as appropriate mechanisms for relaxation and discharge of tension.

The clinician should work to teach the family constructive methods of problem solving. Family members should be convinced that blaming one another jeopardizes the family's overall strength. The family should be helped to understand that their strength has already been compromised by the injury and that mutual support and teamwork are required to achieve stability. Communication skills training that partly focuses on assertiveness is helpful in teaching families to appropriately label their blaming behavior and seek more constructive alternatives. Where conflicts exist over the assumption of responsibilities, the clinician can act as a mediator to assure that responsibilities are shared equally. To eliminate confusion and potential arguments, a contract may be necessary to clearly indicate the responsibilities of individual family members. Sometimes family members complain about having too many responsibilities, yet they may be reluctant to give them up. Occasionally, family members feel guilty about asking others for help. A frank discussion of each family member's responsibilities, needs, and stress levels typically improves empathy, interpersonal sensitivity, and communication.

Family members should be persuaded to accept that guilt is usually inappropriate and self-defeating. A logical reasoning process should be applied to help reduce guilt. Questioning family members about what and how much they have done for the person with traumatic brain injury and how much they have done for themselves is important. Lezak (1978) has stressed the notion that family members must take care of their own needs. The clinician may be required to reassure family members that they must meet their own needs to retain their strength. Without their strength they cannot effectively help the client or support healthy family members. Frequent encouragement and reminders to family members that they have done their best and done as much as anyone can ask also help to effectively reduce inappropriate guilt.

Education regarding the neurophysiological and normal psychological changes following injury may help relieve inappropriate guilt on the part of family members and blame directed toward the injured person. Education and problem solving with the clinician can also help families be realistic about their ability to influence the client's behavior. Nevertheless, the ultimate goal of therapy is the assumption of personal control and responsibility by the person with head injury. As the injured person improves and regains the potential to exert greater control over his or her behavior, parental assumption of responsibility for the client's inappropriate behaviors can only contribute to regression and unwillingness to act as an adult. Under these circumstances, the clinician must especially remember that the family members' efforts may be misdirected, but their intentions are good.

Overprotectiveness

Overprotectiveness is especially common when patients are discharged to parents' homes. Following a lengthy period of hospitalization, the injured person may be perceived as extremely fragile. Uncertainties about appropriate care also contribute to extreme carefulness. Although their beliefs may be illogical, families often feel some responsibility for the initial accident. Overprotectiveness provides parents with an opportunity to partially relieve their guilt by preventing a second injury. Gardner (1973) has suggested that guilt and overprotectiveness help families to feel a greater sense of control. Parents' levels of guilt and overprotectiveness undoubtedly are interrelated.

Gordon (1975) has discussed the dangers of parents' not allowing children the opportunity to test their skills. His ideas can be applied to persons with head injury who are cared for and supervised by parents. Gordon's work suggests that parents must acknowledge that brain-injured individuals can learn by both failures and successes. Overprotectiveness denies clients the opportunity to benefit from potentially valuable learning experiences. Parents who restrict their children may inadvertently convey feelings that the child is incompetent, inadequate, or untrustworthy. For the person with head injury, even

subtle messages can contribute to already existing feelings of inadequacy and poor self-worth. Additionally, Gordon suggests that parents use passive listening and nonintervention as nonverbal methods of conveying acceptance and approval of their children whenever possible.

Difficulties in community integration inherently contribute to the likelihood that parents will be overprotective. No parent enjoys watching his or her child fail, especially a child who nearly died as a result of an accident. Failures in community integration typically include loss of friends, inability to gain or maintain employment, and academic underachievement. parents are naturally inclined to protect their children, no matter how old, from additional failures.

Overprotectiveness can be diminished in a number of ways. Professionals should convey the results of evaluations in positive terms, acknowledging limitations but focusing on strengths. Providers of ongoing therapy should focus on progress, placing lesser emphasis on areas that have shown regression or little improvement. Frequent contact with rehabilitation staff and direct opportunities to view the client's progress allow parents to develop more realistic perceptions of changes. It is often beneficial to negotiate with the family increasing levels of responsibility for the person with traumatic brain injury. Clinicians should outline a series of steps that must be mastered. As each step is mastered, privileges and responsibilities can be increased.

At the opposite end of the spectrum from overprotectiveness is permissiveness. Parents' guilt sometimes leads them to be overly permissive. Permissiveness may be an attractive alternative, especially for insecure parents. Parents may feel apprehensive about assuming an authoritarian role, especially if the person with head injury reacts aggressively. Restricting privileges inevitably creates conflict and parents may choose permissiveness to reduce tension and conflict. However, permissiveness also can be dangerous. Many persons initially suffered a head injury as a consequence of risk-taking behaviors, especially driving under the influence of alcohol. Poor judgment, partly due to brain injury, may result in a postinjury resumption of risk-taking behaviors. Additionally, children may perceive overly permissive parents to be unconcerned or uncaring.

Regardless of age, children with head injury must pass through a series of steps during the recovery process. Clients and parents ideally should develop realistic guidelines for assumption of privileges based on responsibilities, strengths, and skills. Frequent reassurance and explanations into the need for restrictions are usually helpful. Convincing persons with traumatic brain injury that restrictions are well intended and in their best interests represents a formidable but worthy challenge. Overprotectiveness and overpermissiveness are likely to surface numerous times during the process of community integration. However, the negative impact on client and family functioning can be limited through regular negotiations between clients, parents, and experienced rehabilitation professionals.

Aggressive Behavior

Aggressive behavior on the part of the person with traumatic brain injury contributes to family conflicts, stresses, and resentment toward the client, and diminishes family members' ability to express affection toward the client and provide mutual support. Brooks, Campsie, Symington, Beattie, & McKinley (1986) in their 5-year follow-up study found that one fifth of relatives had been physically assaulted by a brain injured family member. Nearly two thirds of clients in their sample were described by relatives as having a bad temper. Problems with temper actually appeared to increase over time.

Among the inappropriate behaviors demonstrated by persons with traumatic brain injury, aggression ranks among the most likely to create family disturbance. Consider the situation in which a husband with traumatic brain injury behaves aggressively toward his wife and children. The wife and children learn to fear the client. The wife is less likely to rely on the husband for emotional support, and may increasingly rely on younger children and friends. Beneficial emotional support is reduced or removed from the client. Reductions in emotional support may increase the head-injured person's frustration, anger, and depression. The client may sometimes become a scapegoat for all family problems. The problem creates emotional conflict for wives and children who are expected to be loving and supportive.

McKinlay and Hickox (1988) have described an apparently successful system for working with family members as co-therapists in an effort to reduce aggressive behavior. Treatment is implemented in the home and involves assertiveness training in conjunction with a behavior management program. Components of the behavioral program include identification of situations likely to trigger aggressive responses, teaching sensitivity to signals of increasing anger, and responding alternatively using relaxation procedures. Those who have difficulty following the sequence of alternative steps are encouraged to remove themselves from the anger-arousing situation. Furthermore, to enhance the possibility of learning from experience, records are kept of the head-injured person's responses in each situation and are later reviewed. McKinlay and Hickox's program can be adapted to help reduce other forms of inappropriate behavior. The authors have noted that working with families to assist the person with traumatic brain injury in the home environment helps eliminate uncertainties about generalization of therapeutic benefits to real-life settings.

Given the apparent frequency and potentially harmful effects of violence directed at family members, psychiatric approaches to behavior control have received considerable attention. If outpatient behavioral and pharmacological approaches do not yield acceptable results, involuntary commitment in a psychiatric hospital may remain the only feasible alternative. Cooperation to have a head-injured relative involuntarily committed may increase a family's sense of guilt. Consequently, families often benefit from appropriate reassurance that hospitalization is temporary and was selected as a last alternative.

FAMILY ASSESSMENT

The authors have suggested that clinicians utilize a variety of structured intervention techniques to enhance family functioning during the process of community integration following traumatic brain injury. They have also delineated a set of common family problems and suggested solutions for resolving these problems. The selection of a particular intervention evolves from an initial assessment process that incorporates interview, history taking, and when possible, quantitative measurement. Considering the dynamics of recovery and adaptation, assessment is necessarily an ongoing process and continues during therapy. To assist clinicians, the authors have outlined a general assessment approach intended to help in determining which families are at risk for development of dysfunction and to help identify which families are adapting poorly. Discussion also focuses on a mechanism for establishing family needs and priorities for addressing needs.

Traumatic brain injury obviously places significant stress on family members. Stress levels vary as clients improve, new services are offered, and therapies are terminated. Families that were dysfunctional prior to injury certainly are at greater risk for postinjury problems than previously well-adjusted families. Clinicians are encouraged to solicit a thorough family history during the intake process. The information provided helps establish the family's level of preinjury stability and establishes a baseline against which progress or regression can be measured.

Information regarding history of divorce, separation, marital disputes, and number of prior marriages will aid in the determination of preinjury stability. Animosities existing prior to the injury often carry over and affect the ability of family members to act cooperatively during community integration. Other preinjury factors to assess include the nature of relationships among members of the immediate family, in-laws, and extended family members. The clinician should obtain similar information pertaining to postinjury history for comparative purposes, inquire about perceived changes and attributed sources of change in relationships, and establish the family's plans for the future.

A prior history of psychiatric hospitalization for any family member is suggestive of po-

tential family instability. Family members with prior emotional problems may have difficulty providing support to the head-injured family member and sharing the burden of additional roles arising as a consequence of the injured person's disabilities. Information should also be obtained about postinjury symptoms of emotional disturbance, and psychological or psychiatric treatment. Clinicians should be alert to symptoms of sleep and appetite disturbance, persistent dysphoria, and blunted or inappropriate affect. Family outcome research by Livingston, Brooks, and Bond (1985a, 1985b) indicates that the incidence of psychiatric disturbance in caregiving relatives ranges from 40% to 45%.

Clinicians additionally are encouraged to routinely obtain historical information about substance abuse, sexual abuse, and physical abuse. Rehabilitation professionals may feel uncomfortable asking adolescent and adult family members about alcohol and drug use. However, evidence suggests that family members of head-injured persons often have histories of heavy alcohol use or abuse of prescription drugs. First, the incidence of alcohol abuse and dependency in the United States is high, with estimates ranging from 10 million to 13 million people (Heinemann, Keen, Donohue, & Schnoll, 1988). Second, many brain-injured persons have substance abuse histories (Rimel, Giordani, Barth, & Jane, 1982). The drinking patterns of children, their parents, and siblings are often interrelated. Therefore, the incidence of substance abuse problems in families of persons with head injury may be higher than the normal population. Third, family outcome research suggests that parents may use alcohol as a means of coping with stresses arising from the injury (Mauss-Clum & Ryan, 1981). Family members with substance abuse problems are typically less capable of providing support to clients and may even interfere with or encumber the rehabilitation process. Many rehabilitation professionals recommend abstinence from alcohol and drugs following brain injury because of potentially negative effects on outcome. Unfortunately, family members with substance abuse problems may be less willing or able to support such abstinence. Furthermore, the ready availability of alcohol and permissive attitudes in the home environment may be conducive to heavy drinking.

Difficulties in community integration and characterological changes in the client may not be the only stresses on family members. Clinicians should query about other potential sources of stress, including financial instability and debt, forced unemployment, difficulty finding housing, and physical illness. Parents sometimes assume caregiving responsibilities for adult head-injured children in addition to elderly parents who are ailing. The results of family outcome research suggest that the stresses of head injury contribute to high rates of psychosomatic and medical illness among caregiving family members (Oddy, Humphrey, & Uttley, 1978). Physically ill family members cannot participate fully in rehabilitation and further burden the family unit. Finally, a chronic lack of available services for especially needy clients can cause major family stress.

The perceived impact of the client's injury on children in the family should be discussed with the family. Inquiry should address changes in behavior, sociability, sleep patterns, appetite, and academic performance. Encopresis and enuresis may develop following the client's injury. Because children often do not have well-developed verbal and cognitive skills they are more likely to express their anxieties behaviorally rather than verbally. When possible, children should be directly questioned to assess their knowledge of what happened to the injured family member. Many adults have difficulty understanding the reasons for behavioral and cognitive changes arising from brain injury. Children certainly have even greater difficulty. Both their feelings about the changes to the injured person and their feelings about themselves should be examined.

Family members should be questioned about their beliefs over the effects of injury and their expectations for improvement. Significant disparities among family members' opinions suggests the need for a series of family discussions. Knowledge of community resources also should be assessed. With this information, clinicians can develop appropriate educational programs for the family and determine the need for advocacy. Depending on the specific effects of injury and family members' levels of education, clinicians can select appropriate reading materials from the office, community support agency, and National Head Injury Foundation libraries.

Clinicians have valuable opportunities to observe family interactions during the interview and history-taking process. The individual who answers most of the questions may also hold most of the family's power. Attendance at therapy meetings and adherence to recommendations will be enhanced by gaining this individual's trust. However, the family member who interrupts others or otherwise interferes with their expressing opinions is likely to be resented by other family members. The clinician should deliberately attempt to solicit relevant information from each family member. The process of giving each family member a turn to speak reinforces the belief that all family members are important.

Minuchin (1974) has suggested that seating arrangements offer clues about family members' feelings toward one another. As such, family members should be encouraged to choose their own seats. Persons who sit near one another may be closely affiliated. Those who sit farther apart, even facing away, may be in a state of conflict. Clinicians can generate hypotheses based on seating positions and confirm their feelings through interpretation of body language and speech content. Antagonism is often communicated directly. For example, family members may say, "He doesn't even try, why should we help him?" or "Given all the abuse we've taken, the best we can do is protect ourselves from him." Preexisting rivalries among siblings may have been exacerbated during the process of providing increased attention to the person with head injury and his or her problems. Predominantly positive or negative statements about an individual also provide insights about how each family member is perceived by others.

Information should be obtained from family members about controversial issues and personal responsibility for family conflict. Clinicians must be sensitive to the head-injured person's potential placement in the role of scapegoat. Family members sometimes blame themselves for the client's problems, although they have little or no responsibility for these problems. In other cases, clients are seen as helpless to control their behavior "because of the head injury." Due to their naiveté, children are often very honest, and disclose a wealth of information that adults are uncomfortable providing.

The reader may wish to employ quantitative assessment procedures to evaluate family functioning. Bishop and Miller (1988) have described the validity and reliability characteristics of a number of assessment scales including the Family Environment Scale (FES), the McMaster Family Assessment Device (FAD; Epstein, Baldwin, & Bishop, 1983), and the Family Adaptation and Cohesiveness Evaluation Scales (FACES). These instruments primarily have been applied to families representing other populations, such as families of stroke and psychiatric clients. Their value for families of persons with traumatic brain injury appears promising and will be determined through systematic research in the years ahead. Interested readers are encouraged to use these measures for assessment along with thorough clinical and history-taking interviews, and to make their own decisions regarding clinical value.

Included in the Appendices to this chapter are two measures the authors and others have developed and found useful for family assessment: the General Health and History Questionnaire (Appendix A, this chapter; Kreutzer, Leininger, Doherty, & Waaland, 1987) and the Family Needs Questionnaire (Appendix B, this chapter; Kreutzer, Camplair, & Waaland, 1988). The General Health and History Questionnaire was developed to provide information similar to the General Health Questionnaire used extensively by Brooks and colleagues (e.g., Livingston et al., 1985a, 1985b). The questionnaire, typically completed by a family member, has been used extensively in supported employment outcome research (e.g., Wehman et al., 1988; Wehman, Kreutzer, Wood, et al., 1989). The form can be mailed, completed at home, and later reviewed with the family. A parallel form was developed for administration to the client.

Completion of the General Health and History Questionnaire (Kreutzer et al., 1987) prior to the first appointment allows clinicians to routinely obtain comprehensive information, saving time for discussion of other issues during intake. Information about the client's injury, employment history, living situation, alcohol and illicit drug use, criminal behavior, and prior medical illness is elicited. An important element of the questionnaire is the problem checklist that inquires about the frequency of somatic, thinking, behavior, communication, and social problems demonstrated by the client. The family's perception of the head-injured person's cognitive and personality attributes provides a useful indication of potential sources of family stress (Lezak, 1978). Brooks, Campsie, Symington, Beattie, and McKinley (1986, 1987) have demonstrated that family burden is related to the type and intensity of the client's problems arising from injury.

The Family Needs Questionnaire (Kreutzer et al., 1988) was designed to be used as a research and clinical needs assessment instrument. Items were selected based on interviews with family members and a review of the needs assessment literature (e.g., Mauss-Clum & Ryan, 1981; Molter, 1979). Forty items were included that represent the diverse needs that may appear during acute rehabilitation and postdischarge. Family members are asked to make two independent ratings. First, an indication of the importance of each perceived need is rated on a four-point scale ranging from not important to very important. Second, the family member rates the extent to which each need has been met. Data collected from a sample of 57 family members (Camplair & Kreutzer, 1989) suggest that the measure is easily completed by family members and provides a valid index of need importance and satisfaction. The Family Needs Questionnaire can be used to develop individualized educational and therapy programs tailored to family members' stated needs. Furthermore, completion of the questionnaire prior to and following intervention helps provide an index of intervention effectiveness and also provides a mechanism for closely following changes in the dynamic process of community integration.

CONCLUSIONS

The complexities and difficulties of community integration following traumatic brain injury inherently arise from the fact that success is dependent upon appropriate interactions among various community systems. The composition of systems varies from community to community, but typically includes the family, rehabilitation team, third-party payers, and community support groups. Each system influences other systems and the functioning of each system is also dependent upon its components. Ideally, family intervention includes working with system components and systems proactively to ensure communication and complementary functioning.

Systems and their components can influence one another both positively and negatively. Negative interactions among systems and the dangers of not working proactively are illustrated by the following example: The depressed client who is verbally aggressive toward family members finds they eventually become fearful and withdraw emotional support. Family members' motivation to expend effort to help the client diminishes and they decide to invest little effort in finding services. Although limited services are available, they are unwilling to invest substantial time lobbying with third-party payers who are reluctant to provide coverage for outpatient cognitive remediation and psychotherapy. Third-party payers' repeated failure to provide compensation for head injury services contributes to reductions in the number of service providers and the number and quality of services available. Because family members choose not to attend support group meetings, they are unable to take advantage of social, advocacy, recreational, and respite opportunities. Diminished contributions due to poor attendance at support group meetings contributes to financial strains on the volunteer organization, which further limits the availability of services. The injured person's continuing behavioral problems and the chronic absence of respite escalates existing family stresses.

Some readers may describe the sequence of events in the preceding example as unlikely. Regardless, the critical point is that effective intervention requires assessment of community and family resources and multiple types of family interventions, which often must be applied simultaneously. Clinicians must be sensitive to the complex interactions within individual service delivery systems and among systems. Effective family intervention initially may require referral to the local head injury support group in conjunction with family therapy sessions. Later, clinicians may need to facilitate meetings with support group members and third-party payers to lobby for coverage of family therapy or transitional living services. Intervention is ultimately a dynamic process in appreciation of the dynamic nature of recovery and changes in community systems. Assessment is also an ongoing process that aids in the rational selection of appropriate intervention strategies.

The authors of this chapter wish to remind the reader that family intervention is not the sine qua non for ameliorating emotional problems following head trauma. Their bias is that clients can best be helped by working in close cooperation with family members. Family members usually are good co-therapists because they know the client well, have relatively frequent contact, and consequently exert considerable influence. Furthermore, many problem behaviors occur in the home environment, which has a negative impact on family members. Some families function well despite serious physical and personality changes in the head-injured individual. For these families, referral to a community support group, offering of educational materials, and occasional phone contacts may meet all their needs. In some cases, families may be unwilling to participate in interventions directed toward improving their well-being. Anxieties about self-examination or guilt arising from failure to attend entirely to the head-injured person's needs may explain their reluctance. In other situations, animosity among family members may be so great that each person chooses to participate in individual psychotherapy.

This chapter has suggested that clinicians remind family members, when necessary, that they are human, and inherently have personal needs and limitations. Clinicians must occasionally be given a similar reminder. Family intervention is often a difficult and long-term process characterized by both failures and successes. Success and progress are relative and must be measured against a baseline rather than an ideal. Furthermore, the most valuable family interven-

tion skills cannot be learned simply by reading books. Patience, common sense, interpersonal sensitivity, and active listening skills can be developed with effort, but arise almost naturally from caring about others.

REFERENCES

Ben-Yishay, Y., Silver, S.M., Piasetsky, E., & Rattok, J. (1987). Relationship between employability and vocational outcome after intensive holistic cognitive rehabilitation. *Journal of Head Trauma Rehabilitation, 2,* 35–48.

Bishop, D., & Miller, I. (1988). Traumatic brain injury: Empirical family assessment techniques. *Journal of Head Trauma Rehabilitation, 3*(1), 16–30.

Brooks, D.N., Campsie, L., Symington, C., Beattie, A., & McKinley, W. (1986). The five year outcome of severe blunt head injury: A relative's view. *Journal of Neurology, Neurosurgery, & Psychiatry, 49,* 764–770.

Brooks, N. Campsie, L., Symington, C., Beattie, A., & McKinlay, W. (1987). The effects of head injury on patient and relative within seven years of injury. *Journal of Head Trauma Rehabilitation, 2*(3), 1–13.

Camplair, P., & Kreutzer, J. (1989, June). *Psychosocial needs of families of adult head injury survivors.* Paper presented at the 13th Annual Postgraduate Course on the Rehabilitation of the Brain Injured Adult and Child, Williamsburg, VA.

Ducharme, S., Gill, K., Biener-Bergman, S., & Feritta, L. (1988). Sexual functioning: Medical and psychological aspects. In J. Delisa (Ed.), *Rehabilitation medicine* (pp. 519–536). Philadelphia: J.B. Lippincott.

Eisner, J., & Kreutzer, J. (1988). A family information system for education following traumatic brain injury. *Brain Injury, 3*(1), 79–90.

Epstein, N.B., Baldwin, L.M., & Bishop, D.S. (1983). The McMaster Family Assessment Device. *Journal of Marital and Family Therapy, 9*(2), 171–180.

Fawber, H., & Wachter, J. (1987). Job placement as a treatment component of the vocational rehabilitation process. *Journal of Head Trauma Rehabilitation, 2*(1), 27–33.

Frankowski, R.F., Annegers, J.F., & Whitman, S. (1985). The descriptive epidemiology of head trauma in the United States. In D.P. Becker and J.T. Povlishock (Eds.), *Central nervous system trauma status report* (GPO: 1988-520-149/00028). Washington, DC: National Institutes of Health, National Institute of Neurological and Communicative Disorders and Stroke.

Gardner, R.A. (1973). *The family book about minimal brain dysfunction.* New York: Jason Aronson.

Goldfried, M., & Davison, G. (1976). *Clinical behavior therapy.* New York: Holt, Rinehart & Winston.

Gordon, T. (1975). *Parent effectiveness training.* New York: The New American Library.

Heinemann, A., Keen, M., Donohue, R., & Schnoll, S. (1988). Alcohol use by persons with recent spinal cord injury. *Archives of Physical Medicine and Rehabilitation, 69,* 619–624.

Jackson, D.D. (1972). Family rules: Marital quid pro quo. In G. Erickson & T. Hogan (Eds.), *Family therapy: An introduction to theory and technique* (pp. 76–85). Monterey, CA: Wadsworth.

Jacobs, H.E. (1988). The Los Angeles Head Injury Survey: Procedures and initial findings. *Archives of Physical Medicine and Rehabilitation, 69,* 425–431.

Kozloff, R. (1987). Networks of social support and the outcome from severe head injury. *Journal of Head Trauma Rehabilitation, 2*(3), 14–23.

Kreutzer, J., Camplair, P., & Waaland, P. (1988). *Family Needs Questionnaire.* Richmond: Medical College of Virginia, Rehabilitation Research and Training Center on Severe Traumatic Brain Injury.

Kreutzer, J., Leininger, B., Doherty, K., & Waaland, P. (1987). *General Health and History Questionnaire.* Richmond: Medical College of Virginia, Rehabilitation Research and Training Center on Severe Traumatic Brain Injury.

Kreutzer, J.S., & Zasler, N. (1989). Psychosexual dysfunction following traumatic brain injury: Methodology and preliminary findings. *Brain Injury, 3*(2), 177–186.

Kurtzke, J.F. (1982). The current neurological burden of illness and injury in the United States. *Neurology, 32,* 1207–1210.

Leske, J. (1986). Needs of relatives of critically ill patients: A follow-up. *Heart and Lung, 15,* 189–193.

Lezak, M.D. (1978). Living with the characterologically altered brain-injured patient. *Journal of Clinical Psychiatry, 39,* 592–598.

Lezak, M.D. (1986). Psychological implications of traumatic brain damage for the patient's family. *Rehabilitation Psychology, 31,* 241–250.

Livingston, M., Brooks, D., & Bond, M. (1985a). Patient outcome in the year following severe head injury and relatives' psychiatric and social functioning. *Journal of Neurology, Neurosurgery, & Psychiatry, 48,* 876–881.

Livingston, M., Brooks, D., & Bond, M. (1985b). Three months after severe head injury: Psychiatric and social impact on relatives. *Journal of Neurology, Neurosurgery, & Psychiatry, 48,* 870–875.

Mauss-Clum, N., & Ryan, M. (1981). Brain injury and the family. *Journal of Neurosurgical Nursing, 13,* 165–169.

McKinlay, W., & Hickox, A. (1988). How can families help in the rehabilitation of the head injured? *Journal of Head Trauma Rehabilitation, 3*(4), 64–72.

Minuchin, S. (1974). *Families and family therapy.* New York: Basic Books.

Molter, N.C. (1979). Needs of relatives of critically ill patients: A descriptive study. *Heart and Lung, 8,* 332–337.

National Head Injury Foundation. (1988). *Catalog of educational materials.* Framingham, MA: Author.

Neistadt, M.E., & Freda, M. (1987). *A guide to sex counseling with physically disabled adults.* Malibar, FL: Robert E. Kreiger.

Norris, L.D., & Grove, S.K. (1986). Investigation of selected psychosocial needs of family members of critically ill adult patients. *Heart and Lung, 15,* 194–199.

Oddy, M., Humphrey, M., & Uttley, D. (1978). Stresses upon the relatives of head-injured patients. *British Journal of Psychiatry, 133,* 507–513.

Panting, A., & Merry, P. (1972). The long term rehabilitation of severe head injuries with particular reference to the need for social and medical support for the patient's family. *Journal of Rehabilitation, 38,* 33–37.

Rimel, R., Girodani, B., Barth, J., & Jane, J. (1982). Moderate head injury: Completing the clinical spectrum of brain trauma. *Neurosurgery, 11*(3), 344–351.

Rogers, P.M., & Kreutzer, J.S. (1984). Family crises following head injury: A network intervention strategy. *Journal of Neurosurgical Nursing, 16,* 343–346.

Rosenthal, M., & Young, T. (1988). Effective family intervention after traumatic brain injury: Theory and practice. *Journal of Head Trauma Rehabilitation, 3*(4), 42–50.

Rueveni, U. (1979). *Networking families in crisis.* New York: Human Sciences Press.

Satir, V. (1972). Family systems and approaches to family therapy. In G. Erickson & T. Hogan (Eds.), *Family therapy: An introduction to theory and technique* (pp. 211–221). Monterey, CA: Wadsworth.

Speck, R., & Attenave, C. (1973). *Family networks.* New York: Pantheon Books.

Terkelson, K. (1980). Toward a theory of the family life cycle. In E. Carter & M. McGoldrick (Eds.), *The family life cycle: A framework for family therapy* (pp. 21–52). New York: Gardner Press.

Thomas, J.P. (1988). The evolution of model systems of care in traumatic brain injury. *Journal of Head Trauma Rehabilitation, 3*(4), 1–5.

Thomsen, I.V (1974). The patient with severe head injury and his family. *Scandinavian Journal of Rehabilitation Medicine, 6,* 180–183.

Thomsen, I.V. (1984). Late outcome of severe blunt head trauma: A 10–15 year follow-up. *Journal of Neurology, Neurosurgery, and Psychiatry, 47,* 260–268.

Waaland, P., & Kretuzer, J.S. (1988). Family response to childhood traumatic brain injury. *Journal of Head Trauma Rehabilitation, 3*(4), 51–63.

Wehman, P., Kreutzer, J., Sale, P., Morton, M., Diambra, J., & West, M. (1989). Cognitive impairment and remediation: Implications for employment following traumatic brain injury. *Journal of Head Trauma Rehabilitation, 4*(3).

Wehman, P., Kreutzer, J., Stonnington, H., Wood, W., Sherron, P., Diambra, J., Fry, R., & Groah, C. (1988). Supported employment for persons with traumatic brain injury: A preliminary report. *Journal of Head Trauma Rehabilitation, 3*(4), 82–94.

Wehman, P., Kreutzer, J., Wood, W., Stonnington, H., Diambra, J., & Morton, M.V. (1989). Helping traumatically brain injured patients return to work with supported employment: Three case studies. *Archives of Physical Medicine and Rehabilitation, 70,* 109–113.

General Health and History Questionnaire

A MODEL PROJECT FOR COMPREHENSIVE REHABILITATIVE SERVICES TO INDIVIDUALS WITH TRAUMATIC BRAIN INJURY

Rehabilitation Psychology and Neuropsychology Service
Medical College of Virginia
Box 677 MCV Station
Richmond, Virginia 23298-0677
(804) 786-0200

GENERAL HEALTH AND HISTORY QUESTIONNAIRE (GHHQ/FAM/MCVEXT/LF)

PART I

DIRECTIONS: We are interested in how the patient has changed because of his/her head injury. Your answers to this form will help us understand problems related to the patient's injury and provide the best treatment. All information will be kept **confidential**. Please answer **all** questions. We realize you may be uncertain about some of the information you provide. We ask you to please be as **accurate as possible.**

Your Name: _____   Date ____-____-____

Address: _____

_____

Phone Number: (___)_____

Patient's Name: _____

Patient's Social Security Number: __ __ __-__ __-__ __ __ __

1. **Your** relationship to the patient (circle one):
    mother   father   wife   husband   brother   sister   son
    daughter   friend   girl/boyfriend   other _____
                                                    (please write in)

2. What is **your** date of birth? (please write in):
    Month: _____; Date: _____; Year: 19 _____

3. **CURRENTLY**, are **you** working? (circle one):
    full time   part time   not working
    If Yes, please write in **your** occupation _____

4. **CURRENTLY**, are **you** in school? (circle one):
    full time   part time   not in school

5. What is the highest grade **you** completed in school? (circle one):
    none   1–8 years   some high school   high school graduate
    some college   college graduate   postgraduate   unknown

6. Please indicate as accurately as possible the **date, month, and year** when the patient was hurt:
    Month: _____; Date: _____; Year 19_____

7. What is the patient's date of birth?
    Month: _____; Date: _____; Year 19_____

(continued)

8. How long was the patient unconscious or in coma? Please give your best estimate as to the number of minutes, hours, days, or months:
   _____ Minutes   _____ Hours   _____ Days   _____ Months
   _____ Never unconscious   _____ Unknown

9. **CURRENTLY**, is the patient taking medications for seizures? (circle one):
   Yes   No

   If yes, please list **all** medications, including those for seizures, the patient takes on a regular basis:
   1. _____   4. _____
   2. _____   5. _____
   3. _____   6. _____

10. **CURRENTLY**, do you live with the patient? (circle one):
    Yes   No

11. **CURRENTLY**, where does the patient live? (circle one):
    home/apartment   hospital   rehabilitation center/hospital
    nursing home   adult home/transitional living center
    other _____
           (please write in)

12. **CURRENTLY**, who lives with the patient? (circle all that apply):
    mother   father   wife   husband   brother   sister   son
    daughter   friend   girl/boyfriend   other _____
                                         (please write in)

13. If the patient is **CURRENTLY** living at home, how **comfortable do you feel about** leaving him/her at home alone? (circle one):
    1 ---------------------- 2 ---------------------- 3 ---------------------- 4 ----------------------5
    very   a little   very
    uncomfortable   uncomfortable   comfortable

14. **CURRENTLY**, is the patient medically restricted from driving? (circle one):
    Yes   No

    If the patient is not medically restricted for driving, does he/she have a valid drivers license? (circle one):
    Yes   No

15. **CURRENTLY**, what is the patient's marital status? (circle one):
    single   married   steady relationship   separated
    engaged   divorced   unmarried/living with mate   widowed
    If married, how many years has he/she been married? _____

16. **BEFORE** the injury, was the patient working? (circle one):
    full time   20–39 hours/week   1–19 hours/week   not working

17. **BEFORE** the injury, was the patient in school? (circle one):
    full time   part time   not in school

18. **CURRENTLY**, is the patient in school? (circle one):
    full time   part time   not in school

19. **CURRENTLY**, is the patient working? (circle one):
    full time   20–39 hours/week   1–19 hours/week   not working

20. **CURRENTLY**, what is the highest grade completed by the patient? (circle one):
    none   1–8 years   some high school   high school graduate
    some college   college graduate   postgraduate   unknown

(continued)

General Health and History Questionnaire (*continued*)

21. List the jobs the patient held **BEFORE** the injury, the number of hours worked per week, and the starting and finishing dates of each job. If you are unsure of the exact dates, please give your **best estimate**. Where needed, describe the position held. Only include those jobs in which the patient earned at least minimum wage. **List his/her most recent job on line #1:**

Type of Job	Average Number of Hours Per Week	Month/Day/Year Started	Finished
1. _____	____ hrs.	___/___/___	___/___/___
2. _____	____ hrs.	___/___/___	___/___/___
3. _____	____ hrs.	___/___/___	___/___/___
4. _____	____ hrs.	___/___/___	___/___/___
5. _____	____ hrs.	___/___/___	___/___/___
6. _____	____ hrs.	___/___/___	___/___/___

22. List the jobs the patient has held **SINCE** the injury, the number of hours worked per week, and the starting and finishing dates of each job. If you are unsure of the exact dates, please give your **best estimate**. Where needed, describe the position held by the patient. Only include those jobs in which the patient earned at least minimum wage. **List his/her most recent job on line #1.**

Type of Job	Average Number of Hours Per Week	Month/Day/Year Started	Finished
1. _____	____ hrs.	___/___/___	___/___/___
2. _____	____ hrs.	___/___/___	___/___/___
3. _____	____ hrs.	___/___/___	___/___/___
4. _____	____ hrs.	___/___/___	___/___/___
5. _____	____ hrs.	___/___/___	___/___/___
6. _____	____ hrs.	___/___/___	___/___/___

23. **CURRENTLY**, is the patient working in a sheltered workshop? (circle one):

Yes   No

24. If the patient is **not CURRENTLY** a full-time student or is **not** working full time, which of the following **prevent or interfere** with employment. Put a check in the blank next to the items that apply:

_____ no transportation   _____ can't speak properly
_____ bad temper   _____ can't understand speech
_____ no motivation/doesn't care   _____ memory
_____ no pep or energy   _____ seizures
_____ can't walk/climb stairs   _____ medically ill, sick
_____depression   _____ thinking problems
_____poor vision   _____ trouble using hands, arms, legs

List any other problems that you feel get in the way:

_____
_____

25. **BEFORE** the injury, did the patient ever have any of the following medical problems? Please check all that apply:

_____ heart attack   _____ senility   _____ diabetes
_____ stroke   _____ other (please write in) _____

(*continued*)

26. **SINCE** the injury, did the patient ever have any of the following medical problems? Please check all that apply:

_____ heart attack _____ senility _____ diabetes

_____ stroke _____ other (please write in) _____

27. For how many head injuries has the patient received medical treatment? Be sure to include the patient's most recent injury. (write in the number of head injuries):

\# _____

28. **BEFORE** the injury, was the patient ever treated by a psychiatrist or psychologist? (circle one):

Yes   No

If yes, please check the following reasons that apply:

_____ depression _____ schizophrenia _____ nerves/tension

_____ drug/alcohol problem _____ other (please write in) _____

29. **SINCE** the injury, has the patient been treated by a psychiatrist or psychologist? (circle one):

Yes   No

If yes, please check the following reasons that apply:

_____ depression _____ schizophrenia _____ nerves/tension

_____ drug/alcohol problem _____ other _____
              specify

30. **BEFORE** the injury, was the patient ever held back a grade in school because of learning problems in reading, writing, and/or arithmetic? (circle one):

Yes   No

31. **SINCE** the injury, has the patient been held back a grade in school because of learning problems in reading, writing, and/or arithmetic? Do not include rehabilitation classes. (circle one):

Yes   No

32 **BEFORE** the injury, was the patient ever placed in special classes for problems in reading, writing, and/or arithmetic? (circle one):

Yes   No

33. **SINCE** the injury, has the patient been placed in special classes for problems in reading, writing, and/or arithmetic? Do not include rehabilitation classes. (circle one):

Yes   No

34. **BEFORE** the injury, was the patient a nondrinker (never drank alcoholic beverages)? (circle one):

Yes   No

35. **BEFORE** the injury, did the patient have a drinking problem? (circle one):

Yes   No

36. **CURRENTLY**, does the patient drink alcohol? (circle one):

Yes   No

37. **CURRENTLY**, does the patient have a drinking problem? (circle one):

Yes   No

38. **BEFORE** the injury, did the patient use illegal drugs? (circle one):

Yes   No

39. Please indicate the drugs that were used **BEFORE** the injury:

marijuana   cocaine   other (please write in) _____

40. **CURRENTLY**, does the patient use illegal drugs? (circle one):

Yes   No

(continued)

General Health and History Questionnaire (*continued*)

41. Please indicate the drugs **CURRENTLY** being used:
    marijuana   cocaine   other (please write in) _____

42. **BEFORE** the injury, was the patient ever arrested? (circle one):
    Yes   No
    If Yes, please explain each arrest:
    _____
    _____
    _____
    _____

43. **BEFORE** the injury, was he/she convicted? (circle one):
    Yes   No
    If Yes, please explain each conviction:
    _____
    _____
    _____
    _____

44. **SINCE** his/her injury, has the patient been arrested? (circle one):
    Yes   No
    If Yes, please explain each arrest:
    _____
    _____
    _____
    _____

45. **SINCE** the injury, has he/she been convicted? (circle one):
    Yes   No
    If Yes, please explain each conviction:
    _____
    _____
    _____
    _____

46. Place a check next to the services listed below that the patient is **CURRENTLY** receiving. If the patient is not receiving any services, leave question blank:
    ____ physical therapy   ____ vocational training
    ____ psychotherapy   ____ occupational therapy
    ____ Virginia Department of   ____ transportation
         Rehabilitative Services (DRS) ____ speech therapy
    ____ cognitive retraining   ____ work adjustment/hardening
    other (please specify): _____
    _____
    _____

PART II

PROBLEM CHECKLIST

DIRECTIONS: We would like to know if the patient **CURRENTLY** has any of the problems listed below, and if so, how often. Please place an "X" in the box under the label ("never," "sometimes," "often," or "always") that best describes how often each problem occurs. **PLEASE ANSWER ALL ITEMS.**

	NEVER	SOMETIMES	OFTEN	ALWAYS	DOES NOT APPLY
SOMATIC					
01. Blackout spells	[ ]	[ ]	[ ]	[ ]	
02. Difficulty lifting heavy objects	[ ]	[ ]	[ ]	[ ]	
03. Dizzy	[ ]	[ ]	[ ]	[ ]	
04. Difficulty smelling things	[ ]	[ ]	[ ]	[ ]	
05. Double vision	[ ]	[ ]	[ ]	[ ]	[ ]
06. Drops things	[ ]	[ ]	[ ]	[ ]	
07. Eats too much	[ ]	[ ]	[ ]	[ ]	
08. Food doesn't taste right	[ ]	[ ]	[ ]	[ ]	
09. Headaches	[ ]	[ ]	[ ]	[ ]	
10. Loses balance	[ ]	[ ]	[ ]	[ ]	[ ]
11. Moves slowly	[ ]	[ ]	[ ]	[ ]	
12. Muscles ache	[ ]	[ ]	[ ]	[ ]	
13. Muscles numb	[ ]	[ ]	[ ]	[ ]	
14. Muscles tingle or twitch	[ ]	[ ]	[ ]	[ ]	
15. Nauseous	[ ]	[ ]	[ ]	[ ]	
16. Nightmares	[ ]	[ ]	[ ]	[ ]	
17. Poor appetite	[ ]	[ ]	[ ]	[ ]	
18. Picks nose or skin	[ ]	[ ]	[ ]	[ ]	
19. Ringing in ears	[ ]	[ ]	[ ]	[ ]	
20. Seizures	[ ]	[ ]	[ ]	[ ]	
21. Stomach bloated or gassy	[ ]	[ ]	[ ]	[ ]	
22. Stomach hurts	[ ]	[ ]	[ ]	[ ]	
23. Tired	[ ]	[ ]	[ ]	[ ]	
24. Trips over things	[ ]	[ ]	[ ]	[ ]	
25. Trouble falling asleep	[ ]	[ ]	[ ]	[ ]	
26. Trouble hearing	[ ]	[ ]	[ ]	[ ]	
27. Trouble staying awake	[ ]	[ ]	[ ]	[ ]	
28. Trouble waking up	[ ]	[ ]	[ ]	[ ]	
29. Vision blurred	[ ]	[ ]	[ ]	[ ]	[ ]
30. Weak	[ ]	[ ]	[ ]	[ ]	
THINKING					
31. Difficulty handling money	[ ]	[ ]	[ ]	[ ]	[ ]
32. Can't get mind off certain thoughts	[ ]	[ ]	[ ]	[ ]	
33. Difficulty performing chores	[ ]	[ ]	[ ]	[ ]	[ ]
34. Difficulty attending work or school	[ ]	[ ]	[ ]	[ ]	[ ]
35. Concentration is poor	[ ]	[ ]	[ ]	[ ]	
36. Confused	[ ]	[ ]	[ ]	[ ]	

(continued)

General Health and History Questionnaire (*continued*)

	NEVER	SOMETIMES	OFTEN	ALWAYS	DOES NOT APPLY
37. Drives dangerously	[ ]	[ ]	[ ]	[ ]	[ ]
38. Easily distracted	[ ]	[ ]	[ ]	[ ]	
39. Forgets or misses appointments	[ ]	[ ]	[ ]	[ ]	[ ]
40. Forgets people's names	[ ]	[ ]	[ ]	[ ]	
41. Forgets phone numbers	[ ]	[ ]	[ ]	[ ]	
42. Forgets to do chores or work	[ ]	[ ]	[ ]	[ ]	[ ]
43. Forgets to eat	[ ]	[ ]	[ ]	[ ]	
44. Forgets to take medications	[ ]	[ ]	[ ]	[ ]	[ ]
45. Forgets yesterday's events	[ ]	[ ]	[ ]	[ ]	
46. Forgets what he/she reads	[ ]	[ ]	[ ]	[ ]	[ ]
47. Friends or relatives are unfamiliar	[ ]	[ ]	[ ]	[ ]	[ ]
48. Late for appointments	[ ]	[ ]	[ ]	[ ]	[ ]
49. Learns slowly	[ ]	[ ]	[ ]	[ ]	
50. Loses track of time, day, or date	[ ]	[ ]	[ ]	[ ]	
51. Loses way, gets lost	[ ]	[ ]	[ ]	[ ]	[ ]
52. Makes mistakes doing arithmetic	[ ]	[ ]	[ ]	[ ]	[ ]
53. Misplaces things	[ ]	[ ]	[ ]	[ ]	
54. Reads slowly	[ ]	[ ]	[ ]	[ ]	
55. Thinks slowly	[ ]	[ ]	[ ]	[ ]	
56. Trouble making decisions	[ ]	[ ]	[ ]	[ ]	
57. Trouble following instructions	[ ]	[ ]	[ ]	[ ]	
58. Loses train of thought	[ ]	[ ]	[ ]	[ ]	
59. Forgets if he/she has done things	[ ]	[ ]	[ ]	[ ]	
60. Forgets to turn off appliances	[ ]	[ ]	[ ]	[ ]	

BEHAVIOR

	NEVER	SOMETIMES	OFTEN	ALWAYS	
61. Bored	[ ]	[ ]	[ ]	[ ]	
62. Breaks or throws things	[ ]	[ ]	[ ]	[ ]	
63. Complains	[ ]	[ ]	[ ]	[ ]	
64. Cries	[ ]	[ ]	[ ]	[ ]	
65. Curses at others	[ ]	[ ]	[ ]	[ ]	
66. Curses at self	[ ]	[ ]	[ ]	[ ]	
67. Difficulty understanding jokes	[ ]	[ ]	[ ]	[ ]	
68. Disorganized	[ ]	[ ]	[ ]	[ ]	
69. Difficulty enjoying activities	[ ]	[ ]	[ ]	[ ]	
70. Feels hopeless	[ ]	[ ]	[ ]	[ ]	
71. Feels worthless	[ ]	[ ]	[ ]	[ ]	
72. Frustrated	[ ]	[ ]	[ ]	[ ]	
73. Hard to get started on things	[ ]	[ ]	[ ]	[ ]	
74. Hits or pushes others	[ ]	[ ]	[ ]	[ ]	
75. Impatient	[ ]	[ ]	[ ]	[ ]	
76. Inappropriate comments/behavior	[ ]	[ ]	[ ]	[ ]	
77. Jumpy, irritable	[ ]	[ ]	[ ]	[ ]	
78. Laughs for no reason	[ ]	[ ]	[ ]	[ ]	
79. Lonely	[ ]	[ ]	[ ]	[ ]	
80. Misunderstood by others	[ ]	[ ]	[ ]	[ ]	

(*continued*)

		NEVER	SOMETIMES	OFTEN	ALWAYS	DOES NOT APPLY
81.	Nervous	[ ]	[ ]	[ ]	[ ]	
82.	No confidence	[ ]	[ ]	[ ]	[ ]	
83.	Restless	[ ]	[ ]	[ ]	[ ]	
84.	Sad, blue	[ ]	[ ]	[ ]	[ ]	
85.	Scared or frightened	[ ]	[ ]	[ ]	[ ]	
86.	Screams or yells	[ ]	[ ]	[ ]	[ ]	
87.	Sits with nothing to do	[ ]	[ ]	[ ]	[ ]	
88.	Threatens to hurt others	[ ]	[ ]	[ ]	[ ]	
89.	Threatens to hurt self	[ ]	[ ]	[ ]	[ ]	

COMMUNICATION

		NEVER	SOMETIMES	OFTEN	ALWAYS	DOES NOT APPLY
90.	Difficulty thinking of right word	[ ]	[ ]	[ ]	[ ]	
91.	Difficulty pronouncing words	[ ]	[ ]	[ ]	[ ]	
92.	Difficulty making conversation	[ ]	[ ]	[ ]	[ ]	
93.	Makes spelling mistakes	[ ]	[ ]	[ ]	[ ]	[ ]
94.	Repeats what others say	[ ]	[ ]	[ ]	[ ]	
95.	Speech doesn't make sense	[ ]	[ ]	[ ]	[ ]	
96.	Talks too fast or slow	[ ]	[ ]	[ ]	[ ]	
97.	Trouble understanding conversation ..	[ ]	[ ]	[ ]	[ ]	
98.	Writes slowly	[ ]	[ ]	[ ]	[ ]	
99.	(His/her)Writing is hard to read	[ ]	[ ]	[ ]	[ ]	

SOCIAL

		NEVER	SOMETIMES	OFTEN	ALWAYS	DOES NOT APPLY
100.	Argues	[ ]	[ ]	[ ]	[ ]	
101.	Avoids family members	[ ]	[ ]	[ ]	[ ]	
102.	Avoids friends	[ ]	[ ]	[ ]	[ ]	
103.	Doesn't participate in sports	[ ]	[ ]	[ ]	[ ]	
104.	Rude to others	[ ]	[ ]	[ ]	[ ]	
105.	Uncomfortable around others	[ ]	[ ]	[ ]	[ ]	

106. How much stress have you felt because of the changes in your relative/friend since the injury? (circle one number):

   0 --------------- 1 --------------- 2 --------------- 3 --------------- 4 --------------- 5 --------------- 6
   No   Moderate   Severe
   Stress   Stress   Stress

107. How <u>accurate</u> are your answers to this questionnaire? (circle one number):

   0 -------------------------- ---- 1 ---------------------------- --- 2 -------------------------- -- 3
   not at all   somewhat   mostly   very
   accurate   accurate   accurate   accurate

REMINDER: Please <u>check</u> to make sure that you have <u>not skipped</u> any items.

Source: Kreutzer, J., Leininger, B., Doherty, K., & Waaland, P. (1987). *General Health and History Question-naire.* Richmond: Medical College of Virginia, Rehabilitation Research and Training Center on Severe Traumatic Brain Injury; reprinted with permission.

Family Needs Questionnaire

Your Name: _____   Date: ____-____-____

DIRECTIONS: The following statements describe needs that friends and relatives of people with head injury sometimes have. These needs normally change over time. We are interested in knowing how important they are to you at the present time and whether they are being met. The information you provide will help us to understand the needs of your family and other families of head injury survivors.

1. Show how important you feel these needs are by using the scale below and placing a circle around the number that best describes your answer. If a certain need does not apply to your situation, circle "N/A" for "not applicable":

N/A	1 -------------- 2 -------------- 3 -------------- 4
Not	Not Slightly Important Very
Applicable	Important Important Important

2. Use this scale to tell us whether each need is being met by circling: Y (Yes), P (Partly), or N (No). Make these ratings only for items that apply to your situation (only if you rated them from 1 to 4):

Y ------------------ P ------------------ N
Yes   Partly   No

Examples:

1. I need to get enough rest or sleep.   N/A | 1 ②3 4   Ⓨ P N

    (this person rated the need as currently being "Slightly Important," and feels it is currently being met)

2. I need to have help keeping the house (e.g., shopping, cleaning, cooking).   Ⓝ/Ⓐ | 1 2 3 4   Y P N

    (this person felt the item didn't apply to her situation, so she circled "N/A" and went on to the next question)

N/A	1 --------------- 2 --------------- 3 --------------- 4	Y --------- P ---------- N
Not	Not Slightly Important Very	Yes Partly No
Applicable	Important Important Important	

I NEED . . .:		HOW IMPORTANT?	NEED MET?
1. to be shown that medical, educational, or rehabilitation staff respect the patient's needs or wishes.	N/A	1 2 3 4	Y P N
2. to be told daily what is being done with or for the patient.	N/A	1 2 3 4	Y P N
3. to give my opinions daily to others involved in the patient's care, rehabilitation, or education.	N/A	1 2 3 4	Y P N
4. to be told about all changes in the patient's medical status.	N/A	1 2 3 4	Y P N
5. to be assured that the best possible medical care is being given to the patient.	N/A	1 2 3 4	Y P N
6. to have explanations from professionals given in terms I can understand.	N/A	1 2 3 4	Y P N
7. to have my questions answered honestly.	N/A	1 2 3 4	Y P N

(continued)

N/A	1 --------------- 2 --------------- 3 --------------- 4	Y --------- P ---------- N
Not	Not	Slightly	Important	Very	Yes	Partly	No
Applicable	Important	Important		Important			

		HOW IMPORTANT?	NEED MET?
I NEED . . . :			
8.	to be shown that my opinions are used in planning the patient's treatment, rehabilitation, or education.	N/A 1 2 3 4	Y P N
9.	to have a professional to turn to for advice or services when the patient needs help.	N/A 1 2 3 4	Y P N
10.	to have different staff members agree on the best way to help the patient.	N/A 1 2 3 4	Y P N
11.	to have complex information on the medical care of head injuries (e.g., medications, injections, or surgery).	N/A 1 2 3 4	Y P N
12.	to have complete information on the patient's physical problems (e.g., weakness, headaches, dizziness, problems with vision or walking).	N/A 1 2 3 4	Y P N
13.	to have complete information on the patient's problems in thinking (e.g., confusion, memory, or communication).	N/A 1 2 3 4	Y P N
14.	to have complete information on drug or alcohol problems and treatment.	N/A 1 2 3 4	Y P N
15.	to be told why the patient acts in ways that are different, difficult, or strange.	N/A 1 2 3 4	Y P N
16.	to be told how long each of the patient's problems is expected to last.	N/A 1 2 3 4	Y P N
17.	to be shown what to do when the patient is upset or acting strange.	N/A 1 2 3 4	Y P N
18.	to have information on the patient's rehabilitative or educational progress.	N/A 1 2 3 4	Y P N
19.	to have help in deciding how much to let the patient do by himself/herself.	N/A 1 2 3 4	Y P N
20.	to have enough resources for the patient (e.g., rehabilitation programs, physical therapy, counseling, job counseling).	N/A 1 2 3 4	Y P N
21.	to have enough resources for myself or the family (e.g., financial or legal counseling, respite care, counseling, nursing or day care).	N/A 1 2 3 4	Y P N
22.	to have help keeping the house (e.g., shopping, cleaning, cooking).	N/A 1 2 3 4	Y P N
23.	to have help from other members of the family in taking care of the patient.	N/A 1 2 3 4	Y P N
24.	to get enough rest or sleep.	N/A 1 2 3 4	Y P N
25.	to get a break from my problems and responsibilities.	N/A 1 2 3 4	Y P N
26.	to spend time with my friends.	N/A 1 2 3 4	Y P N
27.	to pay attention to my own needs, job, or interests.	N/A 1 2 3 4	Y P N
28.	to be told if I am making the best possible decisions about the patient.	N/A 1 2 3 4	Y P N
29.	to have my spouse understand how difficult it is for me.	N/A 1 2 3 4	Y P N
30.	to have other family members understand how difficult it is for me.	N/A 1 2 3 4	Y P N

(continued)

Family Needs Questionnaire (*continued*)

N/A	1 --------------- 2 --------------- 3 --------------- 4				Y --------- P ---------- N
Not	Not	Slightly	Important	Very	Yes Partly No
Applicable	Important	Important		Important	

		HOW IMPORTANT?	NEED MET?
I NEED . . .:			
31.	to have other family members understand the patient's problems.	N/A 1 2 3 4	Y P N
32.	to have the patient's friends understand his/her problems.	N/A 1 2 3 4	Y P N
33.	to have the patient's employer, co-workers, or teachers understand his/her problems.	N/A 1 2 3 4	Y P N
34.	to discuss my feelings about the patient with someone who has gone through the same experience.	N/A 1 2 3 4	Y P N
35.	to discuss my feelings about the patient with other friends or family.	N/A 1 2 3 4	Y P N
36.	to be reassured that it is usual to have strong negative feelings about the patient.	N/A 1 2 3 4	Y P N
37.	help getting over my doubts and fears about the future.	N/A 1 2 3 4	Y P N
38.	help in remaining hopeful about the patient's future.	N/A 1 2 3 4	Y P N
39.	help preparing for the worst.	N/A 1 2 3 4	Y P N
40.	to be encouraged to ask others to help out.	N/A 1 2 3 4	Y P N

If there are other needs that were not included on this questionnaire, please write them in on the lines below:

1. _____

2. _____

3. _____

Source: Kreutzer, J., Camplair, P., & Waaland, P. (1988). *Family Needs Questionnaire.* Richmond: Medical College of Virginia, Rehabilitation Research and Training Center on Severe Traumatic Brain Injury; reprinted with permission.

SECTION VI
Children's Issues

CHAPTER 17

The Rehabilitation of Children with Traumatic Brain Injury
Coma to Community

Janice L. Cockrell, Jeffrey Chase, and Eloise Cobb

In the United States each year approximately 165,000 children and youth are estimated to suffer head injuries severe enough to result in hospitalization (Savage, 1987), yet relatively few rehabilitation programs that are geared to the specific needs of head injured children exist. While the sequelae of head injury in children are often similar to those observed in adults, factors that have proved useful to prognosticate ultimate outcome in adults have not been found to be reliable in pediatric head injury. Most outcome research suggests that the overall recovery from traumatic brain injury is better in preschool or school-age children than in young infants and adults (Bruce, Schut, Bruno, Wood, & Sutton, 1978; Kraus, Fife, & Conroy, 1987; Stover & Zeiger, 1976). Yet one group has found no correlation between age and outcome (Johnston & Mellets, 1980). Certainly motoric outcome is better in the pediatric age group: Brink, Imbus, and Woo-San (1980) found that 73% of 344 severely injured patients less than 18 years of age "regained physical independence."

The reason for poor outcome in very young children has been subject to debate. It has been thought by some individuals to be due to immaturity of the organism (Rutter, Chadwick, & Shaffer, 1983), while others have hypothesized a relationship between the closing of the fontanels and the ability of the cranial vault to protect the brain from injury (Raimondi & Hirschauer, 1984). Yet others have felt that under age 2 the premorbid life repertoire is so limited that the child with brain injury has little to draw on to develop compensatory strategies (Ewing-Cobbs, Fletcher, & Levin, 1985). Certainly the type or cause of injury plays a role (Sprum, Tupper, Risson, Tuokko, & Edgell, 1984). In children below the age of 2 years, traumatic brain injury is often not accidental and may be the result of chronic abuse. In school-age children, pedistrian–motor vehicle, bicycle, and off-the-road vehicle accidents are most common. In adolescents 16 years and older, involvement in high-speed motor vehicle accidents is the most common etiology. An additional problem in comparing outcome studies is that because the neurosurgical management for traumatic brain injury has changed drastically over the past 20 years, older studies are not useful predictors of current outcome.

The issue of the plasticity of a child's brain as compared to the adult brain continues to generate controversy. Indeed it appears that the recovery curve in children is steeper and it plateaus later than in adults. Several studies have documented outcome in children with prolonged unconsciousness from brain injury, and found that 20%–30% became independent in self-care (Brink et al., 1980; Kriel, Krach, & Sheehan, 1988; Pagni, Signoroni, Crotti, & Tombi, 1975). Unfortunately many of the outcome studies have focused primarily on motoric outcome, which, as stated previously, tends to be excellent. Cog-

287

nitive capacity is more difficult to evaluate. Neuropsychological instruments are not available to assess very young children, and even in school-age children higher level cognitive functioning cannot be reliably tested until age 13.

The pediatric head injury program is challenged by the necessity of returning the child to a learning environment. While an adult can return to a previously learned work or home routine, the child must return to school where he or she is expected to learn new material, and it is the ability for new learning that is most affected by head injury. Heiskanen and Kaste (1974) have stated that as many as 50% of children with coma lasting more than 24 hours but less than 2 weeks may have impaired performance in school. In addition, the return to the learning environment is often hindered by distractibility and acquired attention disorder. School is a highly distracting environment, and children with auditory processing or attention deficit disorders secondary to head injury have a great deal of difficulty in this setting. Many rehabilitation programs do not evaluate the child in a distractible environment prior to discharge, and therefore may not prepare the family for these problems at school.

The pediatric rehabilitation specialist is fortunate in that, with the exception of some abuse cases, the child's family invariably is concerned, supportive, and anxious to care for the child in the home environment. It is important that the rehabilitation personnel take advantage of this concern, and avoid any appearance of a judgmental attitude when families may have alternative life-styles. It is important to incorporate family values and concerns into the child's program to enhance parental motivation and participation, as well as long-term generalization of therapy.

INPATIENT REHABILITATION

Goals

While the goals of inpatient rehabilitation are numerous, their interdependence requires that all components be addressed if the patient's long-term adjustment is to be maximized. Inpatient rehabilitation goals include: prevention of secondary medical complications; achievement of maximum physical function and independence within the appropriate developmental framework; education of caregivers, school personnel, and primary physicians regarding the probable sequelae; proper school placement; assisting siblings and parents in coping with their loss and accompanying guilt; and, ultimately, the return to home and community. Unless all of these areas are addressed, the inpatient rehabilitation program is incomplete. Returning a child to a family that is overwhelmed with grief or guilt is a prescription for disaster. Returning a child to a school that is not anticipating either cognitive or behavioral difficulties will result in a child who is frustrated, family members who are angry, and a school system that feels impotent and that lacks investment in the child's recovery.

Inpatient Pediatric Rehabilitation Team

A pediatrician and a physiatrist, preferably one trained in pediatrics, should be readily available to every patient on a pediatric rehabilitation unit. Pediatric subspecialty consultations should be easily accessible, including neurosurgery, general surgery, othropedics, gastroenterology, and neurology.

As in adult head injury rehabilitation programs, a physical therapist, occupational therapist, and speech pathologist are members of the team, but all should be skilled in working with children and be capable of incorporating play into the program. They need to be knowledgeable of the developmental stages of childhood and how to tailor therapy to individual needs. Therapy environments should have a large selection of toys and equipment of various sizes. Because younger children are not always able to work independently, a higher therapist-to-patient ratio is typically required in a pediatric program than in an adult rehabilitation program.

A clinical child psychologist, preferably with an extensive neuropsychological background, should be available to provide not only support to both the child and his or her family, but appropriate testing and counseling as well. A social worker who is skilled in working with families can assist with family counseling, as well as with identification of financial resources and community support systems.

Educational services are an integral part of any pediatric rehabilitation program. The educational consultant needs to be capable of dealing with children with special needs and knowledgeable of technical innovations in education such as alternative computer inputs, and should have an excellent relationship with the local school systems.

A pediatric audiologist is also an important member of the team. The authors have found a fairly high incidence of auditory problems as well as central auditory processing difficulties in children with head injury (Cockrell, Gregory, & Zuparro, in press). Identification of these deficits is vital for a child who plans to return to school, because poor hearing or auditory distractibility can cause great difficulty in the learning environment, as well as confusion for school personnel.

It is commonly said that "play is the work of children." In a pediatric rehabilitation center, recreational therapy should be readily available to all children. Children's Hospital, Richmond, Virginia, where the authors work, feels so strongly about this that it does not charge for recreational therapy services. All children participate at least one time daily in the child life program, where they have opportunities to express themselves in a nonthreatening environment and to improve leisure skills. The playroom is a "safe environment" where the child may not receive any type of medical treatment. An additional advantage of the child life area is that it is a highly distracting environment, and thus allows the staff to test and retrain the child's capacity to concentrate in the presence of multiple visual and auditory stimuli.

Rehabilitation nursing is the backbone of the program. The nurses must be able to implement behavior programs, carry out interdisciplinary goals, and provide loving structure and discipline to the children. They must be supportive of the parents, provide teaching, demonstrate procedures, and serve as an anchor for a child in an active, multifaceted hospital environment. The nursing service provides some of the most

valuable observations regarding a child's functional capacity and adjustment, as well as family relationships. The nursing staff must be able to develop intimate relationships with the patients and their families without becoming over involved. Primary care nursing should be the goal in order to establish the trust and consistency so vital to recovery.

The parent, one of the most important team members, its frequently overlooked in many programs. No parent is perfect, but each parent is the world's expert on his or her child. Staff must not confuse parental grief, guilt, or denial with an inability to understand the child. The parent is a source of valuable information regarding previous interests, behavior, and motivators. It is difficult to establish an effective behavioral program without input from the parent. The authors find it useful in most cases to include the parent in every team conference, and to provide them with copies of the conference report. In this manner, the parents feel that their input is valuable and so develop self-confidence. Frequently parents feel overwhelmed by the expertise and skill of medical personnel, and bring this lack of confidence to the rehabilitation program. It is important to quickly reassure them that the staff feel that they are competent, and that their input is valuable. One useful strategy is to have a parent spend the night with the child when he or she is transferred to the rehabilitation facility. In this way the agitation that often ensues after a transfer can be quieted by the parent. This restores the parents' confidence in their skills with their child, and involves them directly in the child's care. While the authors do not expect the parents to be present at all times, and indeed this is discouraged, from time to time they are requested to attend various therapies to see their child's progress, and to learn some useful techniques. It should be noted that involvement of the parents in the team and in program planning may be more difficult than anticipated; however, most families are capable of making valuable contributions. The only exceptions are families where substance abuse is a significant detriment, or where overt psychiatric behavior on the part of a parent is present. A parent of very low intelligence is not a contraindication to involvement in the team and posthospitalization care of his or her child.

A very common situation facing the rehabilitation team is the divorced and/or melded family. If overt hostility between the divorced parents is present, the team deals primarily with the legal guardian. When divorced couples are at least tolerant of each other's presence, all parents and stepparents are equally involved in both conferencing and passes.

Depending on the institution, other team members may contribute to the program. Volunteer grandparents can be particularly helpful when the parents live a great distance from the institution and cannot visit frequently. Chaplains can assist with family support. The rehabilitation coordinator plays a major role in focusing the child's program.

Physical Plant

A pediatric rehabilitation facility should include a playroom and youth lounge on the unit that allow for free play, in addition to the recreational therapy area. According to the American Academy of Pediatrics (1960) "a playroom is not a luxury or a place where beds may be placed in an emergency. It is a therapeutic adjunct. . . . It is a necessary part of every pediatric unit" (p. 19). Facilities should be available for parents staying overnight, such as convertible chairs in the rooms, hospitality houses, or arrangements with nearby hotels. A supervised outside playground should be available. This should have safe equipment and nonpoisonous plants and shrubbery. Drinking fountains, toilets, and sinks should be accessible to children. Cartoon murals should be used cautiously as very large ones may distress infants and can offend adolescents (Rappazzo, 1980). Rooms should be simple and children should be allowed to decorate their rooms with favorite items, posters, and drawings. Two outstanding resource books regarding the necessary physical facilities for pediatric care are *Changing Hospital Environments for Children* by Lindheim, Glaser, and Coffin (1972), and the American Academy of Pediatrics (1986) publication *Hospital Care of Children and Youth*.

Rehabilitation in the Intensive Care Unit

If the rehabilitation specialist is fortunate enough to receive consultations while the child is still in the intensive care unit, this is an excellent opportunity to meet with family members and provide them with reassurance and educational information such as information regarding the stages of coma, common sequelae, and the likelihood of a temporary increase in agitation with transfer to another setting, such as the general neurosurgery floor. The rehabilitation specialist can work with the intensive care unit in trying to decrease the amount of stimulation in the intensive care unit, assure proper positioning, and ensure a smooth transition from the unit to the floor or to the rehabilitation facility. The rehabilitation specialist can also assist the families with transfers to appropriate out-of-town facilities should they reside in another area of the country. As many families are eager to tour the rehabilitation facility at this time, the rehabilitation specialist can make the necessary arrangements for them to do so.

Acute Inpatient Rehabilitation

Transfer to the rehabilitation facility is often a happy time for the families of children with traumatic brain injury. To them it symbolizes the first step toward return to a normal life. This optimism and enthusiasm can be utilized by the rehabilitation team in eliciting the family's involvement with the rehabilitation program. As previously mentioned, a parent or other adult family member is encouraged to stay overnight until the child adjusts to the new environment.

Families are sometimes disappointed that their child appears to regress immediately following transfer to the rehabilitation unit. However, if they are warned of this possibility ahead of time they are usually better able to deal with it. If the child is agitated or wanders extensively, a family member is often willing to supervise the child and thus avoid the necessity of restraints. When a family member cannot be present and the child is so agitated as to need restraints, the parent needs to be called personally by a familiar team member and informed of the restraining order. It is most upsetting for a family member to arrive at the unit and find the child in restraints. Restrained patients must be watched carefully, as they have been known to wriggle free of restraints and become entangled. Children should never be managed with adult-size restraints. In the authors' unit, restraints are rarely used because of parental involvement and because of the utilization of other staff members to observe the children during the day.

Team conferences are scheduled within 1 week of admission to the rehabilitation unit, and every 2 weeks thereafter. Patients under age 13 are usually not invited to team conferences, but those 13 and older are frequently included in the conferences if they so desire. Parents and other significant family members such as grandparents are invited to all team conferences. School personnel from the child's school district are encouraged to attend, as well as other interested parties, such as insurance case managers. The conference includes a listing of all individuals present and their disciplines, a summary from each team member, individualized goals from each team member with a commentary on whether previous goals have been met, and interdisciplinary strategies to achieve these goals.

Use of a milieu program, which is described in the next section of this chapter, has produced outstanding progress in difficult patients. It has become customary in the authors' program to set up a milieu program for most of the patients to provide more consistency. The individualized milieu program is established during the team conference. During the conference the estimated length of stay and home passes are planned.

The team members are encouraged to present their initial reports in language a layperson can understand so that the family immediately feels a part of the team effort. After a week or so, the parents usually pick up team "jargon" and are able to understand more standard presentations. It is useful for the physician or designated staff member to review the initial team findings with the family afterward in order to clarify and amplify specific team concerns. It is important to explain to parents that the initial findings are baseline evaluations, and that these will be used to subsequently assess the rate of improvement in their child. If this is not reviewed with the parents, they may become quite upset by the initial conference and may refuse to come to subsequent ones. A copy of the team conference report is sent to each team member, including the parents. In this way goals are not misunderstood and the intent of the program is clear.

Discharge planning begins as soon as the patient is admitted to the acute rehabilitation setting. Again, a critical aspect of discharge planning is inclusion of the family in the process. School and home visits enable the team to make knowledgeable recommendations for environmental alterations and equipment. Home passes are another important part of discharge planning. Passes are useful in that they help to motivate the patients as well as provide an opportunity for problem solving in the home setting prior to discharge. The authors initially start with a 4–6-hour pass with the parents, either as a visit home in the case of those who live nearby, or a trip in the car to the child's favorite fast-food place. In the latter example, it is suggested that the family stay in the car and utilize the drive-through window, as the distractible environment in the restaurant may be upsetting to the child. If the weather is nice, the family is encouraged to take the food to the park for a picnic in a quiet area. The patient is then advanced to a 12-hour pass, which can be taken either overnight or during the day. Most patients will have one 12-hour pass a week and a 48-hour pass once a month, when appropriate.

Communication between the child's school and the hospital education consultant are vital aspects of the pediatric rehabilitation program. Any hospital treating patients under the age of 18 should have an active hospital education program. The hospital educators should be skilled in doing educational evaluation and utilizing varied teaching methods, as well as have an extensive knowledge of and a good working relationship with the school systems from which come the majority of the patients. The hospital educator generally obtains permission from the family on the day of admission to obtain school records from the child's home school. This is extremely useful in that intelligence testing done by the school, previous grades, and standardized test scores provide quantitative information regarding premorbid cognitive functioning.

Most school districts are willing to accommodate the child who has experienced a tragedy such as head injury. Unfortunately, occasionally a school district will not provide needed services, and in this instance the hospital team can advocate for the child. Educating school personnel on the similarities and differences between children with head injury and children with learning disabilities is paramount if the child is to be successfully reintegrated into his or her local school program. In addition, because cognitive deficits resulting from traumatic brain injury are evolving, the school program must keep up with the child's healing process. During the inpatient rehabilitation stay, this information is communicated to the school district, and is followed up after discharge. Information made available to the school during the summer is often lost. Thus each September it is important to identify all children who have been discharged during the summer, so that another contact can be made with their school districts to be certain that the appropriate measures have been taken.

It is vital that the rehabilitation program for a child or adolescent be set up with the developmental stage of that child in mind. Behaviors that would be pathological in an adult are often normal for adolescents, and behaviors that are acceptable in 2-year-olds are inappropriate in school-age children. All team members must have an intimate acquaintance with developmental stages of children and adolescents, and feel comfortable not only dealing with the children but with their families as well. They must be patient, but simultaneously be able to provide clear limits. They must provide good parental modeling to the families, as many families discipline their children inappropriately. Usually the inappropriate discipline is ignorance of a better way. Most parents are excited to find that there are other ways to control their children besides

screaming and hitting. At the same time the staff does not act judgmental when the family has a life-style outside the norm. An attempt is made to adapt the program as much to the family's life-style as is morally and ethically permissible.

A positive relationship with insurance companies and Medicaid is useful in developing a pediatric rehabilitation program. Unfortunately adult standards are applied to pediatric programs, and many adult criteria are inappropriate for the developmental level of the child in question. An example of this would be the ability of a 2-year-old to dress him or herself, or development of continence in a child who is not yet toilet trained. These incongruities must be dealt with patiently and kindly with the insurance company in order to foster a spirit of cooperation rather than one of antagonism.

Behavioral Program

As head injury rehabilitation has matured there has been an increased awareness of, and appreciation for, the adverse impact that poor social skills have on the individual's overall recovery. Professionals working with persons with acute head injury are all too familiar with the impulsive, disinhibited, and aggressive individual who does not maximize the benefit of the treatment because of behavioral problems. The negative effects of poor behavioral controls on long-term adjustment following head injury have been well documented, with behavioral changes often being reported as equally or more debilitating than cognitive or physical changes (Brooks, 1984; Mauss-Clum & Ryan, 1981). Such findings indicate the need to emphasize behavioral and social skills equally with medical and physical abilities when rehabilitating the person with head injury. The efficacy of behavioral programs to increase patient participation and treatment, increase and enhance prosocial behavior, and enhance long-term outcome has been demonstrated (Eames & Wood, 1985).

A variety of contingency management programs ranging from highly structured to token economies to individualized behavioral modification programs is available to the professional. All contingency management programs are variations on a theme: they promote the teaching of specific, appropriate responses; provide opportunities for the patient to demonstrate these new responses and have them reinforced; and provide a monitoring system for both the patient and staff regarding the patient's progress through the implementation of a consistent structured environment. It is fortuitous that the necessary components for good behavioral management are similar to those needed for head injury rehabilitation in general. Specifically, these include: detailed observations of baseline abilities to determine where the breakdown of specific skills occurs; focused treatment on discrete functions that comprise larger physical and activities of daily living (ADL) skills; opportunities for the patient to demonstrate his or her improved skills; and provision of structured guidelines for caregivers as to how best to respond to the patient in order to maximize his or her independence.

While others have provided a comprehensive overview of learning theory principles on which milieu programs are based (Seron, 1987) it is beyond the scope of this chapter to do so. However, a brief summary follows. Behavior is defined as *any* observable and measurable event. A behavior increases when it is followed by something pleasant or reinforcing. A behavior will also increase if it is associated with the withdrawal of something unpleasant (e.g., throwing things to get the attention of staff who can then get the patient a urinal). A specific behavior decreases when it is associated with something unpleasant or punishing. Unfortunately, from a rehabilitation perspective, a punishment paradigm teaches the patient what not to do, but does not teach the patient the most important thing— what to do. The impact reinforcement and punishment has on behavior is directly related to how quickly they follow the target behavior, and how consistently they are applied. A milieu or environmental program attempts to decrease the random nature of patient and staff behavior in order to increase specific target behaviors. While each behavioral program must be individually tailored, the authors have found that

such a program works best within a framework of a hospital-wide behavior management system.

What Is Needed To Make A Behavioral Program Work?

1. *Staff Team.* An interdisciplinary team that can reach consensus on what behaviors to target is paramount. This sounds easy but often necessitates staff not completing their specific goals during the assessment period because they are appropriately implementing the behavioral program. Thus, without agreement on the importance of a target behavior, many staff members will opt to perform their particular treatment rather than focus on the specific target behavior in the milieu program. Staff need to view themselves as educators and teachers of general functional skills as well as specialists within their particular field.

2. *Staff Training.* For behavior management programs to be most effective, indirect care staff need to be familiar with the general guidelines and principles of the hospital-wide milieu program. Clinical staff need to have a good grounding in basic learning theory and be able to demonstrate this knowledge. In general, the more that people know, and the more that people are aware of the milieu program, the more powerful the program. Since behavior management is based upon the consistency of staff responses to a particular behavior, it is important that all staff be aware of what is the appropriate response.

3. *Clarity.* Target behaviors and appropriate staff responses should be clearly defined so that everyone will be able to know specifically what to observe and how to respond.

4. *Consistency.* Consistency is the fundamental underpinning of any behavior management program. Because large numbers of people come into contact with the patient daily, it is difficult to maintain consistency across staff members without the promulgation of the milieu principles and clarity of the target behaviors.

What Behaviors Should Be Targeted?

Any *agreed-upon* behavior should be targeted. In specifying a target behavior the following factors need to be assessed:

1. Does everyone agree on the problem behavior? This process will usually need to include the patient's parents and family members. If they are not in agreement with the program, the probability of success is severely diminished, and ill will often develops between staff and family members.
2. A complete detailed behavioral analysis of the target behavior (i.e., get a good baseline) is needed. How often does it occur? Where? With whom? How long does it last? What precedes it? What follows it?
3. Do you have the ability to control the environment for the target behavior? Food is an excellent example. Often treats are used as reinforcers, but if the patient can obtain them by purchasing them, from outside visitors, or from friends, then they will have little impact on the patient's behavior.
4. How does the patient's premorbid personality affect the target behavior? Is there a history of oppositional behavior or depression?
5. How does the patient's premorbid neurological status affect the target behavior? (e.g., Was the patient already diagnosed as having attention deficit hyperactivity disorder?)
6. How supportive will family members be in altering the specific behavior? With education, will they help implement the program?
7. Does the patient's current medical status or medication affect the target behavior (e.g., arousal)?
8. How does the patient's current cognitive deficits affect the target behavior (e.g., memory)?

Such issues are best addressed during patient conferences in which all pertinent professional staff and family members are present. An atmosphere in which all people feel comfortable discussing the relative merits of the behavioral program is necessary in order to ensure later compliance and consistency.

Pragmatics of the Program

In the authors' program they have found it useful for the patients to be responsible for their own milieu "blue book" and to carry it from treatment to treatment. This often necessitates that a book bag be provided and attached to the patient's wheelchair. The blue book contains daily sheets indicating specific times of day, treatment areas, and therapist seen. The daily behavior log has general categories for cooperation, degree of effort, and level of orientation. Blank areas are left for specific, individualized, target behaviors. The target behaviors are structured for success so that the patient has a high probability of successfully completing them and reaping the benefits of his or her achievement. At the end of each day, a specified group or individual, in the authors' case a recreational therapist, summarizes the daily log and provides a percentage of success for the patient. If the patient achieves an 80% success rate he or she obtains daily rewards. If the patient obtains between a 60% and 80% success rate nothing occurs, and below 60% certain privileges may be withheld. The patient may also obtain larger weekly rewards (e.g., home pass, field trip) based on the number of successful days. The authors have found that the process of providing individualized feedback following each treatment and completing the daily behavior log takes only 1–2 minutes.

In conclusion, a behavioral milieu program dovetails well with head injury rehabilitation because it provides for many of the needs that all children with head injury have. Such programs offer structure, consistency, and a system for the patient and staff to monitor progress, increase the staff's sense of control, increase the patient's self-esteem through a highly reinforcing environment, increase the patient's motivation, and model appropriate responses for the family as to how best to interact with the patient.

DAY HOSPITAL PROGRAMS FOR CHILDREN

Because of the extensive supervision that can usually be provided to a child or adolescent by his or her parents or other family members, it is often possible to send the pediatric patient home even in the midst of his or her intensive rehabilitation program. For families who live within an hour's drive of the hospital, the day hospital program is made available as soon as possible. Day treatment offers several advantages. The parent drops the child off at the hospital in the morning and picks him or her up in the evening. The child can spend the night and weekends in his or her own environment; improvements in orientation, emotional stability, and motivation are often observed by staff and parents shortly after transfer to day hospital status.

Funding of day hospitalization is sometimes a difficult problem. Some insurance companies refuse to recognize the existence of day hospitalization. However, this can often be negotiated with the insurance company with the emphasis on the fact that the child would remain an inpatient if day hospitalization were not made available. This actually represents a large savings to the insurance company (e.g., approximately $200 a day in Children's Hospital, Richmond, VA). With some education most insurance companies are quite amenable to the concept.

Day hospitalization is not to be confused with outpatient therapy. The criteria for day hospital status at Children's Hospital includes the necessity for at least 2 hours per day of physical therapy, occupational therapy, and/or speech therapy services, as well as continued need for psychological, educational, and/or recreational therapy intervention, and/or rehabilitation nursing services.

Typically the patient with severe motoric involvement receives 5–6 hours per day of therapy, while the less motorically involved person receives approximately 4 hours of services. Because of the patient's fatigue level, these therapies cannot be delivered sequentially, and must be spaced over a 6–7 hour period. Conferences are still scheduled every other week, and it is during this time that the family members generally become cognizant of the types of issues with which they are going to be dealing on a long-term basis.

During this phase of rehabilitation, preparation for removal of the extensive support services provided by the hospital begins. Reevaluations by all disciplines are performed and appropriate school resources and local services are clearly identified. Local resources may include mental health follow-up for patients and their families.

Often at this time the adolescent patient notes that friends become scarce. The patient's slowed or deficient motor skills, impulsive behavior, and memory deficits are difficult for other adolescents to accept. This loss of important friendships often exacerbates behavioral problems at home. The patient may begin to identify staff and other patients as his or her new friends. This type of reaction may make weaning from the hospital setting even more difficult for the patient and his or her family. The adolescent must be encouraged at this time to find new social outlets, as well as to work on impulse control and socially acceptable compensatory strategies for memory deficits in order to increase social desirability. At this point, adolescent group therapy is quite useful, with other adolescents providing feedback to the patient. Social skills training can also be facilitated by the use of videotape recordings of patients' interactions.

Return to the school setting for the child of any age is now the goal. Up to this point, the patient has been doing his or her lessons under ideal circumstances: on a one-to-one basis in a nondistracting environment. Toward the last 2–3 weeks of the day hospital stay, the child is placed in more distracting environments in order to evaluate his or her capacity to adjust to a typical school setting. If the child is observed to have difficulty functioning in a more school-like environment, a variety of interventions are tried. If visual distractibility is the problem, then the patient is oriented toward a wall while doing lessons. If auditory distractibility is a major problem, a trial of an auditory trainer is indicated. If any of these interventions prove successful, the child's school is notified, and its willingness to utilize the interventions is assessed. In the case of the adolescent with a severe head injury, vocational goals must be reassessed. Pursuit of higher education, while still feasible, is a more complex issue beyond the scope of this chapter.

Approximately 3 weeks before the patient's discharge, the school is notified that the child will be returning to school on a given date. Appropriate reports are forwarded to the school via the educational liaison. These reports include physical therapy, occupational therapy, speech pathology, and medical summaries. Pertinent psychological evaluations are also forwarded, as well as a report from the educational consultant on the child's current educational testing and functioning.

In most cases school personnel can attend team conferences prior to the patient's discharge, and can participate in the planning of educational goals and type of program that would best suit the child. Particularly if there is severe motoric impairment, or if the school personnel are unable to attend conferences prior to discharge, a school visit will be made. Usually the rehabilitation coordinator, social worker, and a physical or occupational therapist participates in the school visit. At this time they instruct the appropriate school personnel in medical procedures such as gastrostomy tube feedings, suctioning tracheostomies, positioning, and feeding. In addition the school is expected to try to identify physical barriers that might interfere with the child's ability to attend school. The school visit should be made at least several weeks prior to the patient's discharge, because of the possibility that some change in the physical environment may need to be brought about. It is also appropriate at that time to discuss the transportation of the child with the school personnel and to make certain that appropriate and safe transportation is available.

The school is usually delighted to receive a visit and suggestions from hospital personnel. If the school is inaccessible, and the team feels that the child should be in a center-based program, it is important for the team to point out that the school is required by law to make the appropriate adjustments in the physical environment to accommodate the handicapped child (PL 94-142). The team can assist the school in planning these modifications. Most schools are aware of their legal duties toward the children in their district. However, some rural school systems really have no money for appropriate services. Again, it should be pointed out to the school system that it will be receiving a stipend from the federal government for each disabled child in the system. It is the school system's obligation to utilize the stipend for the education of the child with a disability, and not place it in the general educational fund.

Because the child's strength and endurance have increased during day hospital to the point of being able to tolerate an entire day of therapy with only a brief rest in the middle of the day, it is advisable to return the child to the school system immediately if at all possible. Homebound instruction only serves to allow the child to decondition for 2 or 3 weeks as well as to keep him or her out of the social milieu. In certain instances a half-day school program with an afternoon of tutoring assistance can be arranged by the school system. This is often an ideal transitional method, although very few school systems are willing to provide these services. Special academic programming and transportation must be arranged for half days of school, and these types of issues must be kept in mind by the team when recommending unusual transitions. The authors generally find that after 1–2 weeks of half-day schooling the child is eager to return to school full time.

OUTPATIENT SERVICES

Once the child with traumatic brain injury is able to move to a less intensive program consisting of one or two therapies several times a week, he or she is placed on outpatient status. As discussed in the previous section, it is at this time that the child returns to school and an attempt is made to have most of the needed services delivered by the school system during the school year. Due to PL 94-142 most school systems comply with the recommendations made by the team. However, when this is not occurring, or when the school delays more than 65 days for evaluation and establishment of the individualized education program (IEP) required by law, the hospital team must attempt to intervene. If the school continues to be unresponsive, the school board must be approached. This should be done jointly by the parents and the hospital team. If the school system continues to be unresponsive, then the parents should be encouraged to contact the state office for the rights of persons with disabilities. Generally one phone call to this office results in a rapid evaluation and placement for the child.

In most cases, the school district will gladly accept the evaluations of the hospital team if they are up to date; however, some school systems may prefer to perform their own evaluations. As discussed in the previous section, suggestions for appropriate transportation as well as additional tutoring may be made by the hospital team. At times the family may wish to contract for independent tutoring services on its own.

Due to the long-term nature of head injury recovery, regular follow-up is necessary. One useful approach is an outpatient head injury clinic consisting of representatives from each discipline, with the primary emphasis on medical, educational, and psychosocial services. The child is initially followed on a monthly basis until he or she is well settled into the educational system. After that the child is followed in 6-month intervals. In most cases the rehabilitation team will receive regular reports from the therapists in the school setting.

Frequently a school visit is made by one team member several weeks after the child has started school. In this way some observation of classroom behavior can be made and additional information can be obtained from the school personnel. It is important to foster a feeling of mutual cooperation between the school and the hospital team. In addition the parents must be encouraged to advocate for their child in a positive fashion.

During the summer it is useful for all the children with head injury to participate in structured programs such as camps and, when indicated, summer school. Participation in organized sports is encouraged, with the exception of contact sports. This serves to improve gross motor skills as well as promote cooperative behavior. Depending on the type of injury that has been suffered and the residual deficit, a specific sport may be prescribed for a head-injured child, such as gymnastics, track, tennis, or swimming. This provides the child with an appropriate physical outlet as well as a sense of accomplishment.

Frequently the child moves out of his or her previous social circle and experiences several months of loneliness. The team encourages the parents and the child to identify new activities so the child can reestablish a circle of friends, which may or may not include previous friends. It appears that teenagers especially often have difficulty accepting a head-injured peer back into their midst, particularly if the peer has maladapative social skills, verbal slowing, or motor slowing. It is vital for the child to begin to resocialize within a few weeks after discharge from inpatient or day-patient status. This must be monitored closely by team members, who should intervene when appropriate. Resocialization can be facilitated through recreation programs, church groups, support groups, and camping experiences.

Usually within a few weeks after the child has reentered school, the parents receive reports from the school of problems with behavior, academics, or peer relationships. This is a difficult time for the family, because the child frequently looks as if he or she has made outstanding progress upon discharge and the parental expectations for school achievement are higher than they should be, in spite of extensive counseling from the rehabilitation team. It is at this time that the appropriate team members, such as the psychologist, physician, social worker, or educational consultant, should be readily available to the family and the child. If the problem can be identified, and appropriate interventions made, the child can achieve some success in school. Interventions may include: decreasing the academic load, resource help, resource classrooms, tutoring, or counseling. Often education of the school personnel regarding the consequences of head injury must be repeated.

During the acute hospitalization, the child's siblings generally experience a great deal of remorse and guilt because of the injury to their sibling. Younger children often feel that they have caused the injury to their siblings through previous angry thoughts. Others feel that they should have been injured instead. However, after discharge, once the family attempts to resume a normal life-style, this guilt often turns to anger. The head-injured child is often difficult to deal with, and it is not easy for the sibling to understand the head-injured child's impulsivity and immature behavior. At this time, siblings are often brought in for several sessions of family counseling in an attempt to ease the transition into a new family life-style. However, one must remember that these sessions in themselves are somewhat punitive to the siblings, because they must give up their own time and activities to participate in counseling sessions brought on by the perceived bad behavior of the child with head injury. This may result in even stronger feelings of anger toward the head-injured sibling. These feelings must be identified and dealt with as quickly as possible.

At discharge it is important that all the hospital information be provided to the primary care physician so that the physician may resume his or her previous role. During outpatient follow-up recommendations of the team should likewise be shared with the primary care physician.

VOCATIONAL PLANNING

Vocational planning must be begun after head injury in young people age 13 and above. Vocational interests must be identified, and approximately 12 months after the patient emerges from coma, a vocational assessment must be performed. At that time the educational program and the vocational capabilities should be matched. In children and young people with disabilities, education for the sake of education is rarely useful. However, if a child can identify a vocational goal, and can relate the academic process to that goal, he or she will often become more motivated in his or her schoolwork. Many school systems do have vocational training programs, and if the head-injured child is not planning to go on to higher education, he or she should become involved with a vocational program. Unfortunately school vocational programs are often limited in the types of work for which they can train, but typing skills, job-seeking skills, organizational skills, and such skills as the use of tools can be successfully applied to a variety of vocational settings. The state department of rehabilitative services should become involved when the child becomes 16, but in most states, the rehabilitative services are most successful with severely impaired persons. It has been the authors' experience that the head injury

team has a better feeling for the types of jobs in which an individual would be successful and that he or she would enjoy. This is particularly true if a rehabilitation counselor is a member of the team. Because most pediatric programs do have a great many adolescent patients, it is certainly worthwhile to have a rehabilitation counselor who can do job skills training and vocational testing, and who can act as a liaison with the state department of rehabilitative services.

A group home with an emphasis on independent living skills, money management, social skills development, and job training in a closely chaperoned and supervised environment would be an ideal transitional program for adolescents. Unfortunately, very few such programs are in existence and most of them are for young adults and are inappropriate for many adolescents.

SPECIAL ISSUES

In the pediatric population (under age 18) consent of parent or guardian is needed for medical services. If a child is transferred to the rehabilitation service, a parent or guardian must accompany him or her. In melded families it is extremely important to find out who the legal guardian is. It is often useful to have the legal documentation in the body of the chart, as occasionally a parent or other relative will purport to have guardianship, particularly on evenings or weekends when the primary team is not present.

In the case of a child who has sustained head injury due to parental abuse or neglect, removal of parental rights has usually occurred prior to transfer to the rehabilitation service. If child protective services has not been notified, this must be done by the rehabilitation team. Again, careful clarification of guardianship, whether it be the local welfare department, the state, or a foster parent is essential. Some antisocial families may bring drugs, alcohol, or weapons onto the unit. This is handled in the same manner as on an adult rehabilitation unit, with intervention of hospital security and limitation of visitation rights if necessary.

Financial resources are somewhat different for children than adults. Often the children with head injury come from young, healthy families, who are enrolled in health maintenance organizations. It is important to negotiate with the health maintenance organization for the optimal type of program for the child. State Medicaid and crippled children services can also be good sources of funding for equipment and needed services. Criteria and eligibility vary from state to state. Many states have children's hospitals that offer services regardless of ability to pay. The hospital social worker must be intimately acquainted with pediatric funding issues as well as other appropriate programs for children and young people.

Adult head injury transitional programs are often unsuitable for adolescents. Transitional programs for adolescents must be identified in the area, and if these programs are absent, the pediatric rehabilitation program should attempt to establish one.

CONCLUSION

In conclusion, a child or adolescent cannot expect to achieve maximum recovery when placed within a standard adult rehabilitation setting. A large body of literature reconfirms the need for specialized programs and environments for hospitalized children, and this can rarely be achieved outside of a specialized pediatric unit. The child's developmental stage must be a constant consideration, and with that the child's interpretation of the meaning of suffering. The child and his or her family must be treated with love and concern, as well as with dignity, in order to maximize function and adjustment in a new life-style. The child or adolescent must then be transitioned into an age-appropriate academic or vocational setting as quickly as possible but must be followed up on a long-term basis, so that the natural developmental process can be facilitated through appropriate interventions on the part of the rehabilitation personnel.

This chapter has provided an overview of a *model system of care* for children with traumatic brain injury. Characteristics of the model system include smooth transitions through stages of rehabilitation, established service delivery systems that specifically address the unique needs of children with head injury, cooperative interactions among agencies and professionals, and involvement of families in development and implementation of treatment programs. Unfortunately, in the United States, rehabilitation systems for children have not developed as rapidly as those for adults. The needs of many children with head injury remain unrecognized and in many cases service delivery systems are inadequate. Over time however, the advocacy efforts of family members, rehabilitation professionals, and academic professionals are becoming increasingly effective and provide assurance that the special needs of children with head injury can and will ultimately be met.

REFERENCES

American Academy of Pediatrics. (1960). *Hospital care of children and youth.* Evanston, IL: Author.

American Academy of Pediatrics. (1986). *Hospital care of children and youth.* Evanston, IL: Author.

Brink, J.D., Imbus, C., & Woo-Sam, J. (1980). Physical recovery after severe closed head trauma in children and adolescents. *Journal of Pediatrics, 97,* 721–727.

Brooks, N. (1984). *Closed head injury: Psychological, social, and family, consequences.* New York: Oxford University Press.

Bruce, D.A., Schut, L., Bruno, L.A., Wood, J.H., & Sutton, L.N. (1978). Outcome following severe head injuries in children. *Journal of Neurosurgery, 48,* 679–688.

Cockrell, J. L., Gregory, S., & Zuparro, J. (in press). *Audiologic deficits in brain injured children and adolescents.* Manuscript submitted for publication.

Eames, P., & Wood, R. (1985). Rehabilitation after severe brain injury: A follow-up study of a behavior modification approach. *Journal of Neurology, Neurosurgery, and Psychiatry, 48,* 613–619.

Ewing-Cobbs, L., Fletcher, J.M., & Levin, H.S. (1985). Neuropsychological sequelae following pediatric head injury. In M. Ylvisaker (Ed.), *Head injury rehabilitation: Children and adolescents* (pp. 71–90). San Diego: College-Hill Press.

Heiskanen, O., & Kaste, M. (1974). Late prognosis of severe brain injury in children. *Developmental Medicine and Child Neurology, 16,* 11–14.

Johnston, R.N., & Mellets, F.D. (1980). Pediatric coma: Prognosis and outcome. *Developmental Medicine and Child Neurology, 22,* 3–12.

Kraus, J.F., Fife, D., & Conroy, C. (1987). Pediatric brain injuries: The nature, clinical course, and early outcomes in a defined United States population. *Pediatrics, 79,* 501–507.

Kriel, R.L., Krach, L.E., & Sheehan, M. (1988). Pediatric closed head injury: Outcome following prolonged unconsciousness. *Archives of Physical Medicine and Rehabilitation, 69,* 678–681.

Lindheim, R., Glaser, H.H., & Coffin, C. (1972). *Changing hospital environments for children.* Cambridge, MA: Harvard University Press.

Mauss-Clum, N., & Ryan, M. (1981). Brain injury and the family. *Journal of Neurosurgical Nursing, 13,* 165–169.

Pagni, C.A., Signorni, G., Crotti, F., & Tombi, G. (1975). Severe traumatic coma in infancy and childhood: Results after surgery and resuscitation. *Journal of Neurology and Science, 19,* 120–128.

Raimondi, A.J., & Hirschauer, J. (1984). Head injury in infants and toddlers: Coma scoring and outcome scale. *Child's Brain, 11,* 12–35.

Rappazzo, J.A. (1980). Psychoesthetic environmental design for pediatric care facilities. *Journal of the Association for the Care of Children's Health, 8,* 85–93.

Rutter, M., Chadwick, O., & Shaffer, D. (1983). Head injury. In Rutter (Ed.), *Developmental neuropsychiatry* (pp. 83–111). New York: Guilford Press.

Savage, R.C. (1987). Educational issues for the head injured adolescent and young adult. *Journal of Head Trauma and Rehabilitation, 2,* 1–10.

Seron, X. (1987). Operant procedures and neuropsychological rehabilitation. In M. Benton & A. Diller (Eds.), *Neuropsychological rehabilitation* (pp. 132–161). New York: Guilford Press.

Sprum, O., Tupper, D., Risson, A., Tuokko, H., & Edgell, D. (1984). *Human developmental neuropsychology.* New York: Oxford University Press.

Stover, S.L., & Zeiger, H.E. (1976). Head injury in children and teenagers: Functional recovery correlated with the duration of coma. *Archives of Physical Medicine and Rehabilitation, 57,* 201–205.

CHAPTER 18

Community and School Integration from a Developmental Perspective

Ellen Lehr and Ronald C. Savage

Traumatic brain injury in infants, children, and adolescents is essentially a community issue. Children are predominantly injured in their communities—whether at home, at school, while playing in neighborhood playgrounds, while crossing streets in the neighborhood, while riding bicycles, or while learning to drive. They are likely to be treated by community medical resources, either by their own pediatricians or by local hospitals and emergency facilities. Rehabilitation and educational intervention is also likely to be provided through nearby programs and through community school resources. Their injuries are also likely to raise community concern for the safety of neighborhood streets and playground equipment, with community impetus to prevent future injuries by installing stop signs or signals, by removing unsafe playground equipment, by reducing speed limits where children play, by encouraging use of bicycle helmets, by changing the age and/or procedures by which adolescents can receive driver's licenses, and by reducing drinking and driving in adolescents.

There are several reasons why children are more likely than adults to be managed in their immediate community after traumatic brain injury. Since children are so reliant and dependent upon their families for support and development, it is very difficult and often contraindicated to separate children from their families after injury. If severely injured children require inpatient rehabilitation, families and professionals often face a "no-win" situation. The scarcity of pediatric rehabilitation programs that can appropri-

ately serve children after head injuries means that very few children are able to participate in such programs without substantial separation from their families. This involves not only the necessary separation of living in the hospital, but also the limited visiting that families can manage when their homes are long distances away.

In addition to geographical limitations, there also may be financial restrictions. Children often have fewer funding resources available to pay for rehabilitation services than those available to provide for intervention with adults. This is especially true for outpatient cognitive rehabilitation services, which are often perceived as "educational" rather than "medical" and therefore not covered by insurance carriers. However, children also have the advantage of possibly having a wide range of community-based educational services available to them and legislation mandating their access to these services. Very few educational programs and services, though, are designed to meet the unique needs of children and adolescents after traumatic brain injury.

UNIQUE PEDIATRIC ISSUES

Incidence and Extent of the Problem

Even though traumatic brain injury is the leading cause of death and disability in children between the ages of 1 and 14 years (National Center for Health Statistics, 1982), very little attention has been focused on this public health problem by either community medical or community educational professionals. When incidence data are considered cumulatively, by the time children are in the middle school years, it is likely that 1 in 20 children has experienced a head injury that has caused sufficient concern to seek medical attention.

Approximately 5% of children admitted to hospitals had sustained severe traumatic brain injuries (Annegers, Grabow, Kurland, & Laws, 1980; Kraus, Fife, Cox, Ramstein, & Conroy, 1986). The majority of injuries were mild in nature (over 85%), with many children experiencing no loss of consciousness (Kraus et al., 1986). Interestingly, many of the children, even those with severe injuries, were transported to the hospital in private, nonemergency vehicles rather than by ambulance or other emergency medical means (Kraus et al., 1986).

Injury Effects

Despite their rapid and more complete physical recovery after severe traumatic brain injuries (Brink, Garrett, Hale, Woo-Sam, & Nickel, 1970; Brink, Imbus, & Woo-Sam, 1980), research data are accumulating that indicate that children are not spared cognitive and psychosocial sequelae (Ewing-Cobbs, Fletcher, Landry, & Levin, 1985; Klonoff, Low, & Clark, 1977; Levin, Eisenberg, Wigg, & Kobayashi, 1982; Rutter, Chadwick, & Shaffer, 1983). Sparing of function depends on a variety of interacting factors, including: age at injury, injury size and location, prior and subsequent experience, and the time when a function appears during the normal course of development. In general, simple or automatic functions are more likely to be spared than complex functions.

Children, by their nature, are undergoing the combined processes of brain growth and development along with experiential learning that shapes the individual in terms of personality and dealing with the environment. Alterations in their neurological intactness not only affects their current abilities but also their capacity to continue to develop and learn. The long-term effects of traumatic brain injury must take into account the possible cumulative impact of deficits on development during childhood and ado-

lescence. For example, the primary effect of a traumatic brain injury may be on the rate and process of learning, rather than on a specific ability. In this case, the effect of injury on development can only be appreciated over many years. Children who have sustained significant injuries also experience an immediate loss of developmental time while they are in coma, in the hospital, and before they recover to the point of being able to begin to learn again.

Unique to pediatric traumatic brain injury is the possibility of delayed onset of deficits. Since an injury may affect parts of the child's brain that are in the process of developing or are not expected to be fully functioning for a long period of time after injury, it is possible for injury effects to not be apparent for even many years after onset. For example, if a 5-year-old child sustains a severe injury to the frontal parts of his or her brain, the full effects of this injury may not be demonstrated until late childhood or early adolescence when abstract reasoning, more mature judgment, and other "executive" functions are expected to emerge. Teuber and Rudel (1962) described three patterns for the appearance of functional deficits after traumatic brain injury of the developing brain: 1) deficits may be apparent shortly after injury and then disappear (other parts of the brain "take over"), 2) deficits are apparent after injury and persist, and 3) deficits may appear only after a delay. Because of the progressive nature of both development and recovery from injury, as well as the possibility of delayed injury effects, it is clear that most of the concerns about a child's functioning after traumatic brain injury are likely to occur after the period of onset and acute hospitalization.

DEVELOPMENTAL PERSPECTIVE

The process of community and school integration for children and adolescents after traumatic brain injury varies according to the developmental needs and recovery/improvement progress of the affected individuals. Depending on the individual's age and developmental status, traumatic brain injury affects different beings, with different neurological organization, who are facing different developmental tasks. Obviously, the needs of an injured infant will be quite different immediately after injury than when he or she formally enters school at age 5 or 6. The needs of two 10-year-old children, one who was injured several years before and one who has been recently injured, will also be quite different. Pediatric traumatic brain injury involves alterations in a "work in progress." Unlike in adults, traumatic brain injury in children involves understanding two processes that are occurring simultaneously—the process of recovery/ improvement from injury superimposed on the overall process of development (Lehr, 1989).

The challenges and difficulties that children and adolescents face after traumatic brain injury must be considered from a developmental perspective. The child's ability to confront and meet the normal challenges of development depends on physical, cognitive, and language skills; personality; temperament; and behavioral mastery of him or herself and the environment. Traumatic brain injury can alter all or some of these areas. Development also takes place within a social context involving the family, friends, teachers, and neighbors, within the home, school, and neighborhood.

Infants and Toddlers

The primary causes of traumatic brain injury in the infant and toddler years are falls, motor vehicle accidents (especially if they are unrestrained or improperly restrained), and child abuse. Almost all injuries occur either at home, in the immediate neighborhood, or with family members when away from home. As the infant begins to move around more independently, the possibility of injury becomes a daily, if not hourly possibility. Toddlers are characterized by the ability to move independently and rapidly through the environment, sampling and exploring virtually everything in their path, but with little awareness of the possible hazards of doing so. The normal attitude of a parent or caregiver of a mobile toddler approaches that of an air traffic controller in maintaining sustained alertness for impending danger and keeping the immediate environment risk free.

Infants and toddlers appear to be at exceptionally high risk for both death and disability after traumatic brain injury. The prognosis for children injured under 2 years of age is less favorable than it is for children who are injured during the school-age years (Kaiser, Rudenberg, Fankhauser, & Zumbuhl, 1986). Apparently this is related to the increased vulnerability of the brain during a period of rapid growth, differences in skull strength and protection before the sutures between the bones close, and differences in brain structure and physiology, including large head size in relation to body size and blood-vessel fragility (Dobbing & Smart, 1974; Raimondi & Hirschauer, 1984). In fact, infants and young toddlers can sustain significant traumatic brain injuries by being severely shaken, with few external indications of abuse (Duhaime et al., 1987).

Developmentally, this is a period of very rapid changes as the infant progresses from complete dependence on others to understand and provide for his or her needs into a much more autonomous toddler who is capable of independent mobility, self-assertion, communication through spoken language, and social interaction. The specific facets of functioning (e.g., sensory, motor, language, emotional, behavioral, and social) are highly interdependent on each other during this period. Interruption of functioning or impairment in any one area is likely to have repercussions on other facets and can jeopardize the developmental course of the child during this period of rapid growth. Traumatic brain injury can also interfere with the ability to learn from experience, to make connections between objects or actions, to attend and respond to demands, and to have the energy or ability to explore. Although these kinds of alterations may be difficult to quantify, their impact on development can be pervasive and extensive.

Parents usually report extensive feelings of guilt and responsibility for their infant's or toddler's injury (Klonoff, 1971). Siblings also can share this guilt, especially if they are older and have had responsibility in caring for the infant or toddler. Rarely are infants and children treated apart from their families, in either acute care or rehabilitation settings. Instead it is common for family members to be present literally 24 hours a day during hospitalization and to assume as much of the infant's or toddler's care as is medically safe or feasible.

Even if small children are severely disabled, it is likely that they will continue to live at home. This is related not only to their size and the relative ease of caring for them, but also the scarcity of pediatric nursing homes or long-term care facilities for infants and young children. However, after the family takes the injured infant or toddler home, therapeutic services may be difficult to obtain. If there are obvious physical impairments, the parents will likely be referred to therapy services through agencies such as Easter Seals or United Cerebral Palsy that are primarily designed for the treatment of congenitally involved children from birth to 3 years of age. Although intervention services are now mandated by federal law for infants and toddlers (PL 99-457), in many areas of the country these services are just beginning to be readily available. Those infants and toddlers who do not have visible impairments or who experience delayed deficits may not receive intervention and their subsequent cognitive, social, and/or behavioral sequelae may not be attributed to their previous traumatic brain injury.

Preschool-Age Children

Preschool-age children are at relatively high risk for injuries as this developmental period has the second highest incidence after adolescence (Hendrick, Harwood-Hashe, & Hudson, 1964; Mannheimer, Dewey, & Melinger, 1966). The primary cause of traumatic brain injury during the preschool-age period continues to be predominantly related to falls, but a growing proportion of severe injuries are due to motor vehicle accidents, in which the child might be a pedestrian or passenger.

Developmentally, preschool-age children are increasingly involved in the larger social world. They are expected to learn to play and share with other children, to master and abide by basic social rules, to engage in most of their own immediate self-care, and to contain some of their emotional and behavior expression. While much

of this development occurs within the family context, preschool-age children are also expected to be able to separate comfortably and function for short periods of time without their parents. This is also a period of rapid cognitive development with laying of the foundation for academic learning that will follow. The preschool child's exuberance and capacity for learning in all settings and practically at all times is probably unmatched. During this period, they experience an explosion in conceptualization, grappling with and mastering the basic concepts of time, size, and quantity, and developing an awareness of self, emotions, and relationships.

Supporting and possibly driving this rapid development in learning is a "supercharged brain." Although the number of brain cells is no longer increasing, the connections between cells are rapidly expanding and are more numerous than in an adult brain (Huttenlocher, 1984). The developing brain is also using twice as much energy as an adult brain (Chugani, Phelps, & Mazziotta, 1987). The effect of injury on this brain in "high gear" is not known since virtually no research studies have focused on injury sustained during the preschool-age period. The greater plasticity during this period may enhance recovery. However, severe injuries during this period are equally as likely to impair the long-term capacity for learning.

Preschool-age children are much more capable of understanding and disliking the alterations in their functioning than an infant or toddler. They are able to revel in their competence, realistically recognize what they are unable to do, and become frustrated when their efforts are not rewarded by success. They are increasingly aware of their bodies, sexuality, and vulnerability to pain and injury. Although play is an integral part of their waking lives, the effects of traumatic brain injury on both physical and cognitive abilities can interfere with this essential aspect of preschool-age children.

As do injured infants and toddlers, preschool-age children usually return home to live with their families after hospital discharge and primarily receive their treatment within their immediate community. Parents may observe behavioral changes in their children after injury, usually described as difficulties with maintaining attention, increased distractibility, perseveration, and hyperactivity or hypoactivity. Those preschool-age children who experience significant impairments after injury are eligible for public school special education services under PL 94-142. However, most classes in this age range are generic or noncategorical and teachers are likely to have little or no experience in working with children who have had traumatic brain injury. In the only study that has been completed to determine the incidence of 3- to 5-year-old children in early childhood special education programs, in Vermont, 25% of the children had a documented head injury in their school records (Savage, 1985).

Elementary and Middle School–Age Children

The years from 6 to 14 are the lowest in terms of traumatic brain injury incidence. Severe injuries are related to motor vehicle accidents, with the child injured either as a passenger, bicycle rider, or pedestrian. Sports-related injuries also become more common during this time. With the increasing community independence exercised by children, injuries are more likely to occur outside of the home and parents or other adults may not be present. Instead, siblings, friends, teachers, or neighbors may witness or be involved in the accidents. Parents also begin to take less direct responsibility for their children's injuries and begin to attribute the cause of injury more frequently to the child's own behavior (Klonoff, 1971).

During the elementary and middle school–age years, the child's brain continues to be "supercharged," supporting the rapid development and learning that occurs during this period. The connections between the two hemispheres of the brain and between areas within each hemisphere become more efficient (Hewitt, 1962). The interconnections between primary sensory/perceptual/motor and association areas increase the ease in learning such academically related activities as reading, spelling, writing, arithmetic, and reasoning.

Children during this period are immersed in learning. However, unlike during the preschool

period, they are expected to do so in a group, away from home, and under the direction of adults other than their family members. Despite the importance of mastery of academic skills, development of competence in social interaction (especially with other children) and self-control/self-confidence is also essential. Traumatic brain injury can interfere not only with academic learning, but also with psychosocial/emotional aspects of functioning during this developmental period. It has been relatively well documented that after a loss of consciousness greater than 24 hours, intellectual deficits can be serious and persistent (Klonoff & Paris, 1974; Levin & Eisenberg, 1979). The effect of traumatic brain injury on academic skill learning may be most significant for younger children who have not yet mastered the basics of reading, writing, and arithmetic prior to injury (Chadwick, Rutter, Thompson, & Shaffer, 1981; Shaffer, Bijur, Chadwick, & Rutter, 1980). Controlled processes that underlie learning, such as attention, memory, and speed of information processing, may be impaired after traumatic brain injury and can directly affect academic learning (Levin & Benton, 1986).

Traumatic brain injuries also interfere with the preferred way that children age 6 to 14 cope with stressful events. During this period, children rely heavily on their cognitive mastery to understand and subsequently feel more in control of what has happened to them. Because the brain itself has been injured, children are less able to mobilize and utilize this cognitively centered coping approach to understand the nature of their injury or the management needed to aid their recovery (Lehr, 1989). However, they are often capable of recognizing their losses and somatic symptoms such as fatigue and headaches. At a time of increasing community independence, the experience and sequelae of traumatic brain injury often results (if only temporarily) in restrictions and the need for adult supervision of the child.

Behaviorally, the most common sequelae of traumatic brain injury in children age 6 to 14 is marked social disinhibition (Rutter et al., 1983). Although this disinhibition is rarely of concern to the head-injured children themselves, other children and adults may have little tolerance for socially embarrassing actions and language. In contrast, the teasing and isolation from other children is often felt keenly by the injured child. If special education services are needed or if the head-injured children's learning is obviously reduced, they may be called "brain damaged" or "retarded" by other children after their return to school. Although the children with traumatic brain injury may not be aware of or in control of behavioral and social changes, they can react emotionally to not feeling accepted and gradually withdraw from interaction outside of the family. Parents may feel powerless to help their children deal with the wider world.

Adolescents

During adolescence the rate of traumatic brain injury increases dramatically, with the number of severe injuries sustained between ages 15 and 19 equal to all of the previous 14 years combined (Gross, Wolf, Kunitz, & Jane, 1985). Most traumatic brain injuries during adolescence are related to motor vehicle accidents. This is the time when adolescents are beginning to get their driver's licenses and are spending much of their time in cars and other vehicles. Experimenting with drugs and alcohol combined with driving increases the possibility of serious accidents during adolescence. It is no longer uncommon for adolescents to have had a friend or classmate who has been killed or injured in an automobile accident. Although this is becoming a major public health issue, it is not clear which aspects of adolescent behavior are implicated or how to prevent traumatic brain injuries during this period.

Neurologically, the brain appears to be going through a major, and perhaps its last, reorganization. It has been known for many years that the frontal area of the brain is myelinated during adolescence. However, recent research has indicated that neurological changes may be more widespread. The increased number of nerve connections or synapses that characterized the earlier stages of development are reduced by as much as half in adolescence (Feinberg, 1982/1983). This appears to be the end of the "supercharged" childhood brain and the beginning of the efficient, stabilized adult brain. Both the changes in the frontal or "executive" part of the brain and the more efficient connections are likely to be related to the emerging ability to sustain logical thought in solving abstract and complex problems.

Adolescents are confronted with rapid physiological changes, including sexual and physical maturation. They are in the process of getting ready to become adults, but are not yet expected to grapple with the demands of adulthood. Along with the development of conceptual thought comes the ability to struggle with issues of self-identity and intimacy. Most adolescents confront the developmental tasks of this period with energy, and with a burgeoning sense of independence, self-sufficiency, and self-confidence. However, they are also more aware of the fragility of life and the reality of death.

Traumatic brain injury can alter the adolescent's sense of physical attractiveness, perception of invulnerability, self-confidence, social appropriateness, and cognitive capacities. Previously mastered academic skills appear to be more resistant to injury effects and intellectual deficits may be less pronounced than in children (Brink et al., 1970; Levin et al., 1982). However, the effect of traumatic brain injury on developing executive functions has rarely been directly studied in adolescence.

Adolescents may resent the perception of being different subsequent to their injuries and may become quite resistant to the need to alter any part of their lives, despite the injury-related necessity. Any loss of school time can present significant difficulty during the high school years, both in terms of academic achievement and in psychosocial relationships. In the latter part of adolescence, the transition to adulthood in terms of vocational planning and training, as well as the development of intimate relationships can be derailed by the effects of traumatic brain injury. The loss or postponement of future plans and dreams can trigger anger, depression, and, possibly, suicidal thoughts or behavior. In an attempt to blunt the personal impact of traumatic brain injury effects, adolescents may resort to alcohol or drug use.

COMMUNITY/SCHOOL TRANSITIONS

There has been considerable interest in addressing the needs of severely injured children who have been treated in rehabilitation hospitals to smooth their transition back home and their return to school. However, probably fewer than 5% of children who sustain traumatic brain injury are admitted to inpatient rehabilitation programs. Even severely injured children are frequently discharged from the acute care hospital directly home and to school. Those children who sustain mild or moderate injuries have received much less attention in terms of the nature of possible deficits, their needs, and their management at home and at school (Boll, 1983).

Transition from Acute Care Medical Settings

Most children and adolescents with significant traumatic brain injury are treated in acute care medical settings, usually within their immediate community. The acute care settings include outpatient or emergency room services, as well as brief or prolonged hospital admissions. Only those children who are most severely injured will be transported to trauma centers that may be many miles away from their homes. Acute care medical personnel have become highly expert in treating and managing the emergency and intensive care medical aspects of traumatic brain injury. However, recognition of possible cognitive or psychosocial impairments is less widespread.

Families rarely receive basic information about the "subtle" aspects of traumatic brain injury in their children in terms of what to look for, and the timing and likelihood of possible sequelae in their child. The materials that have been developed for use with minor head injury in the acute care hospital setting with adults have not been utilized or adapted for use with children and their families (Kay, 1986). One of the few pamphlets designed specifically for families of injured children is most appropriate for those who have sustained more severe injuries and who are being treated in rehabilitation settings (Deaton, 1987). Because of the impression of better recovery in injured children, physicians may underplay or disregard cognitive and psy-

chological aspects of injury. Physicians may also rely on a "wait-and-see" approach, only referring children for evaluation or treatment after they demonstrate definite and troublesome sequelae. In addition, there are very few pediatric traumatic brain injury rehabilitation consultation or treatment services in the acute care medical setting that can directly advise and educate physicians.

The usual scenario for children who are admitted after a traumatic brain injury and who recover rapidly is that of good medical care and quick discharge home as soon as they are medically stable, eating, going to the bathroom, and talking. Return to their normal lives at home is equally as quick, with usually an immediate resumption of education and play/social activities. This is in contrast to the advice to delay return to work that is beginning to be more commonly given to adults, after even minor traumatic brain injury. Although it may well be accurate that children recover best at home, it also can present enormous stress on families if they do not understand what has happened to these children, the time-course of recovery, and possible characterological changes, even if only temporary. It is unlikely that acute care medical personnel will have the time to aid the transition home and back to school for those children who have less severe injuries or who have rapid recovery from severe injuries. Since these children rarely are involved in inpatient rehabilitation programs, the responsibility for their management usually lies with their families and community-based head injury services, if they are available.

Those children who have sustained severe injuries with persistent medical and/or physical impairments are often transferred directly from acute care medical hospitals to acute care rehabilitation hospitals. If a pediatric rehabilitation facility is not available nearby, the child might be admitted to an adult rehabilitation program. This transition can be difficult for those children who are aware that they are going to another hospital instead of going home. Their cooperation and involvement in rehabilitation therapies must be elicited and maintained. Because they are often unaware of the impact of deficits on their functioning, this usually needs to be approached directly but in a way that children can understand during this phase of recovery. Having children experience changes in functioning in a supportive environment with the pervasive belief in improvement and adaptibility can have the dual effect of increasing awareness of impairments while encouraging participation in therapeutic activities. Even young children need a sense of control over their rehabilitation, and it is essential in working with adolescents.

Fewer children are involved in outpatient day treatment programs designed primarily for cognitive and psychosocial rehabilitation. This option, which is beginning to be more commonly available for adults after injury, is less available for adolescents and rarely an option for children. Children, though, may be involved in outpatient physical, occupational, and/or speech /language therapy. However, their individual therapists may not be familiar with the specific deficits frequently seen after traumatic brain injury and may not have treated such children previously.

Transition to and Among School Programs

Unlike injured adults who are commonly advised not to return immediately to work after a traumatic brain injury, children frequently return to school shortly after hospital discharge. School personnel are often unprepared for dealing with children who return to school while they are in acute recovery after a traumatic brain injury. Teachers, principals, and school nurses may not even be aware that the child has been injured, especially if the injury has occurred during a school holiday or during the summer. Changes in the child's learning and behavior may be apparent in the classroom, but the source of these alterations may not be known by the educational staff working with the child.

The decision of when a child is capable of returning to school is a complex one involving both the changing needs of the child and the educational resources available through the school system. For children and adolescents with milder injuries the question of whether they are ready to learn capably in school is rarely even

asked. Rather, it is assumed that they will continue to function as they did prior to injury. If they are experiencing temporary or persistent impairments in information processing, memory, and/or attention/concentration it is likely that they will experience frustration and possibly failure in a demanding academic setting. However, their difficulties may not be attributed to their recent traumatic brain injury.

For children and adolescents who have sustained significant injuries with obvious and persistent sequelae, the probability of being able to return immediately to their preinjury school setting is unlikely. The basic criteria for consideration of involvement in a classroom setting includes: resolution of post-traumatic amnesia and confusion, the ability to attend to a task for 15–20 minutes at a time, and the ability to function in a small class setting (Cohen, 1986). Even with functioning at this level, though, children may be more appropriate for special education settings than regular education programming.

Because of the range of special education services that may be available, the educational and therapy needs of children and adolescents after traumatic brain injury may be able to be at least partially met within the school setting. However, special education services and classes have rarely been designed to meet the specific needs of these children and specific attention must be devoted to making certain that existing services can be adapted to do so. Resources to help the classroom teacher and school-based therapists in working with the child or adolescent after traumatic brain injury are now available (Cohen, Joyce, Rhodes, & Welks, 1985; Savage & Wolcott, 1988). It is especially important to assess how long a child with traumatic brain injury will require special education services and of what kind. Because of children's often rapid recovery/improvement, school programs usually need to be altered frequently, as often as every 3–6 months. The special education system is rarely designed to meet these changing needs, including the transition back to mainstream classes.

Some children and adolescents may not need to be classified as students who require special education services. Instead they may need alterations in their regular school programming to ease their return to school (Savage & Allen, 1987). Such alterations include: one school staff member who coordinates the student's program, reduced course load, access to tutoring, use of learning aids such as audiotape recorders and computers, and a shortened school day or the opportunity of a place to rest in the middle of the day. These changes can sometimes be planned and implemented within the school building with the cooperation of the principal, the student's teachers, and the school nurse. Since school is also a social environment, students may need the support of a counselor or social worker to ease the social return to school.

CONCLUSION

Traumatic brain injury in children and adolescents is a community-based medical and educational challenge. However at the present time, it is primarily an unrecognized one. Few community-based medical and educational professionals are aware of the incidence or the consequences of pediatric traumatic brain injuries. This includes both the short- and long-range implications of traumatic brain injury sustained in the formative years. Very few community professionals have had training in evaluating, intervening, or managing the needs of this ever-increasing population of infants, children, and adolescents. Appropriate community-based services for injured children and adolescents are only now being developed, though they are much more widely available for adults. Because of the changing needs of injured children and adolescents, which are related to both recovery and developmental progress, a long-term perspective must be taken in order to adequately and efficiently manage their care. Without this, their eventual functioning as adults is being jeopardized. Although parents are the primary "case managers" for most injured children and adolescents, they need to be able to collaborate with professionals who have expertise in this area. Prevention of initial and repeat injuries is also a primary community responsibility, through such efforts as bicycle helmet use and Students Against Drunk Driving (SADD) groups.

REFERENCES

Annegers, J.F., Grabow, J.D., Kurland, L.T., & Laws, E.R. (1980). The epidemiology of head trauma in children. In K. Shapiro (Ed.), *Pediatric head trauma*. Mt. Kisco, NY: Futura.

Boll, T.J. (1983). Minor head injury in children: Out of sight but not out of mind. *Journal of Clinical Child Psychology, 12,* 74–80.

Brink, J.D., Garrett, A.L., Hale, W.R., Woo-Sam, J., & Nickel, V.L. (1970). Recovery of motor and intellectual function in children sustaining severe head injuries. *Developmental Medicine and Child Neurology, 12,* 565–571.

Brink, J.D., Imbus, C., & Woo-Sam, J. (1980). Physical recovery after severe closed head trauma in children and adolescents. *Journal of Pediatrics, 97,* 721–727.

Chadwick, O., Rutter, M., Thompson, J., & Shaffer, D. (1981). Intellectual performance and reading skills after localized head injury in childhood. *Journal of Child Psychology and Psychiatry, 22,* 117–139.

Chugani, H.T., Phelps, M.E., & Mazziotta, J.C. (1987). Positron emission tomography study of human brain functional development. *Annals of Neurology, 22,* 487–497.

Cohen, S.B. (1986). Educational reintegration and programming for children with head injuries. *Journal of Head Trauma Rehabilitation, 1,* 22–29.

Cohen, S., Joyce, C., Rhodes, K., & Welks, D. (1985). Educational programming for head injured students. In M. Ylvisaker (Ed.), *Head injury rehabilitation: Children and adolescents.* San Diego: College-Hill Press.

Deaton, A. (1987). *Pediatric head trauma: A guide for families.* New Kent, VA: Cumberland Hospital for Children.

Dobbing, J., & Smart, J.L. (1974). Vulnerability of developing brain and behavior. *British Medical Bulletin, 30,* 164–168.

Duhaime, A., Gennarelli, T.A., Thibault, L.E., Bruce, D.A., Margulies, S.S., & Wiser, R. (1987). The shaken baby syndrome: A clinical, pathological, and biomedical study. *Journal of Neurosurgery, 66,* 409–415.

Ewing-Cobbs, L., Fletcher, J.M., Landry, S.H., & Levin, H.S. (1985). Language disorders after pediatric head injury. In J.K. Darby (Ed.), *Speech and language evaluation in neurology: Childhood disorders.* New York: Grune & Stratton.

Feinberg, I. (1982/1983). Schizophrenia: Caused by a

fault in programmed synaptic elimination during adolescence. *Journal of Psychiatric Research, 17,* 319–334.

Gross, C.R., Wolf, C., Kunitz, S.C., & Jane, J.A. (1985). Pilot traumatic coma data bank: A profile of head injuries in children. In R.G. Dacey, R. Winn, & R. Rimel (Eds.), *Trauma of the central nervous system.* New York: Raven Press.

Hendrick, E.B., Harwood-Hashe, D.C.F., & Hudson, A.R. (1964). Head injuries in children: A survey of 4465 consecutive cases at the Hospital for Sick Children, Toronto, Canada. *Clinical Neurosurgery, 11,* 46–65.

Hewitt, W. (1962). The development of the human corpus callosum. *Journal of Anatomy, 96,* 355–364.

Huttenlocher, P.R. (1984). Synapse elimination and plasticity in developing human cerebral cortex. *American Journal of Mental Deficiency, 88,* 488–496.

Kaiser, G., Rudeberg, A., Fankhauser, I., & Zumbuhl, C. (1986). Rehabilitation medicine following severe head injury in infants and children. In A.J. Raimondi, M. Choux, & C. DiRocco (Eds.), *Head injuries in newborn and infant.* New York: Springer-Verlag.

Kay, T. (1986). *The unseen injury: Minor head trauma.* Southborough, MA: National Head Injury Foundation.

Klonoff, H. (1971). Head injuries in children: Predisposing factors, accident conditions, accident proneness, and sequelae. *American Journal of Public Health, 61,* 2405–2417.

Klonoff, H., Low, M.D., & Clark, C. (1977). Head injuries in children: A prospective five year follow-up. *Journal of Neurology, Neurosurgery, & Psychiatry, 40,* 1211–1219.

Klonoff, H., & Paris, R. (1974). Immediate, short-term and residual effects of acute head injuries in children: Neuropsychological and neurological correlates. In R. Reitan & L. Davison (Eds.), *Clinical neuropsychology: Current status and applications.* New York: John Wiley & Sons, Halstead Press.

Kraus, J.F., Fife, D., Cox, P., Ramstein, K., & Conroy, C. (1986). Incidence, severity, and external causes of pediatric brain injury. *American Journal of Diseases of Childhood, 140,* 687–693.

Lehr, E. (1989). Community integration after traumatic brain injury: Infants and children. In P. Bach-

y-Rita (Ed.), *Traumatic brain injury.* New York: Demos.

Lehr, E. (1990). *Psychological management of traumatic brain injuries in children and adolescents.* Rockville, MD: Aspen Publications.

Levin, H.S., & Benton, A.L. (1986). Developmental and acquired dyscalculia in children. In I. Fleming (Ed.), *Second European Symposium on Developmental Neurology.* Stuttgart, West Germany: Gustav Fisher Verlag.

Levin, H.S., & Eisenberg, H.M. (1979). Neuropsychological impairment after closed head injury in children and adolescents. *Journal of Pediatric Psychology, 4,* 389–402.

Levin, H.S., Eisenberg, H.M., Wigg, N.R., & Kobayashi, K. (1982). Memory and intellectual abilities after head injury in children and adolescents. *Neurosurgery, 11,* 668–673.

Mannheimer, D.I., Dewey, J., & Melinger, G.D. (1966). Fifty thousand child-years of accidental injuries. *Public Health Reports, 81,* 519.

National Center for Health Statistics. (1982). Advance report, final mortality statistics. In *Monthly vital statistics report* (Vol. 31, No. 6, Suppl.; DHHS Publication No. PHS 82-1120). Hyattsville, MD: U.S. Public Health Service.

Raimondi, A.J., & Hirschauer, J. (1984). Head injury in the infant and toddler. *Child's Brain, 11,* 12–35.

Rutter, M., Chadwick, O., & Shaffer, D. (1983). Head injury. In M. Rutter (Ed.), *Developmental neuropsychiatry.* New York: Guilford Press.

Savage, R. (1985). *A survey of traumatically brain injured children within school-based special education programs.* Rutland, VT: Head Injury/Stroke Independence Project.

Savage, R.C., & Allen, M.G. (1987). Educational issues for the traumatically brain injured early adolescent. *The Early Adolescent Magazine, 1,* 23–27.

Savage, R.C., & Wolcott, G.F. (1988). *An educator's manual: What educators need to know about students with traumatic brain injury.* Southborough, MA: National Head Injury Foundation.

Shaffer, D., Bijur, P., Chadwick, O.R.D., & Rutter, M.L. (1980). Head injury and later reading disability. *Journal of the American Academy of Child Psychiatry, 19,* 592–610.

Teuber, H.L., & Rudel, R.G. (1962). Behavior after cerebral lesions in children and adults. *Developmental Medicine and Child Neurology, 4,* 3–20.

SECTION VII
Public Policy Issues

CHAPTER 19

Public Policy Issues Related to Head Injury

Linda C. Veldheer

Public policy is promoted and enacted in a political environment where various interests must compete for scarce resources. In the United States, national and state (and most local) government operates within a politico-administrative system characterized by bureaucracy. Public policy is both the process and the outcome of political bargaining that occurs among pluralist interests (Yates, 1982, chap. 4). This is especially pronounced in the public budgeting process to provide funding for governmental programs. The development and implementation of specific policy and program initiatives by governments are usually achieved slowly and incrementally. They typically result from an effort to respond to political pressure to address a social problem while simultaneously attempting to meet the public demand for administrative efficiency in government.

DISABILITY AND REHABILITATION POLICY

Disability or rehabilitation policy is often regarded to be a topical category or subset within the field of social welfare policy. It has been observed that within government, disability and rehabilitation policy would have to be considered one of the most neglected fields of public administration (Hahn, 1982, p. 385). There are important reasons to address this neglect. The size of the population in the United States with disabilities is substantial and the cost of implementing public policy affecting persons with disabilities is high. Various national estimates place the numbers of persons with disabilities as being 20–50 million; the most commonly used figures

are 35–36 million persons of all ages, including 27–28 million persons age 16 years and over (National Council on the Handicapped, 1988, p. 12). It is also estimated that total disability expenditures in the United States rose from approximately $19.3 billion in 1970 to $169.4 billion in 1986 (Berkowitz, Dean, Hanks, & Portney, 1988, chap. II). Supporting and operating programs and services for persons with disabilities has become a complex intergovernmental enterprise. Beyond pragmatic concerns, however, disability and rehabilitation policy embodies crucial theoretical, ethical, and moral questions concerning how society regards and treats people who are dependent and what should be the responsibility and role of government to assist them. It involves a number of social welfare issues that are highly controversial in the United States and that have dominated many facets of public administration. Such fundamental considerations will certainly influence public policy issues related to persons disabled as a result of traumatic brain injury.

The enactment of disability and rehabilitation policy is influenced both by the competition among disadvantaged groups for public attention and support and by negative attitudes that are prevalent among segments of the public in the United States concerning welfarism and governmental support and spending for social welfare programs. Social welfarism is a normative model that has been a continuous undercurrent for public administration. It is a complex system of beliefs and attitudes concerning the responsibility of society for the welfare of people, especially the welfare of disadvantaged social groups. Welfarism doctrine places much responsibility for the individual and social welfare of its citizens with government (Hochschild, 1981). In this country, public administration reflects a strong heritage of paternalism. There are many constituencies who advocate and lobby actively for government to support policies that provide a variety of direct payments and social programs and services to individuals, families, and other groups with special needs. Public agency budgets are the vehicle to gain sanction and the necessary financial and manpower resources to establish and continue entitlements and social programs. However, because the needs of disadvantaged groups are seemingly infinite while the resources of governments are finite, social welfare policy fosters competition for public support (Thurow, 1981). Welfarism is commonly regarded as a driving force for "uncontrollable" government spending and program expansion. Unfortunately, human services programs frequently do not fare well when subjected to analysis in terms of results and efficiency.

Another factor affecting the formulation and administration of rehabilitation policy is the relativistic nature of the concept and reality of disability. Public policy frequently must attempt to reconcile different moral philosophies, ethical considerations, and socioeconomic realities. Multiple, often conflicting, motives and purposes underlie the provision of programs and services to persons with disabilities. These encompass conceptual and definitional controversies concerning the nature of disabilities and functional limitations. There are currently three distinct theoretical perspectives of disability, including a medical model, an economic model, and a sociopolitical model (Bowe, 1980). Each of these brings different attitudes about and approaches to disability and rehabilitation policy. A serious problem is that all three perspectives are simultaneously held in American society, which often confuses and impedes the development and implementation of policies beneficial to persons with disabilities.

CONCEPTUAL MODELS OF DISABILITY

Perhaps the most commonly held concept of disability is based upon a medical orientation that emphasizes medical criteria and pathological functioning. This "medical model" focuses on impairments as separate diagnostic categories of illness and physical defect or dysfunction (Gliedman & Roth, 1980). People with disabilities are seen as defective or sick. They are considered "patients" who require treatment or care from a medical or clinical perspective. Persons with disabilities are viewed as outside the stream of normal society because they are physically incapable of coping with the requirements of everyday life. They need medical help and protection. Functional limitations are the problem of the specific individual. Physical impediments, if not curable, will relegate individuals to second-class citizenship and dependency. Solutions to problems of persons with medical and physical impairments must be sought primarily through individual, rather than collective, efforts. Persons with disabilities must adjust to society.

The medical model concept of disability seems to correspond most to a libertarian philosophy and a conservative political orientation. Under libertarianism, society would view the problems of people with disabilities as an indication of their individual deficits (Nozick, 1978). Disabled people who cannot maintain themselves and compete in the free marketplace do not have claim to full citizenship. It is not considered legitimate for government to support or specially assist defective or dysfunctional individuals. The approach would be to treat or cure the medical condition or physical problem so that the person can become functional. If this is not possible, then custodial care would fall to the family or to charity.

Another widely accepted view of the concept of disability stresses a health-related limitation on the amount or kind of work that can be performed. Disabilities are defined in terms of an "economic model." Physical limitations and a lack of adequate job skills are perceived as the primary cause for the inability of persons with disabilities to perform many types of jobs. Inability to maintain gainful employment makes them dependent and a burden to society. This has sparked public support for a holistic rehabilitation process aimed at bringing the individual to the highest possible level of functioning for vocational purposes (Berkowitz, Johnson, & Murphy, 1976). The costs of rehabilitation are vindicated by enabling the individual with disabilities to make economic contributions to society, or at least to become less dependent on others. The economic model prescribes vocational rehabilitation or income maintenance programs as the principal solution to the problems facing persons with disabilities. As with the medical model, the economic definition suggests that modification of the individual with disabilities is the most appropriate means for meeting the social and economic needs of the population with disabilities.

This economic model of the concept of disability seems consistent with a utilitarian ethical system and moderate political orientation. Publicly supported training and assistance to improve the vocational capabilities of disadvantaged people are justified (Brandt, 1979). Public policies and financial investment to help persons with disabilities and to relieve the burden for their families are judged and advocated in terms of their remunerative value. Public programs of special education, vocational rehabilitation, and other specialized services to handicapped people and their families reflect a utilitarian approach for addressing a significant social problem (Berkowitz, 1979).

A third, increasingly popular, orientation to the concept of disability is derived from sociological theories of labeling or stigmatization. This "sociopolitical" model highlights societal complicity in the problems experienced by persons with disabilities. It reflects the viewpoint that the primary issue for the individual with disabilities is the failure of a structured social environment to recognize the human rights and to adjust to the needs and aspirations of people with disabilities (Bowe, 1980; Eisenberg, Griggins, & Duval, 1982). This contrasts with the medical and economic models of handicap that highlight the inability of the individual with disabilities to adapt to the demands of society. With the sociopolitical model of disability, people with disabilities are considered a minority group with problems similar to ethnic and racial minorities. They are viewed as being subjected to unfair assumptions of biological inferiority, stereotyping, stigmatizing, segregation, prejudice,

and discrimination. Even compared to other minority groups, persons with disabilities are among the most disadvantaged segments of society. They typically experience high unemployment, poverty, and dependency. Their basic rights have often been deprived and they have experienced greater segregation in schools, housing, transportation, and public accommodation than other minority groups. With the sociopolitical model of disability, these problems are seen as the manifestation of inadequacies in the social and economic order rather than a matter of an individual's physical defect or vocational deficiency.

The socioeconomic concept of disability seems most compatible with Rawlsian philosophy and a liberal political orientation. These feature recognition of the basic human rights of every individual and focus on the legal and moral obligation of society to provide an environment where all citizens are equally capable of asserting their civil rights (Rawls, 1978). The socioeconomic model of disability underlies current trends to support normalization, integration, and independent living for the empowerment of individuals with disabilities. Public support for programs and services to enable them to participate in the mainstream of society are considered moral obligations so that persons with disabilities may exercise their fundamental rights. This corresponds with Rawls's argument that justice requires society to maximize the position of its most disadvantaged members. A socioeconomic perspective would tend to support strong antidiscrimination policies, lenient disability criteria with presumptive entitlement to benefits, income transfer programs, and strong support for provision of comprehensive rehabilitation programs.

The various models of disability highlight the absence of a unifying theoretical framework to facilitate disability and rehabilitation policy, practice, and research. Public policy affecting persons with disabilities will be formulated differently according to the prevailing concept and orientation toward persons with disabilities. The differences and inconsistencies among these approaches become most evident when considering the most severely disabled populations, such as persons with traumatic brain injury. It has been suggested that a new theoretical perspective that encompasses a medical, economic, and sociopolitical understanding of disability would allow for a more integrative and holistic approach to disability and rehabilitation issues (Hahn, 1982). Such a perspective would tend to elevate disability and rehabilitation issues in the public policy arena. The purpose of rehabilitation mirrors the commonly accepted goal of government to provide conditions that allow individuals to achieve their maximum potential, to attain mastery over their environment, and to exercise their rights as citizens.

Traumatic brain injury is an individual and societal issue that is awakening public interest in the United States. Critical to enactment of public policy that will promote the productivity and independence of persons with traumatic brain injury is public acceptance of the importance of this issue. Traumatic brain injury must be recognized as a serious social problem that deserves and requires special public initiatives and financial support. Public initiatives to address social problems are usually activated when one or more of three situations exist (Berkowitz et al., 1976). First, a large number of individuals must directly experience a condition and its side effects, or be potentially threatened by it. Second, the condition must pose an economic concern to a large number of individuals. Third, a significant part of the general population must acknowledge a public responsibility to address the condition. The extent to which persons disabled by traumatic brain injury can meet these criteria is debatable. There is, however, growing recognition that traumatic brain injury is more than a personal or family problem. Promoting the maximum productivity and independence of individuals with traumatic brain injury will enhance the general welfare of communities and states. It will also enhance the opportunity for these citizens to assert their basic human and civil rights.

SERVICES AND PROGRAMS FOR PERSONS WITH TRAUMATIC BRAIN INJURY

Unlike for some disability constituencies in the United States, no special federal policy or pro-

gram initiatives have yet evolved to address specifically and comprehensively the problems of persons disabled as a result of traumatic brain injury (Office of Special Education and Rehabilitative Services [OSERS], 1985). It is presumed that at least some of these individuals participate in programs and services that are intended for other specified constituencies (e.g., persons who are blind, persons with mental illness, persons with mental retardation) or that are directed toward the generic population of persons with disabilities (e.g., special education, vocational rehabilitation, Social Security Disability Insurance). They also may share the same opportunities as others within the general population who are economically disadvantaged to participate in federally assisted programs of social services, housing, employment, and so forth. In addition there is a wide range of programs and services operated by state and local governments, as well as in the nonprofit and private sectors, that may be potentially available to assist persons with head injury. However, there is very limited documentation concerning access, utilization, appropriateness, and effectiveness of currently available entitlements, programs, or services for persons with brain injury.

There are a number of controversial issues involved in determining how service delivery systems can and ought to be structured, administered, and funded to provide a myriad of programs and services that are needed by persons with traumatic brain injury and their families. These questions relate to larger concerns of disability and rehabilitation policy to be responsive to the rights, needs, and desires of many constituencies. While publicly supported efforts to help people with disabilities have increased dramatically in the last 25 years, formal public policy development in the area of comprehensive rehabilitation remains fragmented and intractable (Conley, Noble, & Elder, 1986). For the field of rehabilitation policy and programs, the impetus for state and local efforts to address the needs of persons with disabilities is largely because of a variety of federal mandates, legislation, and funding initiatives. In most states, this has resulted in a service "system" that is fragmented, inconsistent, and inadequate to promote the productivity and independence of many persons who could benefit from comprehensive rehabilitation. Thus, the issue of addressing the needs of persons disabled by traumatic brain injury reflects and is part of a greater problem of persons with significant disabilities who currently do not receive appropriate or sufficient services and other needed assistance.

Public policy initiatives in the United States to assist persons with disabilities has resulted in massive federally assisted programs to provide medical care, income support, social services, special education, and vocational rehabilitation. For many years these major intergovernmental efforts have been criticized for lack of comprehensiveness, lack of coordination, and alleged administrative inefficiency (Conley et al., 1986; Magrab & Elder, 1979). A major problem is that many programs were created and expanded in a piecemeal fashion, often in response to politically timely issues. Therefore, the "system" is really a loose aggregate of independent components that seldom collaborate or coordinate appropriately to achieve desirable social goals. Various agencies and programs were established to deal with specific problems or particular constituencies and are managed independently of each other. The locus of control among various programs may be at federal, state, or local levels. While the existing system is large and complex, many individuals with disabilities still receive inadequate or no services because of eligibility restrictions, insufficient funding levels, manpower inadequacies, and inappropriate policies and program designs. These are major systemic barriers for persons with traumatic brain injury who seek programs and services to assist their comprehensive rehabilitation. It is obvious that there are no simple or quick solutions for making this complex system more responsive and effective.

Several large federal/state programs are commonly regarded as the most relevant public sources or potential resources for obtaining and developing needed services and assistance for adults disabled by traumatic brain injury (OSERS, 1985). Most of these major programs do not specifically recognize or address this constituency. Instead, they broadly target individuals with a variety of types and degrees of disabling conditions. In general, these programs do not provide a coherent system of services so that persons with head injury can receive individualized help that is specialized, comprehensive, and long term.

Income Support

Income support to persons with disabilities is available through the Social Security Disability Insurance (SSDI) program, its adjunct Childhood Disability Beneficiary program (CDB), and the Supplemental Security Income (SSI) program. These are federally funded and administered programs under the Social Security Administration, U.S. Department of Health and Human Services, that provide direct monthly cash payments to eligible recipients (Elder, Conley, & Noble, 1986). The SSDI program was created to provide income protection to qualified working people who become permanently disabled. The CDB program provides similar benefits to adults with disabilities (over age 18 years who become disabled before age 22 years) who are the dependents of a retired, deceased, or disabled worker eligible for Social Security benefits. The SSI program was established to provide a basic benefit to needy persons (limited income and assets) who are aged or disabled but who are not eligible as an individual or as a dependent to receive direct Social Security payments or SSDI/CDB benefits. Some states supplement the federal SSI payment with state-funded welfare payments.

Health and Medical Care

The primary public programs that fund health care and related services to persons with disabilities are Medicare and Medicaid, administered by the Health Care Financing Administration within the U.S. Department of Health and Human Services. Medicare is federally funded and administered but is available only to persons with disabilities who qualify for SSDI/CDB after a 2-year waiting period (unless an eligible retired Social Security beneficiary). Similar to private insurance plans, Medicare has co-payment and deductible provisions that will determine the amount of reimbursement for all specific services. Medicaid is a federally regulated, state-administered program to pay for specific health services for needy people (limited income and assets), including most persons with disabilities who receive SSI. Each state determines its own plan for types and levels of services to be covered by Medicaid and is reimbursed by the federal government for about half the costs for the Medicaid program.

Education

For children and youth who sustain brain injury, the Education for All Handicapped Children Act (PL 94-142) is very important. This federal entitlement requires states and localities to provide all children from ages 3 through 21 years old with a free and appropriate education, regardless of the severity or type of handicapping condition (OSERS, 1988). It also mandates procedural safeguards to protect the rights of children with disabilities and their families. Special education and related services must be provided in the least restrictive setting consistent with the student's needs. This includes availability of and access to all appropriate academic, vocational, and physical education. Federal funds are distributed by the U.S. Department of Education, Office of Special Education and Rehabilitative Services, to states and to local school divisions to fund special education; these are augmented in many states and localities with state and local funds.

Developmental Disabilities Programs

The Administration on Developmental Disabilities in the U.S. Department of Health and Human Services also funds and directs a number of programs that are relevant for persons who become severely disabled prior to age 22 years as a result of traumatic brain injury. The primary purpose of the various developmental disabilities programs is to assist states to develop comprehensive, coordinated, and state-of-the-art services and other assistance for persons with substantial disabilities that begin in childhood and continue throughout life (Elder et al., 1986). Each state receives a Basic State Grant to establish a "State Planning Council" to function as a systems advocate in planning and coordinating services, to promote policy development, and to demonstrate innovative approaches to service

delivery. In addition, each state receives funds to operate a Protection and Advocacy System to secure the civil rights of persons with developmental disabilities. The Administration on Developmental Disabilities also funds University Affiliated Programs that primarily provide interdisciplinary training of personnel who will provide services to persons with developmental disabilities and their families.

Vocational Rehabilitation

The most significant resource for persons with traumatic brain injury is probably the federal/state vocational rehabilitation program. It is a federally funded, state-administered program that provides a wide range of services to persons with disabilities that are focused on assisting people to obtain or to return to employment (OSERS, 1988). This program originated with the Vocational Rehabilitation Act of 1920, which created a system of state vocational rehabilitation agencies. Major revisions were made with adoption of the Vocational Rehabilitation Act in 1954. This was completely rewritten in 1973 (PL 93-112) to place more focus on clients with severe handicaps. In 1978 (PL 95-602) provisions were added to create comprehensive independent living services for persons with severe handicaps. Research activities were also expanded with creation of the National Institute on Disability and Rehabilitation Research. In 1986 (PL 99-506) the emphasis on clients with severe handicaps was strengthened and formal provisions were made for supported employment services. All of the various programs currently designated under the amended Rehabilitation Act are administered by the Office of Special Education and Rehabilitative Services within the U.S. Department of Education.

Although the long-term and broad service needs of persons with severe disabilities has been acknowledged with recent amendments to the Vocational Rehabilitation Act, this federal/state initiative continues to be largely focused on short-term vocational evaluation, specific vocational training, and employment placement as the outcomes for its service delivery system (Whitehead & Marrone, 1986). Thus, the popular general conception of rehabilitation is time limited and vocationally oriented. However, many persons with severe disabilities have very limited potential for gainful employment and may require comprehensive and long-term services to address deficits across all domains of life activities.

There are many problems with attempting to improve and expand traditional vocational rehabilitation services to respond to the many needs of persons with severe and multiple disabilities, such as may result from traumatic brain injury. Paramount is the expenditure of finite resources on clients who need expensive, specialized, long-term services (that are primarily nonvocational) but who are at high risk for unsuccessful vocational rehabilitation (Twelfth Institute on Rehabilitation Issues [TIRI] 1985). In addition to seriously insufficient funding for nontraditional rehabilitation approaches such as independent living services and supported employment services, there is also a lack of trained personnel for such services. While an expanded role for vocational rehabilitation is slowly evolving, there is not yet strong public demand and support for it. However, there is increasing advocacy among individuals with severe disabilities who seek a more meaningful life and among rehabilitation professionals and others to respond more appropriately and equitably to the needs of persons with severe handicaps.

Long-Term Rehabilitation Services

While some services for persons with traumatic brain injury have developed rapidly since 1980, these have been predominantly in the areas of acute medical care and acute rehabilitation. These are much more extensively available and funded than are services that meet later, long-term rehabilitation needs. *The National Directory of Head Injury Rehabilitation Services* issued by the National Head Injury Foundation (1988) provides an indication of the status of services currently available in the United States:

TYPE OF PROGRAM	NUMBER OF PROGRAMS
Coma treatment	102
Acute inpatient rehabilitation	179
Extended inpatient rehabilitation	120
Outpatient rehabilitation	158
Lifelong care	50
Transitional living	103
Independent living	58
Behavior treatment	53
Respite/recreation	36

The coma treatment programs are provided in acute care hospitals or acute rehabilitation facilities. Lifelong care programs are provided in nursing care facilities or other special residential facilities. Independent living programs are services and supports provided in the community. Transitional living programs may be either facility-based or community based. Independent living, behavior treatment, and respite/recreation programs are among long-term rehabilitation services needed by persons with brain injury. This is the least developed part of the evolving spectrum of services. These long-term services are not available everywhere. Many of the programs currently available are concentrated in a few states and a few communities.

Part of the explanation for the slow development of long-term rehabilitation services for persons disabled as a result of traumatic brain injury is the relative "newness" of this disability constituency and the fact that their long-term service needs become apparent with the years following the traumatic event. In some cases, long-term services have developed as an extension or logical next step after acute medical and acute rehabilitation services. A number of large, private providers that created acute treatment and transitional services early in the 1980s have expanded their operations into the development of long-term supported living programs for persons with head injury. Others have appeared as components of preexisting programs for other disability groups. Despite these beginnings, long-term rehabilitation programs remain the least developed component of the array of services needed by persons with traumatic brain injury.

The major reason for limited evolution of community-based residential and support services is the current status of funding for long-term care. There are very few funding mechanisms available for persons with head injury for either community-based or institutional long-term care. Private funding options at this time are limited to workers' compensation, liability settlements, the occasional long-term care insurance coverage, and personal and family financial resources.

Even these options are frequently limited or become exhausted in supporting a variety of programs and services for an indefinite period. For the most part, the long-term programs that have been developed are established in states where public funding mechanisms are more readily available for long-term care services. In some states, this may mean that funding available for elderly citizens is also made available for younger disabled persons for community-based services. In other states, broad Medicaid coverage has made funding available for both nursing home programs and for community-based programs for persons with head injury.

The development of community-based, long-term services for persons with traumatic brain injury is a result of planning, coordination, and the availability of federal, state, and local funding. Although many states have allocated some funding for specific services for persons with head injury, usually for vocational services through the state's vocational rehabilitation agency, only a few states have attempted a broader approach to address long-term, comprehensive rehabilitation needs:

Connecticut In Connecticut, three agencies have been designated to provide services to persons with traumatic brain injury. The Department of Human Resources has funding available for behavioral treatment services. The Department of Rehabilitative Services is involved in vocational training through job coaching and other services. The Department of Income Maintenance provides funding for head-injured persons when eligibility requirements are met. A "hardship release" Medicaid rate, established in 1984, allows for a higher reimbursement rate for the level of care needed by persons with catastrophic brain injury. This has served as an incentive for the development of private services within the state. At the present time, there is no agency that acts to coordinate all

services for persons with head injury in Connecticut (Connecticut Department of Health Services, 1984, January).

Wisconsin In 1983, the governor of Wisconsin directed the Department of Developmental Disabilities to serve persons with traumatic brain injury through its county boards. In 1986, legislation was enacted that provided a statutory inclusion of brain injury in the developmental disabilities definition, rather than the previous inclusion by interpretation. Services for persons with traumatic brain injury have not developed, however, because funding specifically for these services has not been appropriated, and funding to the county boards for all services for developmental disabilities has been cut. A recent interagency task force repeated many of the same recommendations originally made to the governor in 1983 on the need for services for persons with head injury (Wisconsin Department of Health and Social Services, 1986, April).

Missouri Missouri has created a Head Injury Advisory Council to advise the governor of Missouri on the current status of needs and services, and to act as a substitute lead agency for persons with traumatic brain injury. The council conducted a survey and needs assessment of the population and drafted a comprehensive 5-year plan for the development of services in Missouri. This plan has not been implemented because of lack of funding (Missouri Head Injury Advisory Council, 1986, July).

Massachusetts In 1985, Massachusetts developed the Statewide Head Injury Program, known as SHIP, that is administered through the Massachusetts Rehabilitation Commission. SHIP is mandated to provide: 1) case management services; 2) technical assistance and training; 3) program development, and 4) purchase of services as a provider of last resort. SHIP's case management services are available to all persons diagnosed with externally caused traumatic brain injury. The program provides technical assistance and training to other state agencies, to professionals, and to the general public through its staff and through consultants. SHIP is mandated to utilize public and private services whenever possible and to identify and develop needed services not available. SHIP has funds available to purchase services for clients who have no other means of receiving those services (Massachusetts Rehabilitation Commission, 1986, July).

Minnesota   Various agencies in Minnesota help to meet the service needs of persons with head injury. The Department of Human Services and the Department of Vocational Rehabilitation serve persons with traumatic brain injury, although activities are not formally coordinated. Case management is offered through both agencies, but neither one has the capacity to serve all persons with traumatic brain injury. The Department of Human Services provides a personal care attendant program, which has also been adapted to provide staffing for group home facilities for head-injured persons. An extensive Medicaid program provides funding for many of the community-based services needed by persons with traumatic brain injury. The majority of the community-based services in Minnesota have been developed in the Minneapolis–St. Paul area, where local funding has augmented state funds (Minnesota Brain Injury Committee, 1987, September).

California   California's state Medicaid system, MediCal, provides for reimbursement of a number of community-based, as well as institutional, services needed by persons with severe disabilities. This has been an incentive for the development of private services, including services for persons with head injury. California's efforts specifically directed to traumatic brain injury have focused on the creation of a state-wide information and referral system for neurologically impaired persons. Regional centers throughout the state provide information on services that are available in that region, and information on funding sources available in California for these services. Regional centers also provide respite and other family support services (Friss, 1988, Summer).

ADVOCACY EFFORTS

The examples discussed in the previous section reflect the complexity of administrative and funding issues that confront states in attempting to mediate the federal, state, and local roles and functions to respond effectively to the needs of a disability constituency that requires comprehensive, long-term services and support. The fact that there has been significant interest in and activity on behalf of persons with traumatic brain injury during the 1980s must be largely attributed to advocacy efforts of the National Head Injury Foundation (NHIF).

As has happened with a number of disability constituencies, the development and subsequent efforts of advocacy organizations are instrumental in raising awareness and mobilizing action for these causes. Organized advocacy activity on behalf of persons with traumatic brain injury has evolved rapidly during the 1980s. Leadership is provided by NHIF, established in 1980, and its state and local units; all are nonprofit organizations composed of persons with head injury, family members, friends, professionals, service providers, and others concerned with the welfare of persons disabled by traumatic brain injury (E. Horn, personal communication, November 7, 1988). In 1988 there were 34 state associations, 6 state affiliates, and 375 local chapters or support groups in the NHIF advocacy network.

The NHIF federation is concerned with all aspects of traumatic brain injury, from prevention to comprehensive rehabilitation. Major goals include stimulating public and professional awareness of the problem of head injury, providing information and referral resources, developing a network of support groups for persons with head injury and for family members, and promoting the establishment of specialized rehabilitation programs and supportive living arrangements for persons with head injury (NHIF, 1986, September). NHIF also advocates strongly for the establishment of central registries for traumatic brain injury in all states that would be used for epidemiologic studies and would contain basic information on the patient and severity of injury.

In addition to direct assistance to individuals with head injury and their families, the NHIF has been and continues to be aggressively involved in systems advocacy activities at both national and state levels to influence policy and to direct and redirect funding that would benefit persons with head injury and their families (TIRI, 1985). There is ongoing focus by NHIF to have cooperative agreements established among federally assisted programs at national and state levels that would make conventional services more accessible and responsive to persons with head injury. There also is activity to promote the funding of specialized model programs, professional training, basic and applied research, and prevention efforts specific to head injury. There is continuous effort to maximize utilization of Social Security and Medicare/Medicaid benefits by persons with traumatic brain injury. NHIF is also attempting to identify and to draw attention to the problems and gaps in public/private insurance coverage, and to have these appropriately addressed (NHIF, 1988, February).

Particular efforts are being made by the NHIF to expand the scope of traditional vocational rehabilitation and special education programs so that persons with head injury may obtain access to needed comprehensive services. One achievement has been the development of a cooperative agreement between NHIF and the OSERS, U.S. Department of Education, that outlines strategies for making several major programs under this critical government agency more accountable to the educational and vocational/independent living needs of persons with traumatic brain injury (OSERS, 1985). This has resulted in the targeting and funding of several research studies, model service demonstration projects, and personnel training projects that pertain specifically to head injury by the Office of Special Education Programs (OSEP), the Rehabilitation Services Administration (RSA), and the National Institute of Disability Rehabilitation and Research (NIDRR). In addition, the NHIF has itself received a multiyear grant from NIDRR to develop and conduct a national program for public education on traumatic brain injury ("NHIF/NIDRR," 1988, Spring)—Project TAP (Traumatic Head Injury Awareness and Prevention) has focused its efforts on extending access to specialized information about brain trauma through a variety of national and state activities as well as development and dissemination of resource materials. Several minigrants

have been awarded to six states to extend the national programs at the state and local levels.

Recently the NHIF has begun formal lobbying activities to influence federal legislation that can benefit persons with head injury. This involves routine annual budget appropriations for federal programs relevant for persons with head injury (NHIF, 1988, April) as well as special initiatives to increase available resources for head-injured persons, such as through Medicaid reform (NHIF, 1988, March). State and local NHIF units are also becoming increasingly involved in systems and legislative advocacy to improve service opportunities for persons with head injury. Advocacy to influence public policy that will promote the productivity and independence of persons with traumatic brain injury is in an early stage of evolution. Several states, including New York, Connecticut, Minnesota, Texas, Massachusetts, Virginia, Maine, and Wisconsin, have created special task forces or permanent advisory bodies to study the problem of head injury and to make recommendations for improving service delivery to persons with traumatic brain injury. While such activities have raised awareness, there has been limited progress in mobilizing appreciable resources to assist persons with severe disabilities as a result of traumatic brain injury to attain optimal productivity and independence.

There were two very significant results of the advocacy efforts of the National Head Injury Foundation and its federation of state associations, local affiliates, and support groups. One was the conducting of a Senate hearing on issues surrounding head injury ("Senate hearing," 1988, Spring). The hearing conducted on April 12, 1988 by the Senate Subcommittee on the Handicapped is especially noteworthy since this subcommittee seldom conducts a hearing regarding a particular area of disability ("Senate hold historic hearing," 1988, Summer). The purpose of the hearing was to provide subcommittee members with information and perspective that will influence future deliberations on budgets and legislation that might benefit persons with traumatic brain injury.

The other major accomplishment of NHIF was the establishment of a federal Interagency

Head Injury Task Force. In 1987, the U.S. Department of Health and Human Services directed the National Institute on Neurological and Communicative Disorders and Stroke (NINCDS) to organize the federal Interagency Head Injury Task Force to study and address a wide range of issues related to traumatic brain injury. Task force members represent twelve diverse federal agencies, including all major programs with relevance for responding to the needs of persons with head injury. To increase its understanding, the task force solicited public comment and convened a landmark public hearing September 8–9, 1988 to consider testimony from survivors, family members, and service providers ("Interagency task force," 1988, Fall). The task force was expected to prepare a report and submit it in early 1989 to the Secretary of Health and Human Services and to the Appropriations Subcommittee of the Health, Education, and Labor Committee. The report was to address a broad range of concerns, from acute trauma management to comprehensive rehabilitation services.

These two events reflect and are products of the aggressive advocacy efforts of the NHIF and its state associations to bring traumatic brain injury and the persons affected by it to the attention of the public and of governmental decision makers. Much has been achieved since 1980 to promote public and professional interest in the problems and needs of persons with brain injury. However, NHIF recognizes that major barriers exist in current service delivery systems that prevent survivors of head trauma from receiving comprehensive, long-term rehabilitation ("Interagency task force," 1988, Fall). These include failure to formally accept and classify traumatic brain injury as a discrete category of disability, overburdened agendas and budgets in existing federally assisted programs, lack of specialized programs and trained manpower to provide appropriate services to persons with head injury, and lack of funding to expand existing programs or to create new programs and services needed by persons with head injury. NHIF is rapidly

becoming sophisticated in the principles and techniques of systems and legislative advocacy. With its vision and level of activism, NHIF anticipates it can influence public policy and service delivery that will result in improved opportunities for persons disabled as a result of traumatic brain injury.

SUMMARY AND CONCLUSIONS

There are a number of relevant issues related to the development and implementation of public policy related to traumatic brain injury. These involve societal perceptions and attitudes concerning dependent populations, particularly persons with disabilities, and the role of government in assisting them. There is the question of whether traumatic brain injury is yet recognized as an important social problem deserving and requiring special public initiatives and financial support. There are questions about how service delivery systems can and ought to be structured, administered, and funded to provide a myriad of needed programs and services to benefit persons with head injury and their families. Finally, there are questions concerning how advocacy efforts can effectively influence public policy to promote the productivity and independence of persons disabled by traumatic head injury.

An overall conclusion can be made from this review of literature that further research is needed concerning these topics. Both descriptive and empirical research efforts are needed to describe better and to assess more uniformly the functional status and service needs of persons with head injury. Applied research is needed regarding the nature and effectiveness of various rehabilitation approaches, strategies, and settings. Policy research concerning the delivery of rehabilitative services and other assistance must address not only client outcome related to increased independence, productivity, and integration, but also issues of efficiency, accountability, and equity in the allocation and expenditure of public resources.

REFERENCES

Berkowitz, E. (Ed.). (1979). *Disability policies and government programs*. New York: Praeger.

Berkowitz, M., Dean, D., Hanks, D., & Portney, S. (1988, August). *Enhanced understanding of the ec-*

onomics of disability. Richmond: Virginia Department of Rehabilitative Services.

Berkowitz, M., Johnson, W., & Murphy, H. (1976). *Public policy toward disability.* New York: Praeger.

Bowe, F. (1980). *Rehabilitating America: Toward independence for disabled and elderly people.* New York: Harper & Row.

Brandt, R. (1979). *A theory of the good and the right.* New York: Oxford University Press.

Conley, R., Noble, J., & Elder, J. (1986). Problems with the service system. In W.E. Kiernan & J.A. Stark (Eds.), *Pathways to employment for adults with developmental disabilities* (pp. 67–83). Baltimore: Paul H. Brookes Publishing Co.

Connecticut Department of Health Services. (1984, January). *Governor's task force on traumatic brain injury: Final report.* Hartford: Author.

Eisenberg, M., Griggins, C., & Suval, R. (Eds.). (1982). *Disabled people as second-class citizens.* New York: Springer.

Elder, J., Conley, R., & Noble, J. (1986). The service system. In W.E. Kiernan & J.A. Stark (Eds.), *Pathways to employment for adults with developmental disabilities* (pp. 53–63). Baltimore: Paul H. Brookes Publishing Co.

Friss, L. (1988, Summer). *Resource center for families of brain-damaged adults.* San Francisco: Family Survival Project.

Gleidman, J., & Roth, W. (1980). *The unexpected minority: Handicapped children in America.* New York: Harcourt, Brace, & Jovanovich.

Hahn, H. (1982, July/August). Disability and rehabilitation policy: Is paternalistic neglect really benign? *Public Administration Review,* pp. 385–389.

Hochschild, J. (1981). *What's fair.* Cambridge, MA: Harvard University Press.

Interagency task force holds public hearing. (1988, Fall). *NHIF Newsletter,* pp. 1, 8, 12.

Magrab, P., & Elder, J. (Eds.). (1979). *Planning for services to handicapped persons: Community, education, health.* Baltimore: Paul H. Brookes Publishing Co.

Massachusetts Rehabilitation Commission. (1986, July). *The status of people with brain injuries in Massachusetts: Epidemiological aspects and service needs.* Boston: Author.

Minnesota Brain Injury Committee. (1987, September). *FY87 annual report and action plan: Statewide service delivery system.* Minneapolis: Author.

Missouri Head Injury Advisory Council. (1986, July). *Proposed service delivery system for rehabilitation of Missourians with head injury.* St. Louis: Author.

National Council on the Handicapped. (1988, January). *On the threshold of independence: Progress on legislative recommendations from "Toward Independence,"* Washington, DC: Author.

National Head Injury Foundation. (1986, September). *Trauma: The silent epidemic.* Framingham, MA: Author.

National Head Injury Foundation. (1988). *The national directory of head injury rehabilitation services.* Southborough, MA: Author.

National Head Injury Foundation. (1988, February). *Traumatic head injury: A review of gaps and problems in insurance coverage.* Framingham, MA: Author.

National Head Injury Foundation. (1988, March). *Testimony of the National Head Injury Foundation to the Senate Finance Subcommittee on Health relative to the Medicaid Home and Community Quality Services Act of 1989.* Southborough, MA: Author.

National Head Injury Foundation. (1988, April). *Testimony of the National Head Injury Foundation to the House Appropriations Subcommittee on Labor, Health and Human Services. Education relative to fiscal year 1989, appropriations for programs serving persons with head injury.* Southborough, MA: Author.

NHIF/NIDRR project TAP update. (1988, Spring). *NHIF Newsletter,* p. 5.

Nozick, R. (1978). Distributive justice. In J. Arthur & W. Shaw (Eds.), *Justice and economic distribution* (pp. 57–99). Englewood Cliffs, NJ: Prentice-Hall.

Office of Special Education and Rehabilitative Services. (1985). *Report on issues relating to traumatic brain injury* (Program Assistance Circular 85-14). Washington, DC: U.S. Department of Education, Rehabilitation Services Administration.

Office of Special Education and Rehabilitative Services. (1988). *Summary of existing legislation affecting persons with disabilities* (Publication No. E-88-22014). Washington, DC: U.S. Department of Education, Rehabilitation Services Administration.

Public Law 93-112. *The Rehabilitation Act of 1973,* 29 USC 701 (1973).

Public LAW 94-142. *Education for All Handicapped Children Act,* 20 USC 1400 (1975).

Public Law 95-602, *The Rehabilitation, Comprehensive Services and Developmental Disabilities Amendments of 1978,* 29 USC 796 (1978).

Public Law 99-506, *The Rehabilitation Act Amendments of 1986,* 29 USC 732 (1986).

Rawls, J. (1978). A theory of justice. In J. Arthur & W. Shaw (Eds.), *Justice and economic distribution* (pp. 18–52). Englewood Cliffs, NJ: Prentice-Hall.

Senate hearing and interagency task force milestones for NHIF. (1988, Spring). *NHIF Newsletter,* pp. 1, 4.

Senate hold historic hearing on head injury. (1988, Summer). *NHIF Newsletter,* pp. 1–2, 5, 9.

Thurow, L. (1981). *The zero-sum society.* New York: Penguin Books.

Twelfth Institute on Rehabilitation Issues. (1985).

Rehabilitation of traumatic brain injury. Menomonie, WI: Stout Vocational Rehabilitation Institute.

Whitehead, C., & Marrone, J. (1986). Time limited evaluation and training. In W.E. Kiernan & J.A. Stark (Eds.), *Pathways to employment for adults with developmental disabilities* (pp. 163–176). Baltimore: Paul H. Brookes Publishing Co.

Wisconsin Department of Health and Social Services. (1986, April). *Brain injury task force: Final report to the secretary.* Madison: Author.

Yates, D. (1982). *Bureaucratic democracy: The search for democracy and efficiency in American government.* Cambridge, MA: Harvard University Press.

Drug Index

All drugs are listed by their generic names. Trade names follow in parentheses.

Alprazolam (Xanax), 18
Amantadine hydrochloride (Symmetrel), 6
Aminophylline (Theodur), 22
Amitriptyline (Elavil), 16
Atenolol (Tenormin), 24

Baclofen (Lioresal), 9, 22, 23
Bromocriptine mesylate (Parlodel), 6
Buspirone (Buspar), 19

Carbamazepine (Tegretol), 6, 7, 8, 20, 21, 22
Chlorazepate (Tranxene), 18
Chlordiazepoxide (Librium), 18
Chlorpromazine (Thorazine), 6, 17
Cimetidine (Tagamet), 24
Clonazepan (Klonopin), 21
Clonidine (Catapres), 24

Dantrolene sodium (Dantrium), 9, 23
Desipramine (Norpramin), 16
Dextroamphetamine sulfate (Dexedrine), 6
Diazepam (Valium), 9, 18, 23
Dilantin (Phenytoin), 7, 21, 22
L-dopa/Carbidopa (Sinemet), 6
Doxepin (Sinequan), 16

Ethanol (Alcohol), 18
Ethchlorvynol (Placidyl), 18
Ethosuximide (Zarontin), 21
Etidronate disodium (Didronel), 9, 25

Famotidine (Pepcid), 24
Fluoxitane (Prozac), 16
Fluphenazine (Prolixin decanoate), 17

Glutethimide (Doriden), 18

Halazepam (Paxipam), 18
Haloperidol (Haldol), 6, 17
Hydralazine (Apresazide), 24

Imipramine (Tofranil), 16, 26
Indomethacin (Indocin), 25

Lithium (Lithane), 6, 19–20
Lorazepam (Ativan), 18
Loxapine (Loxitane), 17

Maprotilene (Ludiomil), 16
Meperidine (Demerol), 15, 17
Meprobamate (Deprol), 18
Methaqualone (Quaalude), 18
Methyldopa (Aidomet), 24
Methylphenidate (Ritalin), 20
Molindone (Moban), 17
Morphine (Roxanol), 17

Nicotine (Nicorette), 25–26
Nimodipine (Nimotop), 4
Norepinephrine (Livophed Bitrate), 19
Nortriptyline (Pamelor, Aventyl), 16

Oxazepam (Serax), 18

Pemoline (Cylert), 6
Penicillin (Veetids), 22
Pentobarbital (Cafergot), 18
Perphenazine (Trilafon), 17
Phenelzine (Nardil), 16
Phenobarbital (Donnatal), 7, 8, 18, 21, 22
Phenytoin (Dilantin), 7, 21, 22
Prazepam (Centrax), 18
Primidone (Mysoline), 21, 22
Propranolol (Inderal), 24, 26
Protriptyline (Vivactil), 6, 16
Prozac (Fluoxitane), 16

Ranitidine (Zantac), 24
Reserpine (Demi-Regroton), 24

Sucralfate (Carafate), 24, 25

326

This drug index was prepared with assistance from Nathan D. Zasler, M.D.

Subject Index

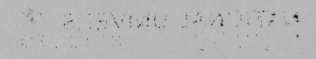